Frontiers in CNS Drug Discovery

(Volume 3)

Edited by

Atta-ur-Rahman, ***FRS***
Honorary Life Fellow, Kings College, University of Cambridge, Cambridge, UK

M. Iqbal Choudhary
H.E.J. Research Institute of Chemistry, International Center for Chemical and Biological Sciences, University of Karachi, Karachi, Pakistan

Frontiers in CNS Drug Discovery

Volume # 3

Editors: Prof. Atta-ur-Rahman and Dr. M. Iqbal Choudhary

ISSN (Online): 1879-6613

ISSN (Print): 2542-5056

ISBN (Online): 978-1-68108-443-5

ISBN (Print): 978-1-68108-444-2

First published in 2017.

General:

1. Any dispute or claim arising out of or in connection with this License Agreement or the Work (including non-contractual disputes or claims) will be governed by and construed in accordance with the laws of the U.A.E. as applied in the Emirate of Dubai. Each party agrees that the courts of the Emirate of Dubai shall have exclusive jurisdiction to settle any dispute or claim arising out of or in connection with this License Agreement or the Work (including non-contractual disputes or claims).
2. Your rights under this License Agreement will automatically terminate without notice and without the need for a court order if at any point you breach any terms of this License Agreement. In no event will any delay or failure by Bentham Science Publishers in enforcing your compliance with this License Agreement constitute a waiver of any of its rights.
3. You acknowledge that you have read this License Agreement, and agree to be bound by its terms and conditions. To the extent that any other terms and conditions presented on any website of Bentham Science Publishers conflict with, or are inconsistent with, the terms and conditions set out in this License Agreement, you acknowledge that the terms and conditions set out in this License Agreement shall prevail.

Bentham Science Publishers Ltd.
Executive Suite Y - 2
PO Box 7917, Saif Zone
Sharjah, U.A.E.
Email: subscriptions@benthamscience.org

BENTHAM SCIENCE

CONTENTS

PREFACE

Central nervous system (CNS) disorders are on the rise globally. Neurological, psychiatric and age-associated neurodegenerative diseases are among the major medical, biomedical, and social problems affecting the health system of many societies. Effective drugs are lacking despite major progress made in the understanding of the CNS diseases at the molecular level. Brain research is the most active area of research in biomedical sciences, and world literature on CNS disorders is expanding rapidly, covering various aspects of CNS disease groups. Thus, there is a strong need of a series of books that provide insights into the latest developments in this important field.

The first two volumes of the series "*Frontiers in CNS Drug Discovery*" have been very well received as a welcome addition to the global literature on this dynamic topic. The present 3rd volume of this internationally recognized books series comprises five invited reviews on various aspects of CNS drug discovery, contributed by leading experts in this field.

The first review contributed by Shibata *et al.* provides a comprehensive account of the major developments in the identification of drug targets for brain tumors, and strategies to treat resistant brain tumors. Unfortunately, prognosis in cancerous brain tumor patients is dismal despite availability of many new classes of drugs and other interventions, such as radiotherapy and surgery. One of the major challenges in the treatment of brain tumors is the emergence of resistance against chemotherapy. The authors have described the molecular characteristics of brain tumors explaining the mechanisms of drug resistance. Modern techniques of genetics, epigenetics, proteomics, transcriptomics, and metabolomics have been used to identify new drug targets in various forms of brain tumors, including glioblastoma. This has led to a better understanding of diseases which can be utilized to develop new strategies for the treatment of the most lethal form of human cancers. Results of recent pre-clinical and clinical studies are also reviewed; some of which have already led to significant improvements in the survival of brain tumor patients.

Hassen *et al.* present a comprehensive review on the role of calpain in various neurodegenerative and neuromuscular diseases in Chapter 2. Calpain is an intracellular Ca^{2+}-dependent cysteine protease. It is among the best-characterized cysteine proteases activated in brain disorders. Extensive research has revealed that the deregulation of calpains activity is a key event in a variety of neurodegenerative disorders. The authors have discussed the role of calpain in neurodegenerative and neuromuscular diseases processes, which led to its identification as a valid target for drug discovery. Targeted calpain inhibition have been successfully studied in animal models. Three new classes of calpain inhibitors have also been presented, with the results of pre-clinical studies on some of them. These studies firmly establish the importance of inhibition of calpain as therapeutic option, and thus open new ways of drug discovery against diseases such as muscular dystrophy and neurodegeneration.

In Chapter 3, Kumar *et al.* focussed on Alzheimer's and Parkinson's diseases, as well as on schizophrenia including molecular basis and novel mechanisms involved in the onset and progression of these complex diseases. These studies have led to the identification of several new targets for drug discovery and development against these diseases. The importance of Tau dysfunction and associated genetic variants is also discussed. Current therapeutic interventions against these devastating neurological disorders are presented.

The review by Verri Jr *et al.* focusses on the role of neuroimmune system in pathological pain and inflammation, and the importance of its regulation as a possible treatment approach.

Chronic pain and inflammation involve complex interactions between sensory neurons and glial cells. The activation of glial cells plays an important role in both the initiation and maintenance of pain. Based on the current understanding of the role glial cells in chronic pain, and associated mechanisms, the authors discuss various therapeutic interventions to manage chronic pain, and inflammation. The results of clinical trials of some modulators of glial cell activation in pain management are also presented.

The importance of cholinesterase inhibition in the treatment of Alzheimer's disease (AD) and other diseases is reemphasized by Potter and Kerecsen in their very well written final chapter. Acetylcholinesterase is among the classical targets for drug discovery and development against AD, and many of the first-generation and second generation blockbuster drugs act through the inhibition of cholinesterases (acetylcholinesterase, and butyrylcholinesterase). The authors have reviewed many classes of cholinesterase inhibitors, their merits and demerits, including toxicity associated with them. The therapeutic role of cholinesterase inhibitors in the treatment of other diseases such as glaucoma, Myasthenia gravis, etc has also been reviewed.

We would like to express our profound gratitude to all the authors of the above cited reviews for their excellent contributions in this vibrant, and exciting area of biomedical and pharmaceutical research. The efforts of Bentham Science Publishers for the timely production of the 3rd volume are deeply appreciated, particularly those of Ms. Faryal Sami (Assistant Manager Publications) and Mr. Mahmood Alam (Director Publications).

Prof. Dr. Atta-ur-Rahman FRS
Honorary Life Fellow,
Kings College,
University of Cambridge,
Cambridge,
UK

Prof. Dr. M. Iqbal Choudhary
H.E.J. Research Institute of Chemistry,
International Center for Chemical and Biological Sciences,
University of Karachi,
Karachi,
Pakistan

List of Contributors

Abraham Shulman	Department of Otorhinolaryngology, SUNY Downstate Medical Center, New York, USA
Alfred Stracher	Department of Emergency Medicine, New York Medical College, Metropolitan Hospital Center, New York, USA
Ana C. Rossaneis	Departamento de Ciências Patológicas, Centro de Ciências Biológicas, Universidade Estadual de Londrina, Rodovia Celso Garcia Cid KM480 PR445, Caixa Postal 10.011, CEP 86057-970, Londrina, Paraná, Brazil
Anil Kumar	School of Biotechnology, Devi Ahilya University,Takshashila Campus, Khandwa Road, INDORE-452001, India
Getaw Worku Hassen	Department of Emergency Medicine, New York Medical College, Metropolitan Hospital Center, New York, USA Center for Drug Delivery Research, SUNY Downstate Medical Center, New York, USA
Kenta Masui	Department of Pathology, Tokyo Women's Medical University, Tokyo 162-8666, Japan
Laszlo Kerecsen	Department of Pharmacology, Arizona College of Osteopathic Medicine, Midwestern University, Glendale, Arizona, USA
Leo Kesner	Department of Emergency Medicine, New York Medical College, Metropolitan Hospital Center, New York, USA
Mariana M. Bertozzi	Departamento de Ciências Patológicas, Centro de Ciências Biológicas, Universidade Estadual de Londrina, Rodovia Celso Garcia Cid KM480 PR445, Caixa Postal 10.011, CEP 86057-970, Londrina, Paraná, Brazil
Mio Harachi	Department of Pathology, Tokyo Women's Medical University, Tokyo 162-8666, Japan
Nikita Chordia	School of Biotechnology, Devi Ahilya University,Takshashila Campus, Khandwa Road, INDORE-452001, India
Noriyuki Shibata	Department of Pathology, Tokyo Women's Medical University, Tokyo 162-8666, Japan
Pamela E. Potter	Department of Pharmacology, Arizona College of Osteopathic Medicine, Midwestern University, Glendale, Arizona, USA
Paul S. Mischel	Ludwig Institute for Cancer Research, University of California San Diego, La Jolla, CA 92093, USA
Sarika Garg	The University of Montreal Hospital Research Centre, CRCHUM R09.476, Tour Viger, 900 Rue St-Denis, Montreal H2X 0A9, Quebec, Canada
Sergio M. Borghi	Departamento de Ciências Patológicas, Centro de Ciências Biológicas, Universidade Estadual de Londrina, Rodovia Celso Garcia Cid KM480 PR445, Caixa Postal 10.011, CEP 86057-970, Londrina, Paraná, Brazil
Thiago M. Cunha	Department of Pharmacology, Ribeirão Preto Medical School, University of São Paulo, Avenida do Café 3900, CEP 14049-900, Ribeirão Preto, São Paulo, Brazil

Tomoko Yamamoto	Department of Pathology, Tokyo Women's Medical University, Tokyo 162-8666, Japan
Victor Fattori	Departamento de Ciências Patológicas, Centro de Ciências Biológicas, Universidade Estadual de Londrina, Rodovia Celso Garcia Cid KM480 PR445, Caixa Postal 10.011, CEP 86057-970, Londrina, Paraná, Brazil
Waldiceu A. Verri	Departamento de Ciências Patológicas, Centro de Ciências Biológicas, Universidade Estadual de Londrina, Rodovia Celso Garcia Cid KM480 PR445, Caixa Postal 10.011, CEP 86057-970, Londrina, Paraná, Brazil

CHAPTER 1

Molecular Targeting of Brain Tumors

Kenta Masui[1], Mio Harachi[1], Paul S. Mischel[2], Tomoko Yamamoto[1] and Noriyuki Shibata[1,*]

[1] *Department of Pathology, Tokyo Women's Medical University, Tokyo 162-8666, Japan*

[2] *Ludwig Institute for Cancer Research, University of California San Diego, La Jolla, CA 92093, USA*

Abstract: An array of molecular underpinnings that dictate brain tumor growth and progression have been unraveled over the past decades. However, brain tumors' resistance to therapeutics remains a basic challenge, and patients with brain tumors still face a dismal prognosis despite an application of extensive surgery, radiotherapy and chemotherapy. Resistance mechanisms of brain tumors to chemotherapy drugs and other kinds of therapeutic molecules range from the failure of drugs to reach their intended sites due to physiological and pathological obstacles through to the molecular circuitry of the cells which can be easily manipulated by cancer cells themselves. Recent advances and knowledge in sequencing technologies of the human genome have made it possible to perform high throughput screening of compounds libraries against biological targets, shedding light on potential new approaches to treat brain tumors. In this chapter, we describe the molecular characteristics of brain tumors which will explain how cancers cleverly resist chemotherapeutics and molecularly targeted therapies, especially focusing on the most common and lethal brain tumor in human, glioblastoma. We then introduce many promising approaches with the preclinical and clinical developments in brain tumor treatments to overcome, circumvent, disrupt or manipulate the physiological and pathological barriers of brain tumors. We lastly depict the emerging new strategies to facilitate the drug discovery through genome, epigenome, transcriptome and proteome approaches, raising new challenges and identifying new leads in brain tumor therapeutics.

Keywords: Biomarker, Cancer metabolism, Chemotherapy, EGFR, Electric-field therapy, Epigenetics, Genetics, Glioblastoma, Glioma, IDH, Immunotherapy, Molecular classification, mTOR, Targeted therapy, Temozolomide, Therapy resistance, WHO.

* **Corresponding author Noriyuki Shibata:** Department of Pathology, Tokyo Women's Medical University, Tokyo 162-8666, Japan; Tel: +81-3-3353-8111; Fax: +81-3-5269-7408; E-mail: shibatan@research.twmu.ac.jp

INTRODUCTION – CANCER DRUG DISCOVERY IN THE ERA OF MOLECULAR GENETICS

Unified comprehension of the intricate molecular mechanisms that regulate tumor development has been introduced over the past years. However, it still remains a fundamental challenge to translate an array of the molecular genetic information on cancer into promising therapeutic strategies, especially for patients with brain cancers. The most successful example of effective anti-cancer drug development was represented by that of chemotherapeutic drugs. These agents could halt cell proliferation and induce cell death in rapidly proliferating cells, but the fundamental problem is that they did not effectively discern tumor cells from normal constituents [1]. Thus, caution should be taken in use of chemotherapeutics, where efficacy can be maximized while non-tumor side-effect can be minimized.

Advances in the knowledge of cancer genomics and epigenomics achieved by next-generation sequencing and large-scale DNA methylation profiling techniques have ushered in a new era of molecular diagnostics, especially represented in the field of brain tumors as "integrated diagnoses" [2, 3]. One of the genomically well-characterized brain tumors is gliomas, a potentially deadly type of brain tumors in human. They have been traditionally classified as astrocytic, oligodendroglial, oligoastrocytic (mixed) or ependymal tumors based on histological characteristics in the World Health Organization (WHO) classification of central nervous system (CNS) tumors [4]. Further, depending on morphologic features of anaplasia including mitotic activities, microvascular proliferation and necrosis, the WHO classification additionally assigns each tumor a histologic grade ranging from WHO grade I to grade IV, reflecting low to high grade of malignancy. The WHO classification and grading system has served as the guidance of post-operative treatment for many decades. However, the current comprehension of molecular genetics in brain tumors have been drastically changing the diagnostic scheme as well as therapeutic strategies against them.

The promising implication of advances in genetics and epigenetics in cancer is their potential to develop "molecularly targeting therapeutics" that specifically target the cancer-relevant genetic and epigenetic lesions, potentially without the major side effects in normal constituents in comparison with chemotherapeutics [5]. Nevertheless, it has become evident that drug resistance to this category of therapy could also occur irrelevant to the target and mechanism of drugs. In spite of the resistance which could hinder the effective cancer treatment, we remain clinically dependent on both chemotherapeutic and molecularly targeting drugs due to their unique advantages for treating cancer. As resistance remains the critical obstacle to success of both types of the drug, the challenge is to determine how to rationally and effectively use and combine these drugs based on the knowledge on molecular genetics.

Understanding the mechanisms by which cancer cells evade drug treatments and at the same time translating this knowledge into more effective treatment strategies will require a thoughtful as well as basic, clinical and translational approach. An empiric approach will not suffice as cancer cells possess too many targetable mutations and activated signaling pathways. Scientifically justified combination of targeted agents will pose significant challenges including cost-effectiveness, intellectual property considerations and cumulative toxicities [6]. Therefore, maximally harnessing the molecular genetic information of tumors and identifying mechanisms of inherent and acquired resistance to cytotoxic and targeted agents could provide potential hints that could guide the next generation of treatments against brain tumors.

This chapter will describe the molecular characteristics of brain tumors which will explain how cancers cleverly resist chemotherapeutics and molecularly targeted therapies, especially focusing on the most common and lethal brain tumor in human, glioblastoma (GBM) because of the breadth of its genomic and epigenomic information [7]. We then introduce many promising approaches with the preclinical and clinical developments in brain tumor treatments to overcome, circumvent, disrupt or manipulate the physiological and pathological barriers of brain tumors. We lastly depict the emerging new strategies to facilitate the drug discovery through genome, epigenome, transcriptome, proteome and metabolome approaches, raising new challenges and identifying new leads in brain cancer therapeutics.

New Molecular Framework for the Classification and Therapeutics of Gliomas

Major cellular constituents in the CNS system are neurons and glial cells including astrocytes, oligodendroglia and microglia. Until recently, most of the brain tumor classifications including gliomas had been based on the purely histological system of the classification scheme developed by Bailey and Cushing in 1926 [A Classification of the Tumors of the Glioma Group on a Histogenetic Basis with a Correlated Study of Prognosis], forming the foundation on which modern pathological diagnosis still rests. Their system relied on the histological resemblance of glioma cells to the normal glial constituents and putative developmental stages of glia. For instance, astrocytoma cells histologically resemble astrocytes in their star-shaped appearance and oligodendroglioma cells are similar to oligodendrocytes with round nuclei and perinuclear halo. Further, malignant transformation of these tumors can be understood as dedifferentiation of these tumor cells to immature states which have similar characteristics of glial progenitors and neural stem cells, normally residing in the specific niches of CNS [8]. The classification of gliomas based on histology thus seemed reasonable, but have in fact caused several problems in the clinic. Firstly, some tumor entities show histological phenotypes overarching several cellular lineages, well exemplified by the existence of mixed gliomas or oligoastrocytomas [4]. Second, glioma classification using histologic criteria suffers from a considerable degree of interobserver variability [9], especially prominent in regard to the detection of oligodendroglioma components. Third, histological classification does not necessarily well correspond to the patients' survival and therapeutic efficacy.

Recent advances in deciphering the genomic landscape of gliomas have begun to reshape the practice of brain tumor diagnosis and classification. Our understanding on glioma pathogenesis and biology have been facilitated by the identification of important genetic, epigenetic and transcriptional aberrations in the various types of gliomas which also revealed that certain molecular alterations are associated with response to therapy and prognosis, while others may serve as diagnostic markers for more accurate classification [10, 11]. Thus, a major goal in current glioma diagnostics, and potentially subsequent therapeutic application, was proposed by incorporating molecular information into routine, primarily histology-oriented tumor classification. For the purpose of achieving that promising goal, 27 neuropathologists from 10 countries gathered in Haarlem, the Netherlands, in May 2014, under the auspices of the International Society of Neuropathology (ISN), and discussed how molecular criteria can be best incorporated into brain tumor diagnostics with improving current patient management. The meeting came up with the "ISN-Haarlem guidelines" proposing that brain tumor diagnostics should be layered, with histology (layer 2), WHO grading (layer 3) and molecular information (layer 4), listed under an integrated diagnosis (layer 1), so that brain tumor entities can be defined as narrowly as possible to improve interobserver compatibility, clinicopathologic predictions and therapeutic strategies [2]. Indeed, feasibility of this integrated diagnostic approach was well demonstrated, achieving a more accurate classification of biologically distinct glioma entities as well as a better prognostic stratification [12]. The ISN-Haarlem concept has been adapted by the updated version of WHO classification 2016, with the major glioma entities now being defined by not only histologic features but also molecular marker profiles [13].

One of the major discoveries that led to the current molecular classification of gliomas was the identification of isocitrate dehydrogenase 1 (*IDH1*) gene mutations as a new hotspot alteration in a subset of GBMs from younger patients and secondary GBMs progressed from pre-existing lower grade gliomas [14]. Since then, the overall concept of gliomas has dramatically changed. *IDH1* or, less common *IDH2* mutations are observed in more than 70% of lower grade (WHO grade II and grade III) astrocytic and oligodendroglial gliomas, as well as in secondary GBMs [15]. Numerous studies have revealed that *IDH* mutation separates gliomas with distinct biology and clinical behavior [10]. Additionally, it has been shown that gliomas occurring in children usually lack *IDH* mutations and can be subdivided into #1) low-grade tumors with circumscribed growth that are frequently associated with *BRAF* abnormalities activating downstream mitogen-activated protein kinase (MAPK) signaling [16, 17], and #2) high-grade gliomas with diffuse growth and frequent mutations in the histone H3 (*H3F3A*) gene [13, 18]. This dynamic transition from histology to molecular genetics enables us not only to sophisticate the classification of gliomas but also to illustrate the potential to transform our approaches towards performing chemotherapies as well as guiding targeted therapies to those patients most likely to benefit from them (Fig. **1**).

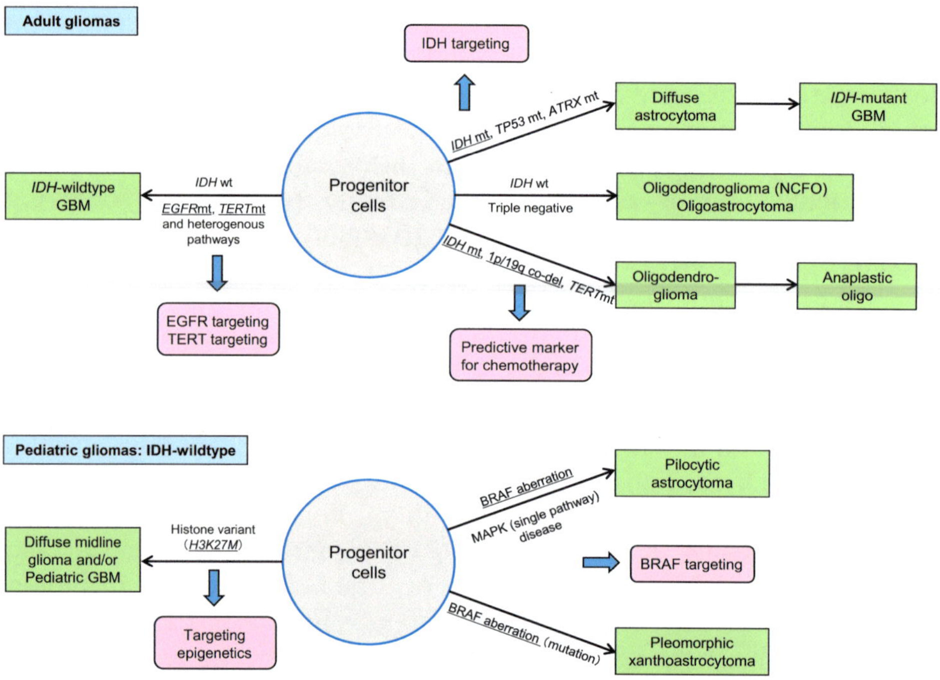

Fig. (1). Molecular classifications of gliomas and relevant therapeutic targets. In adult gliomas, alterations in *IDH*, a very early genetic event in glioma development, are followed by the *p53-ATRX* mutational pathway (astrocytic tumors) or the 1p/19 co-deletion and *TERT* pathway (oligodendroglial tumors). *IDH*-wildtype glioblastomas are characterized by mutations in *EGFR* and *TERT*. Pediatric gliomas are usually *IDH*-independent, and can be classified into benign, localized tumors associated with *BRAF* abnormalities and diffuse midline gliomas with abnormal histone *H3* variant. This molecular information will be available not only for accurate classifications of each entity but for therapeutic strategies specifically targeting each tumor with a distinct genetic background. wt, wild type; mt, mutant; GBM, glioblastoma.

Chemotherapeutics Against Gliomas

Current Standard Chemotherapy of Gliomas

Gliomas are potentially incurable brain tumors, and GBM is the most frequent and devastating primary brain cancer with a median survival in the range of 12-15 months even after the intensive treatment [19, 20]. Treatment options for gliomas include surgery, radiation and chemotherapy, involving neurosurgeons, neuro-oncologists, radiation therapists and pathologists. Surgery is the most commonly performed therapeutic option for gliomas. The extent of the removal of tumor tissue is an important prognostic factor for glioma patients, guided by intraoperative MRI and administration of fluorescent agents such as 5-aminolevulinic acid (5-ALA) [21, 22]. Importantly, surgery can also allow for the precise diagnosis of the tumor by the pathologists. Radiation therapy and chemotherapy usually follow surgery as adjuvant treatments once the diagnosis of the tumor is determined. Radiation therapy generally ranges from whole-brain radiation to stereotactic radiosurgery according to the tumor types, locations and patients' status [23].

The general concept for cancer chemotherapeutics relies on the fact that chemotherapy uses highly potent chemicals that hit rapidly proliferating cells. Tumor cells are especially sensitive to these drug treatments because of their fast growing capability well recognized as one of the hallmarks of cancer [24]. Chemotherapeutic drugs interfere with cell division, often at the level of DNA, and are divided into several classes based on the mechanism [1]. Alkylating agents (*e.g.* carmustine and platinum compounds cisplatin) damage DNA at any phase of the cell cycle, inducing a DNA-damage response (DDR) that leads to apoptosis. Mitotic inhibitors such as the taxanes (paclitaxel, docetaxel) and vinca alkaloids (vinblastine, vincristine) halt cell division by affecting microtubules which are used during cell divisions. Antitumor antibiotics, represented by the anthracyclines such as doxorubicin, interfere with DNA synthesis by intercalating between DNA strands. Topoisomerase inhibitors, such as irinotecan and topotecan, prevent DNA replication by inhibiting the activity of topoisomerases which are involved in the normal replication processes of DNA. Antimetabolites work by substituting for normal constituents of DNA, RNA or other cellular metabolites during the cell cycle where these molecules are synthesized. Administration of these drugs causes macromolecular damage and eventually cell death, and such antimetabolites include the pyrimidine antagonist 5-fluorouracil (5-FU) and capecitabine as well as the folate antagonist methotrexate.

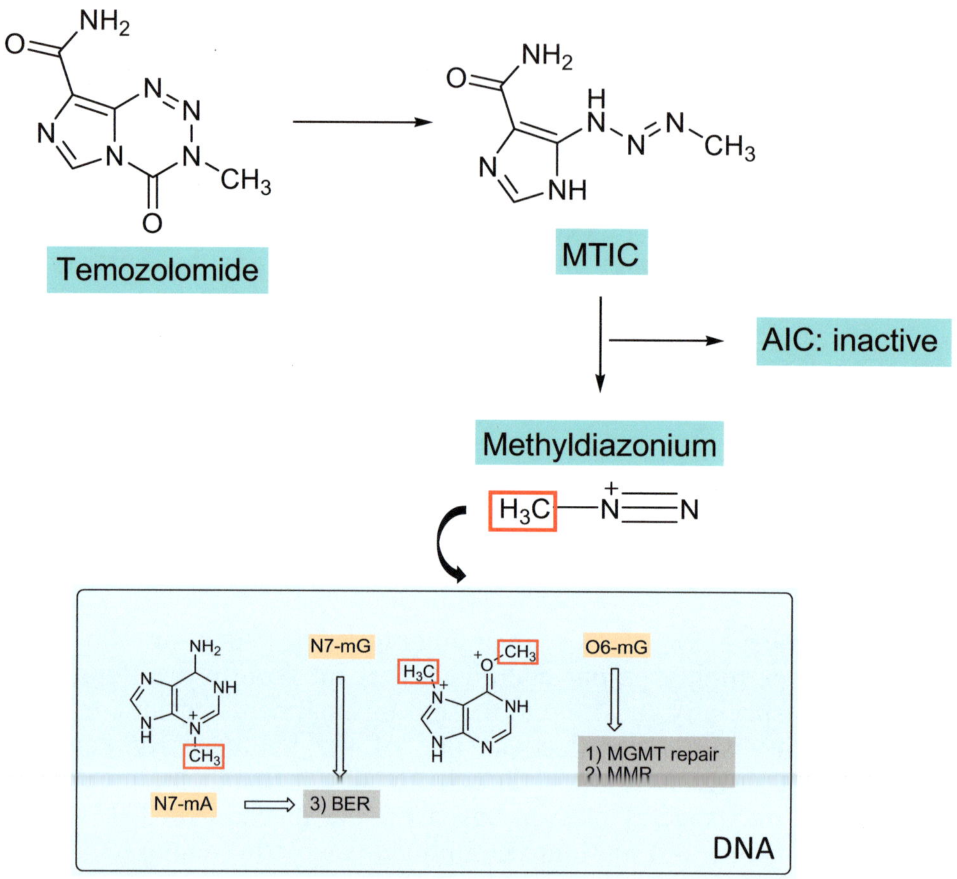

Fig. (2). Mechanisms of TMZ action, repair and resistance. TMZ is spontaneously converted to 3-methyl--(triazen-1-yl)imidazole-4-carboximide (MTIC) which is subsequently broken down to methyldiazonium cation and 5-aminoimidazole-4-carboxamide (AIC). Methyldiazonium ions deliver methyl groups to the purine bases of DNA such as O6-guanine, N7-guanine and N3-adenine, forming O6-methylguanines, N7-methylguanines and N3-methyladenines, respectively [28]. The O6-methylguanine DNA adduct can be removed and restored by MGMT. Alternatively, the mismatched base pair of the persistent O6-methylguanine with thymine is recognized by the mismatch repair (MMR) pathway, resulting in futile repair cycling and cell death. N7-methylguanines and N3-methyladenines of DNA are repaired by the base excision repair (BER) pathway, and they usually do not contribute much to the cytotoxicity of TMZ.

Alkylating agents had been the mainstay of treatment for brain tumors, and despite the development of efficient drug delivery systems such as convection-enhanced delivery (CED) including pressure-driven infusion of chemotherapeutic drug *via* an intracranial catheter [25], the role of chemotherapy in the treatment of gliomas has been controversial for decades until Stupp *et al.* demonstrated the first convincing data that the addition of an alkylating agent temozolomide (TMZ) to radiotherapy increased median survival in comparison with radiation alone, leading to a new "standard of care" for GBM [26]. TMZ is an orally available alkylating agent that is used for patients newly diagnosed with GBM. TMZ belongs to a new class of alkylating agents imidazotetrazines, and it is well applicable to brain tumors because it is lipophilic and crosses the blood-brain barrier (BBB) which is a major hindrance to the use of agents for CNS tumors [27]. TMZ is spontaneously hydrolyzed to the active metabolite 3-methy--(triazen-1-yl)imidazole-4-carboxamide (MTIC), which further breaks down to the reactive methyldiazonium ion. The methyldiazonium ion donates the methyl-group to guanine residues in the DNA, resulting in the formation of O6- and N7-methylguanine, and the O6-methylguanine is primarily responsible for the cytotoxic effects of TMZ [28, 29] (Fig. **2**). TMZ does not chemically cross-link the DNA strands, and thus it is less harmful to the bone marrow than are the nitrosoureas (*i.e.*, carmustine, lomustine), platinum compounds and procarbazine, which do cross-link the DNA. Indeed, various studies have reported that TMZ was well tolerated with a survival benefit in comparison with other alkylating agents. Adjuvant and concomitant use of TMZ with radiation significantly improved the median progression-free survival over radiation alone (6.9 *vs* 5 months), the overall survival (14.6 *vs* 12.1 months), and the likelihood of 2-year survival (26% *vs* 10%) [26].

As for the conventionally used nitrosourea compounds, intraoperatively-performed chemotherapeutic strategies have been developed using bis-chloroethylnitrosourea (BCNU, carmustine)-polymer wafers (Gliadel), which were approved by the U.S. Food and Drug Administration (FDA) in 2003. The wafer is composed of the gel containing BCNU. After removing the tumor tissue, the wafers are intraoperatively placed in the resected space. Placed wafers release BCNU into the area over the next few days, and the wafers eventually dissolve over 2 to 3 weeks [30]. Gliadel wafers for initial treatment have shown a modest increase in median survival over placebo (13.8 *vs* 11.6 months) in the phase III trial, but may also be associated with the leakage of cerebrospinal fluid and increased intracranial pressure secondary to brain edema, especially with the combination of TMZ radio-chemotherapy [31, 32].

Predictive Molecular Markers for Glioma Chemotherapeutics

Recent advances in the molecular diagnostics in gliomas have a profound impact even on predicting the efficacy of glioma chemotherapeutics on each patient basis. The O6-methylguanine-DNA methyltransferase (MGMT) acts as a DNA repair enzyme that can neutralize the efficacy of chemotherapy with TMZ by removing TMZ-induced methylation at the O6-position of guanine residues of the DNA strands (Fig. **2**) [33]. The *MGMT* gene at 10q26 is transcriptionally silenced by aberrant DNA methylation of its 5'-associated CpG island, an epigenetic aberration which is referred to as "*MGMT* promoter methylation", in around 40% of *IDH*-wildtype GBMs as well as the vast majority of *IDH*-mutant gliomas which constitutes specific glioma subgroups, glioma-CpG island methylator phenotype (G-CIMP) [34]. Importantly, GBMs with *MGMT* promoter methylation respond better to treatment with DNA alkylating agents including TMZ [35, 36] and carmustine [34], and survive longer compared to GBMs with unmethylated *MGMT* promoter. Thus, *MGMT* promoter methylation is an important prognostic marker in GBM patients treated with the current standard therapy (*i.e.*, radiotherapy combined with concomitant and adjuvant TMZ chemotherapy). However, combined radiochemotherapy may be too aggressive in the elderly patients with GBM (> 65 years of age). As stated above, *MGMT* promoter methylation is detectable in the vast majority of *IDH*-mutant gliomas, and the predictive power of *MGMT* promoter methylation may be associated with the high coincidence of other prognostic molecular markers in the tumors, including 1p/19q-codeletions [37 - 39] and *IDH* mutations [40 - 42]. The MGMT status is usually tested by methylation-specific PCR or methylation-specific pyrosequencing based on bisulfite conversion of unmethylated cytosines into uracils. Application of other techniques like methylation-specific multiplex ligation-dependent probe amplification (MS-MLPA), combined bisulfite restriction analysis (COBRA) or methylation-specific high resolution melting (HRM) analyses are currently less common in the clinic [43, 44].

In the revised WHO classification 2016, together with *IDH* mutation, codeletion of the whole chromosome arms 1p and 19q serves as an essential diagnostic marker that defines *IDH*-mutant and 1p/19q-codeleted oligodendroglioma (WHO grade II) and anaplastic oligodendroglioma (WHO grade III). Importantly, the phase III trials revealed evidence for a role of 1p/19q-codeletion in predicting patients' survival with oligodendroglial tumors following chemotherapy with procarbazine, 1-(2-chloroethyl)-3-cyclohexyl-1-nitrosourea (CCNU, lomustine) and vincristine, namely PCV chemotherapy [45, 46]. Patients with 1p/19q-codeleted anaplastic oligodendrogliomas had significantly longer median overall survival when treated upfront with radiotherapy plus PCV chemotherapy in comparison with upfront radiotherapy alone. The findings underscore the importance of molecular testing for 1p/19q-codeletion not only for more accurate classification of diffuse gliomas but also for the stratification of patients to the best treatment [47]. Commonly used methods for 1p/19q-codeletion testing include microsatellite analysis for loss of heterozygosity (LOH), fluorescence *in situ* hybridization (FISH) and multiplex ligation-dependent probe amplification (MLPA) [43]. A microarray-based assessment of genome-wide DNA methylation and copy number profiling has been recently developed and used for simultaneous detection of *IDH* mutation/G-CIMP status, 1p/19q-codeletion and MGMT promoter methylation [48].

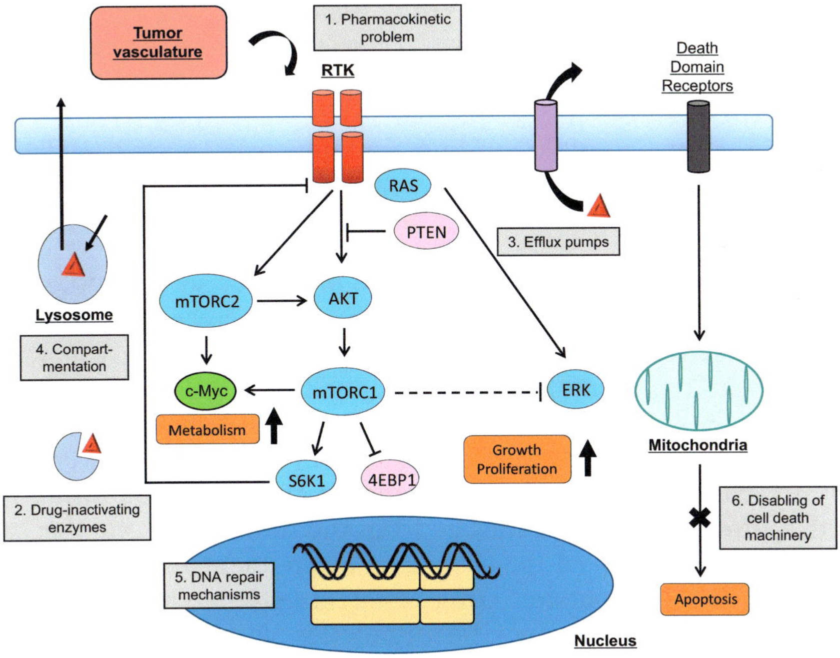

Fig. (3). Resistance mechanism to cytotoxic chemotherapies. Resistance to cytotoxic therapy generally results from a failure of the drug to reach its intended target. This is mediated by pharmacokinetic/pharmacodynamic problems (#1), induction of drug-inactivating enzymes (#2), enhanced activity of drug transporters (#3), sequestration of drugs (#4), induction of rescue genes to promote the repair of damaged DNA (#5), or disruption of mitochondrial-dependent apoptotic pathways (#6). Gray boxes represent the major resistant mechanisms to cytotoxic treatments.

Resistance to Cytotoxic Chemotherapy

Resistance of cancer cells to chemotherapy drugs falls into two categories, extrinsic and intrinsic resistance mechanisms (Fig. **3**). Extrinsic resistance involves the failure of drugs to reach their intended site of action due to pharmacokinetic/pharmacodynamic problems, such as a short half-life or rapid clearance [49]. Alterations in tumor drug metabolism involving such enzymes as cytochrome P450 (CYP) also affect the response to chemotherapy, and genetic polymorphisms of drug-metabolizing enzymes influence the plasma levels of active drug as well as drug sensitivity [50]. In order to circumvent these problems, chemotherapeutics can be conjugated to tumor-related antibodies or loaded into carriers such as liposomes or nanoparticles. These approaches have improved drug uptake and decreased drug-induced toxicity to normal tissue by enhancing specific drug delivery to the tumor. The tumor microenvironment is another emerging component of extrinsic drug resistance. The abnormal vasculature of tumors often prevents the access of chemotherapeutic drugs, and agents to affect the tumor vasculatures can improve drug distribution and delivery. The hypoxic environment of tumors is also known to cause chemoresistance by inhibiting cell proliferation since most chemotherapeutic drugs rest on rapid cell cycles for their efficacy. In addition, the transcriptional shifts induced by hypoxia contribute to resistance [51]. Thus, targeting of hypoxia inducible factor 1 (HIF-1), the major mediator of a hypoxic response, is one of the approaches to restore tumor oxygenation in an effort to increase drug sensitivity and response [52].

Intrinsic resistance mechanisms include the processes such as drug removal from its site of action by increased efflux or decreased uptake, enzymatic modification/inactivation of the drug, and alteration of drug targets within the cell. All the processes represent the ways tumor cells can utilize to acquire multi-drug resistance (MDR), enabling tumor cells to be cross-resistant to several cytotoxic drugs simultaneously. P-glycoprotein family of proteins in the context of MDR [53, 54] are components of the ATP-binding cassette (ABC) transporter efflux pumps that effectively remove drugs from the tumor cell. Another strategy that tumor cells exploit to avoid the effects of chemotherapeutics is to sequester the drug away from its action site. Drug-resistant cells facilitate the localization of chemotherapeutic drugs in specific organelles within the cytoplasm, whereas drug-sensitive cells tend to display nuclear drug localization and a more general distribution throughout the cytosol [55]. It is thought that the weak basic charge of many chemotherapy drugs promotes their trapping within acidic vesicles, followed by secretion from the tumor cells by harnessing normal vesicular trafficking.

As cancer cells depend on DNA synthesis to meet their proliferative demands, most of the chemotherapeutic drugs act in the way of damaging DNA molecules. DNA damage forces repair of the damaged DNA or induction of apoptosis as a means for preventing the cells with damaged DNA from abnormally expanding. The DNA repair machinery is an enzymatic complex which assures the integrity of DNA strands when damaged. DNA damage induces specific repair enzymes such as direct reversal (DR), transcription coupled repair (TCR), mismatch repair (MMR), homologous recombination (HR), Mre11–Rad50–Nbs1 (MRN) complex, base excision repair (BER), nucleotide excision repair (NER), global genome repair (GGR) and non-homologous end joining (NHEJ) [56], which tumor cells usurp to rescue the DNA damage caused by chemotherapy. MGMT promoter methylation-dependent resistant mechanism to TMZ is one of such examples utilized by glioma cells [35]. Another avenue to chemo-resistance is through the reprogramming of apoptotic pathways. Suppression of pro-apoptotic proteins and related pathways is often associated with the emergence of resistance to chemotherapy. The Bcl-2 family of proteins [57], the p53-regulated pro-apoptotic members [58] as well as inhibitor of apoptosis (IAP) family members are necessary for apoptotic cell death in response to DNA damaging agents, or chemotherapies. Therefore, significant effort has been made to overcome chemotherapy-induced resistance to apoptosis by using agents that specifically target the intracellular apoptotic machinery shown above [59]. We will later discuss how we could overcome this clever resistance mechanism of cancer cells against chemotherapies by combining several promising agents with chemotherapeutic drugs.

Molecularly Targeted Therapy Against Gliomas

The Current Status of Molecular Therapies Targeting the EGFR-mTOR Signaling Pathway

The field of the cancer treatment field has evolved considerably over the past decades with the introduction of molecular targeted therapies with higher specificities than chemotherapy, promising the potential for tumor cell eradication with decreased side effects. Cancer cells typically possess multiple mutations, but may develop dependence on a single chief mutation for survival rendering them preferentially susceptible to targeted inhibition [60, 61]. Experimental models and clinical studies support the hypothesis of "oncogene addiction", providing compelling rationale for targeted cancer therapy [62, 63]. Molecularly targeting agents comprise small molecules (usually < 900 daltons) or monoclonal antibodies that block tumor cell proliferation and can induce apoptosis. The small molecules penetrate cellular membranes to reach their intended targets within cells, whereas the monoclonal antibodies are generally directed against cellular surface or extracellular antigens.

Recent progress in large-scale, multi-disciplinary molecular analyses of cancers based on novel array-based DNA methylation profiling and next-generation sequencing approaches have made possible the molecular stratification of GBMs by assessing the combination of molecular genetic signatures, as opposed to evaluating the individual markers [3, 11]. The Cancer Genome Atlas (TCGA) Research Network has been established to make the comprehensive catalog of genomic abnormalities driving tumorigenesis, and has revealed biologically relevant alterations in three core pathways in GBMs: namely, RTK/RAS/PI3K signaling, p53 and Rb pathways [64, 65]. Among these, the genomic characterization of most frequent subtypes of *IDH*-wildtype GBMs reveals frequent genetic alterations of key components of the epidermal growth factor receptor (EGFR)-PI3K-Akt signaling pathway which is integrated into mechanistic target of rapamycin (mTOR) signaling [64, 66] (Fig. **4**).

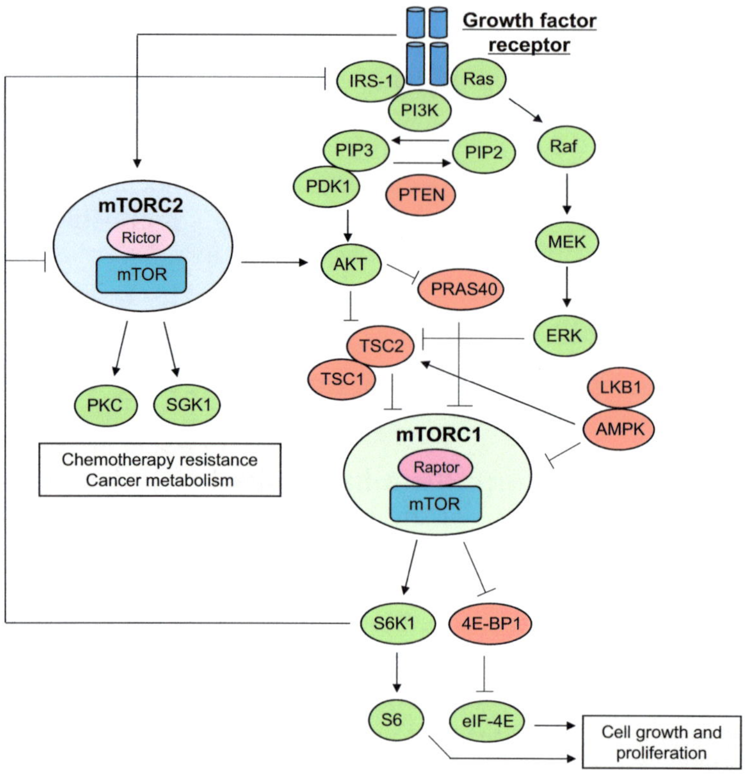

Fig. (4). mTOR complexes are the key integrators of growth factor receptor signaling. mTORC1 and C2 play a key role in integrating signal transduction and metabolic pathways in GBM. Schematic representation shows intricate pathways that regulate or are regulated by mTOR signaling in GBM, which affect the efficacy of molecularly targeting therapies but could be an achele's heel of GBM from a therapeutic point of view.

The fact that most of the GBMs depend on the abnormally activated EGFR-mTOR pathway suggest that they may be quite vulnerable to the inhibition of EGFR-mTOR pathways according to the hypothesis of oncogene addiction. An array of clinical experiences suggests that tumor cell responses to EGFR-mTO--targeting treatments are greatly affected by context-dependent oncogene addiction and an alternative acquired resistance. Our group demonstrated that expression of the constitutively active mutant EGFR variant III (*EGFRvIII*) made tumors sensitive to EGFR inhibitor, but only if the PTEN tumor suppressor protein was intact. In fact, loss of PTEN uncoupled the inhibition of EGFR from the inhibition of downstream PI3K signaling, demonstrating that PTEN loss was a critical factor in promoting resistance to EGFR inhibitors, partly because maintained PI3K signal flux was maintained in PTEN deficient tumors [67]. These studies indicate that intact regulation of PI3K signaling appears to be critical for predicting effective response to EGFR-targeting therapies.

Understanding the complex role of mTOR in regulating signal transduction is essential in developing more effective mTOR-targeted therapies although studies in human patients with recurrent malignant gliomas failed to demonstrate consistent responses to allosteric mTORC1 inhibitor rapamycin and its analogues because of several resistance mechanisms [19, 68]. Combinatorial molecular therapies may be useful to overcome the resistance, and a dual PI3K/mTOR inhibitor was indeed efficacious at halting the growth of GBM cells, independent of PTEN status [69]. Dual PI3K/mTOR inhibitors may also suppress extracellular signal-regulated kinase (ERK) signaling led by mTORC1 inhibition as a remarkable plasticity of tumor cells and their capacity for rewiring [70]. mTORC2 signaling in GBM is less well understood than that in mTORC1. We recently demonstrated that mTORC2 is frequently activated in GBM, resulting in the growth and survival of the tumor cells by activating NF-κB [71]. We also showed that mTORC2 is involved in feedback activation of Akt in rapamycin-treated patients, demonstrating a need to inhibit both mTORC1 and mTORC2 to achieve a better clinical response, and such clinical trials are currently on-going. However, this study also identified a previously unsuspected role for mTORC2 in mediating chemotherapy resistance, and EGFRvIII-expressing GBMs are exquisitely resistant to a platinum compound cisplatin [71]. We will further discuss the resistant mechanisms of tumor cells to molecularly targeting therapies in the following section.

Anti-angiogenic Therapy

One of the hallmarks of malignant gliomas is the capability to promote angiogenesis including microvascular proliferation in GBM [72]. The anti-angiogenic agent bevacizumab (Avastin; Genentech), a humanized monoclonal antibody against vascular endothelial growth factor (VEGF) ligands was approved by the U.S. FDA for recurrent GBM in 2009 [73]. When combined with irinotecan, bevacizumab prolonged 6-month survival in recurrent glioma patients to 46% compared with 21% in patients treated with TMZ [74]. Patients with supratentorial GBM received intravenous bevacizumab or placebo, plus radiotherapy and an oral TMZ, demonstrating that the median progression-free survival was longer in the bevacizumab group than in the placebo group (10.6 months *vs.* 6.2 months). The benefit relevant to progression-free survival was observed across subgroups, but overall survival was not significantly different between each group [75]. Intriguingly, gene expression analyses with the data from TCGA subclassified GBM into 4 transcriptomic groups (classical, proneural, neural and mesenchymal) [76, 77], and a proneural transcriptional signature has been connected to better response to upfront anti-angiogenic treatment with bevacizumab [78]. Anti-angiogenic agents also decrease peritumoral brain edema, potentially reducing the necessity to use corticosteroid. What is more, bevacizumab can improve the efficacy of combined cytotoxic agents through several mechanisms; 1) efficient delivery of cytotoxic drugs to the tumor by normalizing the tumor vasculature, 2) inhibition of rapid re-population of the tumor cells after cytotoxic therapies, and 3) enhancement of the anti-vascular effects of chemotherapeutic agents [79, 80]. However, to the contrary, it also has the potential to foil the effect of the combinatorial therapy by normalizing blood vessels and reconstituting the BBB in brain tumors, thereby preventing the diffusion of anti-cancer drugs.

Resistance to Molecularly Targeted Cancer Therapy

Like chemotherapeutics, resistance to molecular targeted drugs can be subclassified as intrinsic (primary) or acquired (secondary) and often counts on cellular reprogramming that sustain the signaling flux through alteration of downstream effectors, and/or disable the cell death machinery *via* compensatory cell survival pathways (Fig. **5**).

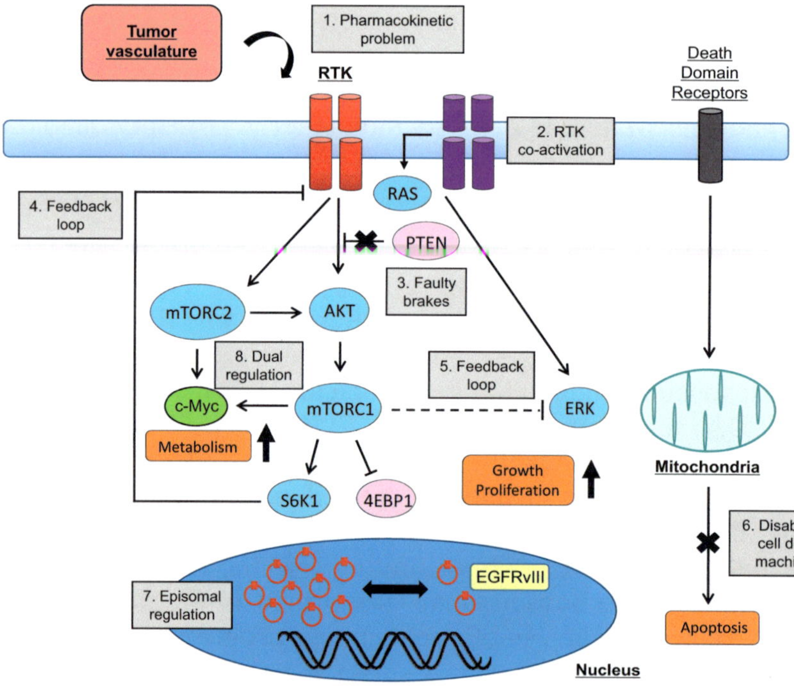

Fig. (5). Resistance mechanism to molecular targeted therapies. The major mechanisms for molecular targeted therapy resistance include pharmacokinetic/pharmacodynamic problems (#1), co-activation of other RTKs (#2), persistence of activated downstream signaling (#3), bypass mechanisms including activation of alternative driver-oncogenes or other downstream signaling pathways (#4, 5), dampening of mitochondrial-dependent apoptotic pathways (#6), genetic alteration/mutation of the target itself including the dynamic regulation of extrachromosomal DNA (episomes) (#7), or mTOR-mediated dual regulation of cancer metabolism (#8). Gray boxes denote resistance mechanisms to target therapies.

One of the most common resistant mechanisms to molecular targeted therapies involves the maintenance of oncogenic signaling *via* downstream pathways in spite of efficient target inhibition by a drug. A typical example for this type of resistance occurs in use of the drug to target the growth factor receptor or receptor tyrosine kinases (RTKs). When treating tumors with RTK inhibitors such as EGFR inhibitors, cancer cells display various resistance mechanisms including co-activation of other RTKs, signaling by physiologically regulated RTKs while mutant RTKs are inhibited, and secondary activating resistance mutations. EGFR tyrosine kinase inhibitors (TKIs) and the allosteric mTOR inhibitor rapamycin (and its derivatives) have failed to display durable efficacy in gliomas despite the rationale for targeting these molecules as aforementioned [67, 68, 81 - 83]. These failures could be explained by the relative ease with which cancer cells develop alternative resistance mechanisms to sustain downstream signaling flux. When treated with EGFR inhibitors, other RTKs including c-MET and/or platelet-derived growth factor receptor (PDGFR) become co-activated, engaging the shared PI3K to maintain downstream pathway activation [84, 85]. Thus, effective targeted therapy may require the combinatorial regimens targeting multiple RTKs simultaneously. Further, Akt inhibition induces the expression and phosphorylation of multiple RTKs, due to mTORC1 inhibition and a subsequent FoxO-dependent transcriptional activation of receptor expression [86]. Additionally, preclinical studies in GBMs have shown that upon EGFR inhibition, compensatory signaling is sustained by fibroblast growth factor (FGF) receptor and Src kinases and involves the inactivating phosphorylation of PTEN at Y240 [87].

Another type of acquired (secondary) drug resistance is facilitated by tumor cells through re-wiring of downstream signaling pathways thereby providing faulty brakes on growth checkpoints, secondary mutations in downstream signaling effectors, and/or feedback loop activation. As loss of chromosome 10 or PTEN is a common event in GBM, expression of EGFRvIII without functional PTEN can be a critical factor to display resistance to an EGFR inhibitor erlotinib due to uncoupled inhibition of EGFR from PTEN-mediated inhibition of downstream PI3K signaling [67]. Consistent with this, patients carrying tumors with high levels of EGFR coupled with low levels of activated Akt were prone to respond better to the TKI treatments [82]. These studies indicate that intact PI3K signaling seems to be critical for effective response to EGFR inhibitors and that efficacy of targeted agents requires consideration of genetic synthetic lethality or complementation for optimal effect. Rapamycin treatment which inhibits mTORC1 activity results in Akt activation by disturbing the negative feedback loop that normally mitigates PI3K signaling and is associated with significantly shorter time to tumor progression [68]. Additionally, it has been increasingly recognized that rapamycin only demonstrates the partial inhibition of the phosphorylation of 4E-BP1, which may explain the resistance to rapamycin treatment in cancer [88].

The failure to cause cell death due to disabling of the cellular death machinery is a mechanism which is involved not only in chemotherapy resistance but also in that of molecularly targeted therapies. For instance, high levels of the pro-apoptotic Bcl-2 family protein Bim expression are necessary for the induction of apoptosis upon TKI exposure [89]. However, the novel Bim isoform found in some cancers lacks the pro-apoptotic Bcl-2 homology domain 3 (BH3), and it is incapable of inducing apoptosis and contributes to poor clinical response to TKI treatment. For these patients, sensitivity to targeted therapy might be heightened by combining TKI and BH3 mimetics [89].

Together, all the examples provide compelling evidences that the approach to achieve the best clinical response to molecular targeted therapy will result from the utilization of molecular genetic information to stratify patients and clinical trials to assess the most effective strategy to inhibit both the driver mutations and the mechanisms that evade drug efficacy. Importantly, several studies with massively parallel sequencing technologies have demonstrated intra-tumoral genetic heterogeneity in solid cancers [90, 91] and revealed that specific mutations, including *PIK3CA* or *PTEN* mutations, may only preside in a subset of tumor cells in a given cancer [92, 93]. Additionally, GBM cells were reported to demonstrate completely unexpected mechanism of resistance mediated through modulation of extrachromosomal DNA of *EGFRvIII* [94]. These observations imply the necessity to develop accurate diagnostic biomarkers to collect representative tumor specimens and personalize therapies throughout the disease course. We will lastly depict the novel strategy to forestall the resistant mechanism which cancer cells exploit, and introduce the emerging effort of drug discovery which may much more effectively and specifically target malignant gliomas.

Next Generation Drug Treatments for Gliomas – Beyond the Genetics

Therapeutic Combination of Cytotoxic and Molecular Targeted Agents

Drug resistance is the dominant factor which prevents the successful application of cytotoxic chemotherapy as well as molecular targeted therapy. The complex biology of cancer cells and tumors prevents the success of both types of the agent. Each therapeutic approach hinges upon an essential dependency: chemotherapies on DNA synthesis/cell division, and molecular targeted treatments on the targeted pathway/addicted oncogene. Like their dependencies, resistance mechanism is reflective of each type of drug. Resistance to cytotoxic therapy generally results from the failure of the drug to reach the target site in an active form within a tumor cell. By contrast, the major mechanisms for resistance to molecular targeted therapy are genetic alteration of the target itself, and subsequent persistent activation of downstream signaling pathways. Analogous to the concept of genetic complementation or synthetic lethality [95], the combination of these two classes of drugs appear to be a promising avenue to overcome the resistance of each drug by complementing each other. However, combinations should be approached rationally and carefully, and not in the opportunistic way in which combinations have been tested and failed to demonstrate clinical benefit. In illuminating this point, it would be helpful to refer to and consider examples of combinatorial approaches that have demonstrated clinical efficacy as a way to inform and achieve the development of future treatment paradigms. For more information, see review [Masui *et al.*, 2013] [6].

Emerging Targeted Therapies and Biomarkers

Important spinoffs derived from the advances in the glioma molecular diagnostics are the development of several molecular markers which may serve as predictive biomarkers for response of malignant gliomas to different types of targeted therapy. These include activating *BRAF V600E* mutation as a predictive marker for response to mutant BRAF inhibitors vemurafenib in anaplastic pleomorphic xanthoastrocytoma [96] and GBM [97 - 99]. Detection of *IDH* mutation in diffuse gliomas may provide predictive information when novel therapeutic strategies are applied such as mutant IDH inhibitors [100] or vaccination against IDH1-R132H [101]. Detection of *FGFR-TACC* fusion genes could identify GBM patients who are susceptible to FGFR kinase inhibition [102]. Subependymal giant cell astrocytoma (SEGA) is a WHO grade I glioma, and usually occur in patients with tuberous sclerosis complex (TSC) with mutations in the *hamartin* gene (TSC1) or the *tuberin* gene (TSC2) which may serve as therapeutic target when using mTOR inhibitors like everolimus [103]. The selectively high frequency of the telomerase reverse transcriptase (*TERT*) promoter mutations was observed among 1p/19q-codeleted oligodendrogliomas and the *IDH*-wildtype GBM [104], and a recently developed, novel TERT-targeting therapy [105, 106] might be a promising therapy to specifically target *IDH*-wildtype GBM with poorer prognosis and fewer effective therapeutics.

Immunotherapy for Gliomas

A promising avenue of clinical research in brain cancer is the use of immune system-targeting therapies including immune checkpoint inhibitors despite the fact that CNS is generally considered as an immune-privileged organ. These treatments act by hitting molecules which serve as brakes on immune responses. By blocking the inhibitory molecules, the treatments are aimed to augment pre-existing anti-cancer immune responses. The efficacy of this type of treatment was well demonstrated in several cancers including melanomas [107], and was also examined in brain cancer using anti-PD-1 (programmed cell death 1) and anti-CTLA-4 (cytotoxic T lymphocyte-associated protein 4) antibodies [108, 109]. Oncolytic virus therapy is another immune system-based strategy to use a modified virus that can force tumor cells to self-destroy and generate a strong immune response against the cancer as well [110, 111]. Several clinical trials are under way. Moreover, in an adoptive cell therapy, including the use of chimeric antigen receptors (CARs) designed to redirect T cells to specific antigens; immune cells taken from a patient are genetically modified or treated with chemicals to enhance their activity, and re-introduced into the patient with the aim to strengthen the immune response to the specific cancer. In this scenario, EGFRvIII may become an important predictive biomarker in GBM when peptide-based vaccination strategies, which recently showed promising activity [112, 113], will eventually enter the clinic.

Electric-field Therapy in Conjunction with Chemotherapy

The recently developed Optune device utilizes low-intensity, intermediate-frequency, alternating electric fields (tumor-treating fields: TTF) in order to hit rapidly dividing cells in GBM whereas not harming normal constituents in the brain. The electrodes are placed on the scalp according to the patient's magnetic resonance imaging, generating the TTFs for the treatment. "Optune" or "NovoTTF-100A System", was approved in 2011 for use in patients with recurrent or progressed GBM. In the first controlled trial, any improvement was not demonstrated in overall survival, but efficacy and activity with the chemotherapy-free device treatment appears to be comparable to chemotherapy regimens for recurrent GBM. Further, TTF was favored in comparison with chemotherapy with respect to toxicity and quality of life [114]. In 2015, the FDA expanded its approval to allow for use of the device in conjunction with TMZ chemotherapy in the first-line option, based on the results of a randomized phase III trial, demonstrating that median overall survival was 19.4 months with use of the device plus TMZ, *versus* 16.6 months with chemotherapy alone [http://www.medscape.com/viewarticle/852196].

Targeting Cancer Metabolism and Epigenetics

A key mechanism to connect the genetic alterations with the glioma biology including epigenetic changes and therapeutics resistance is through metabolic reprogramming by cancer cells [115] (Fig. **6**). The oncogenic transcription factor c-Myc is one of the main regulators of cancer metabolic reprogramming [116]. Studies from our group identify a set of interlacing molecular mechanisms by which EGFRvIII, an activating mutant of EGFR, engages c-Myc to reprogram intracellular metabolism and drive tumor cell proliferation [117 - 119]. Importantly, multiple upstream signaling pathways converge on c-Myc in cancer cells, raising the possibility that bromodomain and extraterminal (BET) bromodomain inhibitors that interfere with c-Myc-dependent target gene expression [120], may have a role in PI3K and mTOR activated tumors including GBM. In addition to the shift in nutrient within the cell, we recently made the novel discovery that exogenous fuel sources, glucose and acetate which are widely available in the brain and readily taken up by cancer cells [121, 122], are required for mutant EGFR signaling, affecting the therapeutic efficacy including chemotherapeutics [123] and molecularly targeted treatments [124 - 126]. This further suggests the importance to targeting cancer metabolism as next generation glioma therapeutics.

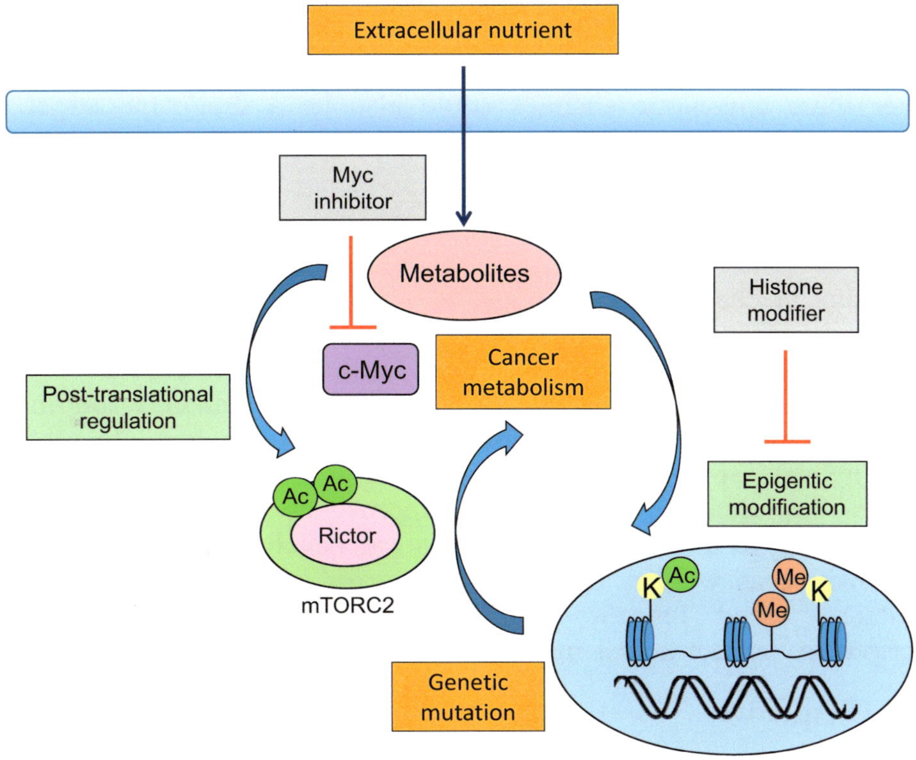

Fig. (6). Interaction of genetics and metabolism, a novel therapeutic target. Metabolic reprogramming in gliomas is driven by mutations in the cardinal genes related to gliomagenesis. Through metabolic reprogramming promoted by genetic aberrations, glioma cells vigorously take up extracellular nutrients and metabolize them into intermediary metabolites which in turn tailor the genetic signaling by altering epigenetics as well as post-translationally modifying oncogenic proteins in the cytoplasm. Targeting Myc-mediated metabolism or epigenetics could be a novel therapeutic strategy against GBMs. Ac, acetyl-group; Me, methyl-group; K, lysine residues.

Diffuse midline glioma H3-K27M mutant (WHO grade IV), is a new WHO entity that is characterized by midline tumor location, including thalamus, brain stem and spinal cord, K27M mutation in either *H3F3A* (encoding histone H3.3) or *HIST1H3B* (encoding histone H3.1), and includes the vast majority of diffuse intrinsic pontine gliomas (DIPG) [18, 127, 128]. *H3-K27M* mutation mechanistically leads to global reduction in H3K27 trimethylation in glioma cells [129], and pharmacologic inhibition of the K27 demethylase JMJD3 with the GSK-J4 inhibitor increased H3K27 trimethylation and demonstrated potent antitumor activity against *H3-K27M* mutant glioma cells [130]. In addition, the multi-histone deacetylase inhibitor panobinostat also showed antitumor activity against *H3-K27M* mutant glioma synergistic with GSK-J4 treatment [131], suggesting promising novel approaches for targeting epigenetics in cancer. Other important regulatory mechanisms of epigenetics in gliomas are through IDH mutations in lower grade gliomas represented by G-CIMP and aberrant histone methylation [132], and through constitutive PI3K and mTOR activation in EGFR-mutant IDH-wildtype GBMs [133]. Future studies are necessary to examine whether these epigenetic changes could also be a druggable target to treat gliomas.

For the effective targeting of cancer metabolism and epigenetics, a new paradigm shift will be required since normal cells and cancer cells generally share the fundamental mechanisms to regulate intracellular metabolism and epigenetics. Thus, the cancer metabolism and epigenetics should be targeted in a genotype-specific and context-dependent fashion. Further, the influence of metabolic heterogeneity and microenvironment in tumor, which potentially contribute to the utilization of metabolic fuels by tumor cells, should be taken into consideration [134]. The state-of-the-art technologies such as peptide-based drug discovery strategies, new qualitative proteomics approaches and nanotechnology-based single-cell analysis tools for drug discovery and development [135] may aid in far more sensitive as well as specific targeting of brain cancer metabolism and epigenetics, based on the fruitful knowledge of genome, epigenome, transcriptome, proteome and metabolome in brain tumors.

Future Perspectives

Rapidly evolving technology will offer a platform for more sophisticated strategies of rational drug discovery against brain tumors. Molecular network analysis and the approach of systems biology, both in silico and in cells and tumor tissue, could provide a way to identify synergistic strategies for drug combinations and new vulnerabilities created on the emergence of drug resistance. The expanding data of cancer genomes, epigenomes, transcriptomes and proteomes will play a role in the design and rationalization of therapies for individuals who will benefit the most; for example, molecular subgroups of GBM based on TCGA data provide information not only on the targetable driver mutations but also on their sensitivity to the treatment [76]. Moreover, it is becoming increasingly clear that the metabolic pathways that link the genetics and cancer biology and are thus of critical importance in influencing tumor behavior represent novel targets for therapy. As a consequence, a personalized, tailor-made medicine approach has been becoming more feasible than before.

To more effectively leverage the new genomic and epigenomic insights towards better outcomes for glioma patients, innovative clinical trial designs will be needed, including adaptive clinical trials [136] and clinical trials that increase our understanding of mechanisms of drug resistance. Non-invasive imaging or serum biomarkers will also need to be established that enable clinicians to determine whether a particular drug crosses the BBB, engages its target and initiates the desired biological effects. These clinical trials may need to incorporate repeated tumor tissue sampling to directly assess target engagement and biological activity. The application of molecular assays that detect new resistance-causing mutations, altered signaling networks, epigenetic alterations and metabolic networks that drive resistance to these longitudinal biopsies may potentially yield valuable insight that can be used to develop more effective and durable treatments.

There are eventually multi-layered complexities under successful clinical application of a rational and simple biological concept. Toxicity of the drug, dose scheduling, and intratumoral molecular heterogeneity are issues related to drug efficacy and resistance. Combining approaches of cytotoxic chemotherapeutics with molecular targeted therapies represent a formidable challenge but also a distinct opportunity. Novel molecular targets in brain tumors have been discovered on a monthly basis. Immunotherapy, with the help of check point inhibitors, has once again enjoyed its prominence in the field of cancer, and targeting metabolism and epigenetics could be a feasible strategy in the upcoming future. The success of the approach requires a careful consideration of what is learned by clinical trial and errors with respect to mechanistic knowledge of therapeutic sensitivity and resistance, and also a thoughtful design of rational future trials with the goal of developing novel and more effective treatment paradigms.

CONFLICT OF INTEREST

The authors declare no conflict of interest, financial or otherwise.

ACKNOWLEDGEMENTS

This work is supported by National Institute for Neurological Diseases and Stroke Grant NS73831; the Defeat GBM Research Collaborative, a subsidiary of National Brain Tumor Society, National Cancer Institute Grant CA119347; The Ben and Catherine Ivy Foundation; generous donations from the Ziering Family Foundation in memory of Sigi Ziering; and a grant provided by The Cell Science Research Foundation, Grant-in-Aid from the Tokyo Biochemical Research Foundation and JSPS KAKENHI Grant Number 15K19067.

REFERENCES

[1] Chabner BA, Roberts TG Jr. Timeline: Chemotherapy and the war on cancer. Nat Rev Cancer 2005; 5(1): 65-72.
[http://dx.doi.org/10.1038/nrc1529] [PMID: 15630416]

[2] Louis DN, Perry A, Burger P, *et al.* International Society Of NeuropathologyHaarlem consensus guidelines for nervous system tumor classification and grading. Brain Pathol 2014; 24(5): 429-35.
[http://dx.doi.org/10.1111/bpa.12171] [PMID: 24990071]

[3] Masui K, Mischel PS, Reifenberger G. Molecular classification of gliomas. Handb Clin Neurol 2016; 134: 97-120.
[http://dx.doi.org/10.1016/B978-0-12-802997-8.00006-2] [PMID: 26948350]

[4] Louis DN, Ohgaki H, Wiestler OD, *et al.* The 2007 WHO classification of tumours of the central nervous system. Acta Neuropathol 2007; 114(2): 97-109.
[http://dx.doi.org/10.1007/s00401-007-0243-4] [PMID: 17618441]

[5] Huang M, Shen A, Ding J, Geng M. Molecularly targeted cancer therapy: some lessons from the past decade. Trends Pharmacol Sci 2014; 35(1): 41-50.
[http://dx.doi.org/10.1016/j.tips.2013.11.004] [PMID: 24361003]

[6] Masui K, Gini B, Wykosky J, *et al.* A tale of two approaches: complementary mechanisms of cytotoxic and targeted therapy resistance may inform next-generation cancer treatments. Carcinogenesis 2013; 34(4): 725-38.
[http://dx.doi.org/10.1093/carcin/bgt086] [PMID: 23455378]

[7] Sturm D, Bender S, Jones DT, *et al.* Paediatric and adult glioblastoma: multiform (epi)genomic culprits emerge. Nat Rev Cancer 2014; 14(2): 92-107.
[http://dx.doi.org/10.1038/nrc3655] [PMID: 24457416]

[8] Zong H, Parada LF, Baker SJ. Cell of origin for malignant gliomas and its implication in therapeutic development. Cold Spring Harb Perspect Biol 2015; 7(5): a020610.
[http://dx.doi.org/10.1101/cshperspect.a020610] [PMID: 25635044]

[9] van den Bent MJ. Interobserver variation of the histopathological diagnosis in clinical trials on glioma: a clinicians perspective. Acta Neuropathol 2010; 120(3): 297-304.
[http://dx.doi.org/10.1007/s00401-010-0725-7] [PMID: 20644945]

[10] Weller M, Weber RG, Willscher E, *et al.* Molecular classification of diffuse cerebral WHO grade II/III gliomas using genome- and transcriptome-wide profiling improves stratification of prognostically distinct patient groups. Acta Neuropathol 2015; 129(5): 679-93.
[http://dx.doi.org/10.1007/s00401-015-1409-0] [PMID: 25783747]

[11] Sturm D, Witt H, Hovestadt V, *et al.* Hotspot mutations in H3F3A and IDH1 define distinct epigenetic and biological subgroups of glioblastoma. Cancer Cell 2012; 22(4): 425-37.
[http://dx.doi.org/10.1016/j.ccr.2012.08.024] [PMID: 23079654]

[12] Reuss DE, Sahm F, Schrimpf D, *et al.* ATRX and IDH1-R132H immunohistochemistry with subsequent copy number analysis and IDH sequencing as a basis for an integrated diagnostic approach for adult astrocytoma, oligodendroglioma and glioblastoma. Acta Neuropathol 2015; 129(1): 133-46. [http://dx.doi.org/10.1007/s00401-014-1370-3] [PMID: 25427834]

[13] Louis DN, Perry A, Reifenberger G, *et al.* The 2016 World Health Organization Classification of Tumors of the Central Nervous System: a summary. Acta Neuropathol 2016; 131(6): 803-20. [http://dx.doi.org/10.1007/s00401-016-1545-1] [PMID: 27157931]

[14] Parsons DW, Jones S, Zhang X, *et al.* An integrated genomic analysis of human glioblastoma multiforme. Science 2008; 321(5897): 1807-12. [http://dx.doi.org/10.1126/science.1164382] [PMID: 18772396]

[15] Yan H, Parsons DW, Jin G, *et al.* IDH1 and IDH2 mutations in gliomas. N Engl J Med 2009; 360(8): 765-73. [http://dx.doi.org/10.1056/NEJMoa0808710] [PMID: 19228619]

[16] Jones DT, Hutter B, Jäger N, *et al.* Recurrent somatic alterations of FGFR1 and NTRK2 in pilocytic astrocytoma. Nat Genet 2013; 45(8): 927-32. [http://dx.doi.org/10.1038/ng.2682] [PMID: 23817572]

[17] Zhang J, Wu G, Miller CP, *et al.* Whole-genome sequencing identifies genetic alterations in pediatric low-grade gliomas. Nat Genet 2013; 45(6): 602-12. [http://dx.doi.org/10.1038/ng.2611] [PMID: 23583981]

[18] Schwartzentruber J, Korshunov A, Liu XY, *et al.* Driver mutations in histone H3.3 and chromatin remodelling genes in paediatric glioblastoma. Nature 2012; 482(7384): 226-31. [http://dx.doi.org/10.1038/nature10833] [PMID: 22286061]

[19] Masui K, Cloughesy TF, Mischel PS. Review: molecular pathology in adult high-grade gliomas: from molecular diagnostics to target therapies. Neuropathol Appl Neurobiol 2012; 38(3): 271-91. [http://dx.doi.org/10.1111/j.1365-2990.2011.01238.x] [PMID: 22098029]

[20] Cloughesy TF, Cavenee WK, Mischel PS. Glioblastoma: from molecular pathology to targeted treatment. Annu Rev Pathol 2014; 9: 1-25. [http://dx.doi.org/10.1146/annurev-pathol-011110-130324] [PMID: 23937436]

[21] Senft C, Bink A, Franz K, Vatter H, Gasser T, Seifert V. Intraoperative MRI guidance and extent of resection in glioma surgery: a randomised, controlled trial. Lancet Oncol 2011; 12(11): 997-1003. [http://dx.doi.org/10.1016/S1470-2045(11)70196-6] [PMID: 21868284]

[22] Stummer W, Pichlmeier U, Meinel T, Wiestler OD, Zanella F, Reulen HJ. Fluorescence-guided surgery with 5-aminolevulinic acid for resection of malignant glioma: a randomised controlled multicentre phase III trial. Lancet Oncol 2006; 7(5): 392-401. [http://dx.doi.org/10.1016/S1470-2045(06)70665-9] [PMID: 16648043]

[23] Fiveash JB, Spencer SA. Role of radiation therapy and radiosurgery in glioblastoma multiforme. Cancer J 2003; 9(3): 222-9. [http://dx.doi.org/10.1097/00130404-200305000-00010] [PMID: 12952307]

[24] Hanahan D, Weinberg RA. Hallmarks of cancer: the next generation. Cell 2011; 144(5): 646-74. [http://dx.doi.org/10.1016/j.cell.2011.02.013] [PMID: 21376230]

[25] Vogelbaum MA, Aghi MK. Convection-enhanced delivery for the treatment of glioblastoma. Neuro-oncol 2015; 17 (Suppl. 2): ii3-8. [http://dx.doi.org/10.1093/neuonc/nou354] [PMID: 25746090]

[26] Stupp R, Mason WP, van den Bent MJ, *et al.* Radiotherapy plus concomitant and adjuvant temozolomide for glioblastoma. N Engl J Med 2005; 352(10): 987-96. [http://dx.doi.org/10.1056/NEJMoa043330] [PMID: 15758009]

[27] Agarwala SS, Kirkwood JM. Temozolomide, a novel alkylating agent with activity in the central

nervous system, may improve the treatment of advanced metastatic melanoma. Oncologist 2000; 5(2): 144-51.
[http://dx.doi.org/10.1634/theoncologist.5-2-144] [PMID: 10794805]

[28] Friedman HS, Kerby T, Calvert H. Temozolomide and treatment of malignant glioma. Clin Cancer Res 2000; 6(7): 2585-97.
[PMID: 10914698]

[29] Stevens MF, Hickman JA, Langdon SP, *et al.* Antitumor activity and pharmacokinetics in mice of 8-carbamoyl-3-methyl-imidazo[5,1-d]-1,2,3,5-tetrazin-4(3H)-one (CCRG 81045; M & B 39831), a novel drug with potential as an alternative to dacarbazine. Cancer Res 1987; 47(22): 5846-52.
[PMID: 3664486]

[30] Perry J, Chambers A, Spithoff K, Laperriere N. Gliadel wafers in the treatment of malignant glioma: a systematic review. Curr Oncol 2007; 14(5): 189-94.
[http://dx.doi.org/10.3747/co.2007.147] [PMID: 17938702]

[31] Westphal M, Ram Z, Riddle V, Hilt D, Bortey E. Gliadel wafer in initial surgery for malignant glioma: long-term follow-up of a multicenter controlled trial. Acta Neurochir (Wien) 2006; 148(3): 269-75.
[http://dx.doi.org/10.1007/s00701-005-0707-z] [PMID: 16482400]

[32] Gutenberg A, Bock HC, Brück W, *et al.* MGMT promoter methylation status and prognosis of patients with primary or recurrent glioblastoma treated with carmustine wafers. Br J Neurosurg 2013; 27(6): 772-8.
[http://dx.doi.org/10.3109/02688697.2013.791664] [PMID: 23662801]

[33] Wick W, Weller M, van den Bent M, *et al.* MGMT testing the challenges for biomarker-based glioma treatment. Nat Rev Neurol 2014; 10(7): 372-85.
[http://dx.doi.org/10.1038/nrneurol.2014.100] [PMID: 24912512]

[34] Esteller M, Garcia-Foncillas J, Andion E, *et al.* Inactivation of the DNA-repair gene MGMT and the clinical response of gliomas to alkylating agents. N Engl J Med 2000; 343(19): 1350-4.
[http://dx.doi.org/10.1056/NEJM200011093431901] [PMID: 11070098]

[35] Hegi ME, Diserens AC, Godard S, *et al.* Clinical trial substantiates the predictive value of O^6-methylguanine-DNA methyltransferase promoter methylation in glioblastoma patients treated with temozolomide. Clin Cancer Res 2004; 10(6): 1871-4.
[http://dx.doi.org/10.1158/1078-0432.CCR-03-0384] [PMID: 15041700]

[36] Hegi ME, Diserens AC, Gorlia T, *et al.* MGMT gene silencing and benefit from temozolomide in glioblastoma. N Engl J Med 2005; 352(10): 997-1003.
[http://dx.doi.org/10.1056/NEJMoa043331] [PMID: 15758010]

[37] van den Bent MJ, Dubbink HJ, Sanson M, *et al.* MGMT promoter methylation is prognostic but not predictive for outcome to adjuvant PCV chemotherapy in anaplastic oligodendroglial tumors: a report from EORTC Brain Tumor Group Study 26951. J Clin Oncol 2009; 27(35): 5881-6.
[http://dx.doi.org/10.1200/JCO.2009.24.1034] [PMID: 19901104]

[38] Möllemann M, Wolter M, Felsberg J, Collins VP, Reifenberger G. Frequent promoter hypermethylation and low expression of the MGMT gene in oligodendroglial tumors. Int J Cancer 2005; 113(3): 379-85.
[http://dx.doi.org/10.1002/ijc.20575] [PMID: 15455350]

[39] Brandes AA, Nicolardi L, Tosoni A, *et al.* Survival following adjuvant PCV or temozolomide for anaplastic astrocytoma. Neuro-oncol 2006; 8(3): 253-60.
[http://dx.doi.org/10.1215/15228517-2006-005] [PMID: 16723632]

[40] Balss J, Meyer J, Mueller W, Korshunov A, Hartmann C, von Deimling A. Analysis of the IDH1 codon 132 mutation in brain tumors. Acta Neuropathol 2008; 116(6): 597-602.
[http://dx.doi.org/10.1007/s00401-008-0455-2] [PMID: 18985363]

[41] Ichimura K, Pearson DM, Kocialkowski S, *et al.* IDH1 mutations are present in the majority of

common adult gliomas but rare in primary glioblastomas. Neuro-oncol 2009; 11(4): 341-7. [http://dx.doi.org/10.1215/15228517-2009-025] [PMID: 19435942]

[42] Wick W, Meisner C, Hentschel B, *et al.* Prognostic or predictive value of MGMT promoter methylation in gliomas depends on IDH1 mutation. Neurology 2013; 81(17): 1515-22. [http://dx.doi.org/10.1212/WNL.0b013e3182a95680] [PMID: 24068788]

[43] Riemenschneider MJ, Jeuken JW, Wesseling P, Reifenberger G. Molecular diagnostics of gliomas: state of the art. Acta Neuropathol 2010; 120(5): 567-84. [http://dx.doi.org/10.1007/s00401-010-0736-4] [PMID: 20714900]

[44] Yang SH, Lee KS, Yang HJ, *et al.* O^6-methylguanine-DNA-methyltransferase promoter methylation assessment by microdissection-assisted methylation-specific PCR and high resolution melting analysis in patients with glioblastomas. J Neurooncol 2012; 106(2): 243-50. [http://dx.doi.org/10.1007/s11060-011-0668-4] [PMID: 21792731]

[45] van den Bent MJ, Brandes AA, Taphoorn MJ, *et al.* Adjuvant procarbazine, lomustine, and vincristine chemotherapy in newly diagnosed anaplastic oligodendroglioma: long-term follow-up of EORTC brain tumor group study 26951. J Clin Oncol 2013; 31(3): 344-50. [http://dx.doi.org/10.1200/JCO.2012.43.2229] [PMID: 23071237]

[46] Cairncross G, Wang M, Shaw E, *et al.* Phase III trial of chemoradiotherapy for anaplastic oligodendroglioma: long-term results of RTOG 9402. J Clin Oncol 2013; 31(3): 337-43. [http://dx.doi.org/10.1200/JCO.2012.43.2674] [PMID: 23071247]

[47] Weller M, van den Bent M, Hopkins K, *et al.* EANO guideline for the diagnosis and treatment of anaplastic gliomas and glioblastoma. Lancet Oncol 2014; 15(9): e395-403. [http://dx.doi.org/10.1016/S1470-2045(14)70011-7] [PMID: 25079102]

[48] Wiestler B, Capper D, Sill M, *et al.* Integrated DNA methylation and copy-number profiling identify three clinically and biologically relevant groups of anaplastic glioma. Acta Neuropathol 2014; 128(4): 561-71. [http://dx.doi.org/10.1007/s00401-014-1315-x] [PMID: 25008768]

[49] Danesi R, De Braud F, Fogli S, Di Paolo A, Del Tacca M. Pharmacogenetic determinants of anti-cancer drug activity and toxicity. Trends Pharmacol Sci 2001; 22(8): 420-6. [http://dx.doi.org/10.1016/S0165-6147(00)01742-9] [PMID: 11479005]

[50] Ingelman-Sundberg M. Pharmacogenetics of cytochrome P450 and its applications in drug therapy: the past, present and future. Trends Pharmacol Sci 2004; 25(4): 193-200. [http://dx.doi.org/10.1016/j.tips.2004.02.007] [PMID: 15063083]

[51] Wilson WR, Hay MP. Targeting hypoxia in cancer therapy. Nat Rev Cancer 2011; 11(6): 393-410. [http://dx.doi.org/10.1038/nrc3064] [PMID: 21606941]

[52] Wang R, Zhou S, Li S. Cancer therapeutic agents targeting hypoxia-inducible factor-1. Curr Med Chem 2011; 18(21): 3168-89. [http://dx.doi.org/10.2174/092986711796391606] [PMID: 21671859]

[53] Kartner N, Riordan JR, Ling V. Cell surface P-glycoprotein associated with multidrug resistance in mammalian cell lines. Science 1983; 221(4617): 1285-8. [http://dx.doi.org/10.1126/science.6137059] [PMID: 6137059]

[54] Chen CJ, Chin JE, Ueda K, *et al.* Internal duplication and homology with bacterial transport proteins in the mdr1 (P-glycoprotein) gene from multidrug-resistant human cells. Cell 1986; 47(3): 381-9. [http://dx.doi.org/10.1016/0092-8674(86)90595-7] [PMID: 2876781]

[55] Hindenburg AA, Gervasoni JE Jr, Krishna S, *et al.* Intracellular distribution and pharmacokinetics of daunorubicin in anthracycline-sensitive and -resistant HL-60 cells. Cancer Res 1989; 49(16): 4607-14. [PMID: 2545346]

[56] Tell G, Wilson DM III. Targeting DNA repair proteins for cancer treatment. Cell Mol Life Sci 2010; 67(21): 3569-72.

[http://dx.doi.org/10.1007/s00018-010-0484-6] [PMID: 20706767]

[57] Adams JM, Cory S. The Bcl-2 apoptotic switch in cancer development and therapy. Oncogene 2007; 26(9): 1324-37.
[http://dx.doi.org/10.1038/sj.onc.1210220] [PMID: 17322918]

[58] Happo L, Cragg MS, Phipson B, *et al.* Maximal killing of lymphoma cells by DNA damage-inducing therapy requires not only the p53 targets Puma and Noxa, but also Bim. Blood 2010; 116(24): 5256-67.
[http://dx.doi.org/10.1182/blood-2010-04-280818] [PMID: 20829369]

[59] Ni Chonghaile T, Letai A. Mimicking the BH3 domain to kill cancer cells. Oncogene 2008; 27 (Suppl. 1): S149-57.
[http://dx.doi.org/10.1038/onc.2009.52] [PMID: 19641500]

[60] Weinstein IB. Cancer. Addiction to oncogenes the Achilles heal of cancer. Science 2002; 297(5578): 63-4.
[http://dx.doi.org/10.1126/science.1073096] [PMID: 12098689]

[61] Weinstein IB, Joe A. Oncogene addiction. Cancer Res 2008; 68(9): 3077-80.
[http://dx.doi.org/10.1158/0008-5472.CAN-07-3293] [PMID: 18451130]

[62] Weinstein IB, Joe AK. Mechanisms of disease: Oncogene addiction a rationale for molecular targeting in cancer therapy. Nat Clin Pract Oncol 2006; 3(8): 448-57.
[http://dx.doi.org/10.1038/ncponc0558] [PMID: 16894390]

[63] Sharma SV, Settleman J. Oncogene addiction: setting the stage for molecularly targeted cancer therapy. Genes Dev 2007; 21(24): 3214-31.
[http://dx.doi.org/10.1101/gad.1609907] [PMID: 18079171]

[64] Brennan CW, Verhaak RG, McKenna A, *et al.* The somatic genomic landscape of glioblastoma. Cell 2013; 155(2): 462-77.
[http://dx.doi.org/10.1016/j.cell.2013.09.034] [PMID: 24120142]

[65] Network CG. Comprehensive genomic characterization defines human glioblastoma genes and core pathways. Nature 2008; 455(7216): 1061-8.
[http://dx.doi.org/10.1038/nature07385] [PMID: 18772890]

[66] Ciriello G, Miller ML, Aksoy BA, Senbabaoglu Y, Schultz N, Sander C. Emerging landscape of oncogenic signatures across human cancers. Nat Genet 2013; 45(10): 1127-33.
[http://dx.doi.org/10.1038/ng.2762] [PMID: 24071851]

[67] Mellinghoff IK, Wang MY, Vivanco I, *et al.* Molecular determinants of the response of glioblastomas to EGFR kinase inhibitors. N Engl J Med 2005; 353(19): 2012-24.
[http://dx.doi.org/10.1056/NEJMoa051918] [PMID: 16282176]

[68] Cloughesy TF, Yoshimoto K, Nghiemphu P, *et al.* Antitumor activity of rapamycin in a Phase I trial for patients with recurrent PTEN-deficient glioblastoma. PLoS Med 2008; 5(1): e8.
[http://dx.doi.org/10.1371/journal.pmed.0050008] [PMID: 18215105]

[69] Fan QW, Knight ZA, Goldenberg DD, *et al.* A dual PI3 kinase/mTOR inhibitor reveals emergent efficacy in glioma. Cancer Cell 2006; 9(5): 341-9.
[http://dx.doi.org/10.1016/j.ccr.2006.03.029] [PMID: 16697955]

[70] Carracedo A, Ma L, Teruya-Feldstein J, *et al.* Inhibition of mTORC1 leads to MAPK pathway activation through a PI3K-dependent feedback loop in human cancer. J Clin Invest 2008; 118(9): 3065-74.
[PMID: 18725988]

[71] Tanaka K, Babic I, Nathanson D, *et al.* Oncogenic EGFR signaling activates an mTORC2-NF-κB pathway that promotes chemotherapy resistance. Cancer Discov 2011; 1(6): 524-38.
[http://dx.doi.org/10.1158/2159-8290.CD-11-0124] [PMID: 22145100]

[72] Zhang M, Ye G, Li J, Wang Y. Recent advance in molecular angiogenesis in glioblastoma: the challenge and hope for anti-angiogenic therapy. Brain Tumor Pathol 2015; 32(4): 229-36. [http://dx.doi.org/10.1007/s10014-015-0233-5] [PMID: 26437643]

[73] Cohen MH, Shen YL, Keegan P, Pazdur R. FDA drug approval summary: bevacizumab (Avastin) as treatment of recurrent glioblastoma multiforme. Oncologist 2009; 14(11): 1131-8. [http://dx.doi.org/10.1634/theoncologist.2009-0121] [PMID: 19897538]

[74] Herrlinger U, Schäfer N, Steinbach JP, *et al.* Bevacizumab Plus Irinotecan *Versus* Temozolomide in Newly Diagnosed O6-Methylguanine-DNA Methyltransferase Nonmethylated Glioblastoma: The Randomized GLARIUS Trial. J Clin Oncol 2016; 34(14): 1611-9. [http://dx.doi.org/10.1200/JCO.2015.63.4691] [PMID: 26976423]

[75] Chinot OL, Wick W, Mason W, *et al.* Bevacizumab plus radiotherapy-temozolomide for newly diagnosed glioblastoma. N Engl J Med 2014; 370(8): 709-22. [http://dx.doi.org/10.1056/NEJMoa1308345] [PMID: 24552318]

[76] Verhaak RG, Hoadley KA, Purdom E, *et al.* Integrated genomic analysis identifies clinically relevant subtypes of glioblastoma characterized by abnormalities in PDGFRA, IDH1, EGFR, and NF1. Cancer Cell 2010; 17(1): 98-110. [http://dx.doi.org/10.1016/j.ccr.2009.12.020] [PMID: 20129251]

[77] Phillips HS, Kharbanda S, Chen R, *et al.* Molecular subclasses of high-grade glioma predict prognosis, delineate a pattern of disease progression, and resemble stages in neurogenesis. Cancer Cell 2006; 9(3): 157-73. [http://dx.doi.org/10.1016/j.ccr.2006.02.019] [PMID: 16530701]

[78] Sandmann T, Bourgon R, Garcia J, *et al.* Patients with proneural glioblastoma may derive overall survival benefit from the addition of bevacizumab to first-line radiotherapy and temozolomide: retrospective analysis of the AVAglio trial. J Clin Oncol 2015; 33(25): 2735-44. [http://dx.doi.org/10.1200/JCO.2015.61.5005] [PMID: 26124478]

[79] Mathieu V, De Nève N, Le Mercier M, *et al.* Combining bevacizumab with temozolomide increases the antitumor efficacy of temozolomide in a human glioblastoma orthotopic xenograft model. Neoplasia 2008; 10(12): 1383-92. [http://dx.doi.org/10.1593/neo.08928] [PMID: 19048117]

[80] Kerbel RS. Antiangiogenic therapy: a universal chemosensitization strategy for cancer? Science 2006; 312(5777): 1171-5. [http://dx.doi.org/10.1126/science.1125950] [PMID: 16728631]

[81] Haas-Kogan DA, Prados MD, Tihan T, *et al.* Epidermal growth factor receptor, protein kinase B/Akt, and glioma response to erlotinib. J Natl Cancer Inst 2005; 97(12): 880-7. [http://dx.doi.org/10.1093/jnci/dji161] [PMID: 15956649]

[82] Kreisl TN, Lassman AB, Mischel PS, *et al.* A pilot study of everolimus and gefitinib in the treatment of recurrent glioblastoma (GBM). J Neurooncol 2009; 92(1): 99-105. [http://dx.doi.org/10.1007/s11060-008-9741-z] [PMID: 19018475]

[83] Reardon DA, Quinn JA, Vredenburgh JJ, *et al.* Phase 1 trial of gefitinib plus sirolimus in adults with recurrent malignant glioma. Clin Cancer Res 2006; 12(3 Pt 1): 860-8. [http://dx.doi.org/10.1158/1078-0432.CCR-05-2215] [PMID: 16467100]

[84] Stommel JM, Kimmelman AC, Ying H, *et al.* Coactivation of receptor tyrosine kinases affects the response of tumor cells to targeted therapies. Science 2007; 318(5848): 287-90. [http://dx.doi.org/10.1126/science.1142946] [PMID: 17872411]

[85] Huang PH, Mukasa A, Bonavia R, *et al.* Quantitative analysis of EGFRvIII cellular signaling networks reveals a combinatorial therapeutic strategy for glioblastoma. Proc Natl Acad Sci USA 2007; 104(31): 12867-72. [http://dx.doi.org/10.1073/pnas.0705158104] [PMID: 17646646]

[86] Chandarlapaty S, Sawai A, Scaltriti M, *et al.* AKT inhibition relieves feedback suppression of receptor tyrosine kinase expression and activity. Cancer Cell 2011; 19(1): 58-71. [http://dx.doi.org/10.1016/j.ccr.2010.10.031] [PMID: 21215704]

[87] Fenton TR, Nathanson D, Ponte de Albuquerque C, *et al.* Resistance to EGF receptor inhibitors in glioblastoma mediated by phosphorylation of the PTEN tumor suppressor at tyrosine 240. Proc Natl Acad Sci USA 2012; 109(35): 14164-9. [http://dx.doi.org/10.1073/pnas.1211962109] [PMID: 22891331]

[88] Thoreen CC, Kang SA, Chang JW, *et al.* An ATP-competitive mammalian target of rapamycin inhibitor reveals rapamycin-resistant functions of mTORC1. J Biol Chem 2009; 284(12): 8023-32. [http://dx.doi.org/10.1074/jbc.M900301200] [PMID: 19150980]

[89] Ng KP, Hillmer AM, Chuah CT, *et al.* A common BIM deletion polymorphism mediates intrinsic resistance and inferior responses to tyrosine kinase inhibitors in cancer. Nat Med 2012; 18(4): 521-8. [http://dx.doi.org/10.1038/nm.2713] [PMID: 22426421]

[90] Turner NC, Reis-Filho JS. Genetic heterogeneity and cancer drug resistance. Lancet Oncol 2012; 13(4): e178-85. [http://dx.doi.org/10.1016/S1470-2045(11)70335-7] [PMID: 22469128]

[91] Yap TA, Gerlinger M, Futreal PA, Pusztai L, Swanton C. Intratumor heterogeneity: seeing the wood for the trees. Sci Transl Med 2012; 4(127): 127ps10. [http://dx.doi.org/10.1126/scitranslmed.3003854] [PMID: 22461637]

[92] Gerlinger M, Rowan AJ, Horswell S, *et al.* Intratumor heterogeneity and branched evolution revealed by multiregion sequencing. N Engl J Med 2012; 366(10): 883-92. [http://dx.doi.org/10.1056/NEJMoa1113205] [PMID: 22397650]

[93] Shah SP, Roth A, Goya R, *et al.* The clonal and mutational evolution spectrum of primary triple-negative breast cancers. Nature 2012; 486(7403): 395-9. [PMID: 22495314]

[94] Nathanson DA, Gini B, Mottahedeh J, *et al.* Targeted therapy resistance mediated by dynamic regulation of extrachromosomal mutant EGFR DNA. Science 2014; 343(6166): 72-6. [http://dx.doi.org/10.1126/science.1241328] [PMID: 24310612]

[95] Szczurek E, Misra N, Vingron M. Synthetic sickness or lethality points at candidate combination therapy targets in glioblastoma. Int J Cancer 2013; 133(9): 2123-32. [http://dx.doi.org/10.1002/ijc.28235] [PMID: 23629686]

[96] Chamberlain MC. Salvage therapy with BRAF inhibitors for recurrent pleomorphic xanthoastrocytoma: a retrospective case series. J Neurooncol 2013; 114(2): 237-40. [http://dx.doi.org/10.1007/s11060-013-1176-5] [PMID: 23756728]

[97] Kleinschmidt-DeMasters BK, Aisner DL, Foreman NK. BRAF VE1 immunoreactivity patterns in epithelioid glioblastomas positive for BRAF V600E mutation. Am J Surg Pathol 2015; 39(4): 528-40. [http://dx.doi.org/10.1097/PAS.0000000000000363] [PMID: 25581727]

[98] Kleinschmidt-DeMasters BK, Aisner DL, Birks DK, Foreman NK. Epithelioid GBMs show a high percentage of BRAF V600E mutation. Am J Surg Pathol 2013; 37(5): 685-98. [http://dx.doi.org/10.1097/PAS.0b013e31827f9c5e] [PMID: 23552385]

[99] Robinson GW, Orr BA, Gajjar A. Complete clinical regression of a BRAF V600E-mutant pediatric glioblastoma multiforme after BRAF inhibitor therapy. BMC Cancer 2014; 14: 258. [http://dx.doi.org/10.1186/1471-2407-14-258] [PMID: 24725538]

[100] Rohle D, Popovici-Muller J, Palaskas N, *et al.* An inhibitor of mutant IDH1 delays growth and promotes differentiation of glioma cells. Science 2013; 340(6132): 626-30. [http://dx.doi.org/10.1126/science.1236062] [PMID: 23558169]

[101] Schumacher T, Bunse L, Pusch S, *et al.* A vaccine targeting mutant IDH1 induces antitumour

immunity. Nature 2014; 512(7514): 324-7.
[http://dx.doi.org/10.1038/nature13387] [PMID: 25043048]

[102] Singh D, Chan JM, Zoppoli P, *et al.* Transforming fusions of FGFR and TACC genes in human glioblastoma. Science 2012; 337(6099): 1231-5.
[http://dx.doi.org/10.1126/science.1220834] [PMID: 22837387]

[103] Krueger DA, Care MM, Holland K, *et al.* Everolimus for subependymal giant-cell astrocytomas in tuberous sclerosis. N Engl J Med 2010; 363(19): 1801-11.
[http://dx.doi.org/10.1056/NEJMoa1001671] [PMID: 21047224]

[104] Arita H, Narita Y, Fukushima S, *et al.* Upregulating mutations in the TERT promoter commonly occur in adult malignant gliomas and are strongly associated with total 1p19q loss. Acta Neuropathol 2013; 126(2): 267-76.
[http://dx.doi.org/10.1007/s00401-013-1141-6] [PMID: 23764841]

[105] Maida Y, Masutomi K. Telomerase reverse transcriptase moonlights: Therapeutic targets beyond telomerase. Cancer Sci 2015; 106(11): 1486-92.
[http://dx.doi.org/10.1111/cas.12806] [PMID: 26331588]

[106] Yamaguchi S, Maida Y, Yasukawa M, Kato T, Yoshida M, Masutomi K. Eribulin mesylate targets human telomerase reverse transcriptase in ovarian cancer cells. PLoS One 2014; 9(11): e112438.
[http://dx.doi.org/10.1371/journal.pone.0112438] [PMID: 25375122]

[107] Ott PA, Hodi FS, Robert C. CTLA-4 and PD-1/PD-L1 blockade: new immunotherapeutic modalities with durable clinical benefit in melanoma patients. Clin Cancer Res 2013; 19(19): 5300-9.
[http://dx.doi.org/10.1158/1078-0432.CCR-13-0143] [PMID: 24089443]

[108] Garber ST, Hashimoto Y, Weathers SP, *et al.* Immune checkpoint blockade as a potential therapeutic target: surveying CNS malignancies. Neuro-oncol 2016; 18(10): 1357-66.
[http://dx.doi.org/10.1093/neuonc/now132] [PMID: 27370400]

[109] Nicholas S, Mathios D, Ruzevick J, Jackson C, Yang I, Lim M. Current trends in glioblastoma multiforme treatment: radiation therapy and immune checkpoint inhibitors. Brain Tumor Res Treat 2013; 1(1): 2-8.
[http://dx.doi.org/10.14791/btrt.2013.1.1.2] [PMID: 24904882]

[110] Kane JR, Miska J, Young JS, Kanojia D, Kim JW, Lesniak MS. Sui generis: gene therapy and delivery systems for the treatment of glioblastoma. Neuro-oncol 2015; 17 (Suppl. 2): ii24-36.
[http://dx.doi.org/10.1093/neuonc/nou355] [PMID: 25746089]

[111] Thomas AA, Brennan CW, DeAngelis LM, Omuro AM. Emerging therapies for glioblastoma. JAMA Neurol 2014; 71(11): 1437-44.
[http://dx.doi.org/10.1001/jamaneurol.2014.1701] [PMID: 25244650]

[112] Schuster J, Lai RK, Recht LD, *et al.* A phase II, multicenter trial of rindopepimut (CDX-110) in newly diagnosed glioblastoma: the ACT III study. Neuro-oncol 2015; 17(6): 854-61.
[http://dx.doi.org/10.1093/neuonc/nou348] [PMID: 25586468]

[113] Reardon DA, Schuster JM, Tran DD, Fink KL, Nabors LB, Li G, *et al.* 107 ReACT: Overall Survival From a Randomized Phase II Study of Rindopepimut (CDX-110) Plus Bevacizumab in Relapsed Glioblastoma. Neurosurgery 2015; 62 (Suppl. 1): 198-9.
[http://dx.doi.org/10.1227/01.neu.0000467069.86811.3f]

[114] Stupp R, Wong ET, Kanner AA, *et al.* NovoTTF-100A *versus* physicians choice chemotherapy in recurrent glioblastoma: a randomised phase III trial of a novel treatment modality. Eur J Cancer 2012; 48(14): 2192-202.
[http://dx.doi.org/10.1016/j.ejca.2012.04.011] [PMID: 22608262]

[115] Masui K, Cavenee WK, Mischel PS. Cancer metabolism as a central driving force of glioma pathogenesis. Brain Tumor Pathol 2016; 33(3): 161-8.
[http://dx.doi.org/10.1007/s10014-016-0265-5] [PMID: 27295313]

[116] Dang CV. MYC, metabolism, cell growth, and tumorigenesis. Cold Spring Harb Perspect Med 2013; 3(8): a014217.
[http://dx.doi.org/10.1101/cshperspect.a014217] [PMID: 23906881]

[117] Babic I, Anderson ES, Tanaka K, *et al.* EGFR mutation-induced alternative splicing of Max contributes to growth of glycolytic tumors in brain cancer. Cell Metab 2013; 17(6): 1000-8.
[http://dx.doi.org/10.1016/j.cmet.2013.04.013] [PMID: 23707073]

[118] Masui K, Tanaka K, Akhavan D, *et al.* mTOR complex 2 controls glycolytic metabolism in glioblastoma through FoxO acetylation and upregulation of c-Myc. Cell Metab 2013; 18(5): 726-39.
[http://dx.doi.org/10.1016/j.cmet.2013.09.013] [PMID: 24140020]

[119] Masui K, Cavenee WK, Mischel PS. mTORC2 in the center of cancer metabolic reprogramming. Trends Endocrinol Metab 2014; 25(7): 364-73.
[http://dx.doi.org/10.1016/j.tem.2014.04.002] [PMID: 24856037]

[120] Delmore JE, Issa GC, Lemieux ME, *et al.* BET bromodomain inhibition as a therapeutic strategy to target c-Myc. Cell 2011; 146(6): 904-17.
[http://dx.doi.org/10.1016/j.cell.2011.08.017] [PMID: 21889194]

[121] Mashimo T, Pichumani K, Vemireddy V, *et al.* Acetate is a bioenergetic substrate for human glioblastoma and brain metastases. Cell 2014; 159(7): 1603-14.
[http://dx.doi.org/10.1016/j.cell.2014.11.025] [PMID: 25525878]

[122] Lyssiotis CA, Cantley LC. Acetate fuels the cancer engine. Cell 2014; 159(7): 1492-4.
[http://dx.doi.org/10.1016/j.cell.2014.12.009] [PMID: 25525870]

[123] Weiler M, Blaes J, Pusch S, *et al.* mTOR target NDRG1 confers MGMT-dependent resistance to alkylating chemotherapy. Proc Natl Acad Sci USA 2014; 111(1): 409-14.
[http://dx.doi.org/10.1073/pnas.1314469111] [PMID: 24367102]

[124] Masui K, Tanaka K, Ikegami S, *et al.* Glucose-dependent acetylation of Rictor promotes targeted cancer therapy resistance. Proc Natl Acad Sci USA 2015; 112(30): 9406-11.
[http://dx.doi.org/10.1073/pnas.1511759112] [PMID: 26170313]

[125] Masui K, Shibata N, Cavenee WK, Mischel PS. mTORC2 activity in brain cancer: Extracellular nutrients are required to maintain oncogenic signaling. BioEssays 2016; 38(9): 839-44.
[http://dx.doi.org/10.1002/bies.201600026] [PMID: 27427440]

[126] Masui K, Cavenee WK, Mischel PS. mTORC2 and Metabolic Reprogramming in GBM: at the Interface of Genetics and Environment. Brain Pathol 2015; 25(6): 755-9.
[http://dx.doi.org/10.1111/bpa.12307] [PMID: 26526943]

[127] Khuong-Quang DA, Buczkowicz P, Rakopoulos P, *et al.* K27M mutation in histone H3.3 defines clinically and biologically distinct subgroups of pediatric diffuse intrinsic pontine gliomas. Acta Neuropathol 2012; 124(3): 439-47.
[http://dx.doi.org/10.1007/s00401-012-0998-0] [PMID: 22661320]

[128] Gessi M, Gielen GH, Dreschmann V, Waha A, Pietsch T. High frequency of H3F3A (K27M) mutations characterizes pediatric and adult high-grade gliomas of the spinal cord. Acta Neuropathol 2015; 130(3): 435-7.
[http://dx.doi.org/10.1007/s00401-015-1463-7] [PMID: 26231952]

[129] Bender S, Tang Y, Lindroth AM, *et al.* Reduced H3K27me3 and DNA hypomethylation are major drivers of gene expression in K27M mutant pediatric high-grade gliomas. Cancer Cell 2013; 24(5): 660-72.
[http://dx.doi.org/10.1016/j.ccr.2013.10.006] [PMID: 24183680]

[130] Hashizume R, Andor N, Ihara Y, *et al.* Pharmacologic inhibition of histone demethylation as a therapy for pediatric brainstem glioma. Nat Med 2014; 20(12): 1394-6.
[http://dx.doi.org/10.1038/nm.3716] [PMID: 25401693]

[131] Grasso CS, Tang Y, Truffaux N, *et al.* Functionally defined therapeutic targets in diffuse intrinsic pontine glioma. Nat Med 2015; 21(6): 555-9. [http://dx.doi.org/10.1038/nm.3855] [PMID: 25939062]

[132] Noushmehr H, Weisenberger DJ, Diefes K, *et al.* Identification of a CpG island methylator phenotype that defines a distinct subgroup of glioma. Cancer Cell 2010; 17(5): 510-22. [http://dx.doi.org/10.1016/j.ccr.2010.03.017] [PMID: 20399149]

[133] Liu F, Hon GC, Villa GR, *et al.* EGFR Mutation Promotes Glioblastoma through Epigenome and Transcription Factor Network Remodeling. Mol Cell 2015; 60(2): 307-18. [http://dx.doi.org/10.1016/j.molcel.2015.09.002] [PMID: 26455392]

[134] Hensley CT, Faubert B, Yuan Q, *et al.* Metabolic Heterogeneity in Human Lung Tumors. Cell 2016; 164(4): 681-94. [http://dx.doi.org/10.1016/j.cell.2015.12.034] [PMID: 26853473]

[135] Heath JR, Ribas A, Mischel PS. Single-cell analysis tools for drug discovery and development. Nat Rev Drug Discov 2016; 15(3): 204-16. [http://dx.doi.org/10.1038/nrd.2015.16] [PMID: 26669673]

[136] Alexander BM, Wen PY, Trippa L, *et al.* Biomarker-based adaptive trials for patients with glioblastomalessons from I-SPY 2. Neuro-oncol 2013; 15(8): 972-8. [http://dx.doi.org/10.1093/neuonc/not088] [PMID: 23857706]

CHAPTER 2

Calpain Inhibition: A Potential Therapeutic Target for Neurodegenerative and Neuromuscular Disorders

Getaw Worku Hassen[1,2,*], **Leo Kesner**[1,+], **Alfred Stracher**[1,+] and **Abraham Shulman**[3]

[1] *Department of Emergency Medicine, New York Medical College, Metropolitan Hospital Center, New York, USA*

[2] *Center for Drug Delivery Research, SUNY Downstate Medical Center, New York, USA*

[3] *Department of Otorhinolaryngology, SUNY Downstate Medical Center, New York, USA*

Abstract: Proteases are involved in different neurodegenerative and neuromuscular disorders. The role of protease inhibitors as therapeutic agents has been the matter of intense research.

Given the role of proteases in these diseases, it is appealing to develop a single agent as a "magic bullet" that would target all the disease states. Calpain inhibitors have been tested with success in animal models of human diseases.

In this review, we summarize the role of calpain in selected neurodegenerative and neuromuscular diseases. We describe the various instances in which calpain has been implicated and discuss the results of calpain inhibition in each disease entity as well as how targeted calpain inhibition could be beneficial. The focus of this review is to highlight the potential role of targeted inhibition as a therapeutic option and to introduce three newer calpain inhibitors with unique characteristics.

Keywords: Calcium, Calpain, Calpain inhibitors, CNS, Cyclin-dependent kinase, Excitotoxicity, Muscular dystrophy, Neurodegeneration, Targeted-calpain inhibition.

INTRODUCTION

Calpains

Calpain is a cysteine protease that plays a significant role in the life and death of

* **Corresponding author Getaw Worku Hassen:** Department of Emergency Medicine, New York Medical College, Metropolitan Hospital Center, 1901 First Avenue, New York, NY, 10029, USA; Tel: 212-4236464; Fax: 212-4236383; E-mail: getawh@yahoo.com

+ Deceased

Atta-ur-Rahman & M. Iqbal Choudhary (Eds.)

mammalian cells including proliferation, differentiation and migration. Under physiological conditions, calpain is inhibited by its natural inhibitor calpastatin [1 - 8].The rise in cytosolic free Ca^{2+} concentration following genetic defects, injury or inflammation activates this proteolytic enzyme by autocleavage of its subunits and degradation of its natural inhibitor calpastatin. The free enzyme then moves to the membrane and exerts its action [9 - 13]. Abnormally activated calpain is associated with different disease conditions and plays a significant role in cell necrosis as well as cellular apoptosis [14 - 18]. There are about 15 different types of calpains. Some are tissue specific while others are ubiquitous. Two of the ubiquitous calpain types present in the central nervous system (CNS) are μ-calpain (calpain 1) and m-calpain (calpain 2). The terms, μ-calpain and m-calpain are derived from their respective requirement of micromolar and milimolar concentrations of calcium to confer catalytic activity *in vitro* [1, 19 - 21]. Inhibition of calpain may ameliorate the symptoms, or help to treat these diseases that resulted from abnormal and/or prolonged activation. Although other proteases are also involved in muscle and neuronal degradation, calpain appears to play a major role, making it an ideal target for therapeutic intervention. Given the role of calpain in different pathological conditions, several calpain inhibitors were developed and tested in both animal models of disease as well as in human trials [22 - 25].

MECHANISMS OF NEURODEGENERATION IN NEURO-DEGENERATIVE AND NEUROMUSCULAR DISORDERS

Different pathways lead to the prolonged and abnormal activation of calpain as a result of increased intracellular calcium. Of the various molecular mechanisms involved, Cyclin-dependent kinase (Cdk) 5 in association with calpain appears to play a central role in most neurodegenerative and neuromuscular disease pathologies and is considered an ideal target for therapeutic intervention. Cyclin-dependent kinase 5 is a small protein serine/threonine kinase with close structural homology to the mitotic Cdks. The p35/Cdk5 kinase is required for neurite growth and lamination and the association of Cdk5 with p35, the regulatory subunit is crucial for kinase activation. It has been shown that various insults known to activate calpain, including ischemia, genetic alterations, excitotoxicity or changes in calcium ion homeostasis, could cause the generation of p25 from p35, a truncated form. The resulting truncated product accumulates in neurons and activates Cdk5 aberrantly, which results in deregulation and mislocalization of the Cdk5/p25 complex, leading to hyperphosphorylation of tau. This process disrupts cytoskeletal elements, degenerates neurons, causes apoptosis and disrupts synaptic plasticity and cognition [26 - 33]. Of note, mechanisms other than abnormal calpain activation contribute to the pathophysiology of neurodegenerative and neuromuscular diseases. Here we will discuss the role of calpain in the pathophysiology of individual diseases.

Alzheimer's Disease (AD)

Different hypotheses exist about mechanisms leading to AD (amyloid cascade and cholinergic hypothesis) and aberrant calpain activation plays central role in the pathophysiology of AD [34 - 37]. Overproduction and extracellular deposition of amyloid β-peptide (Aβ) as well as deposition of neurofibrillary tangles (NFT) intracellularly are believed to initiate the disease process. These depositions play a role as initiating factors for multiple neurotoxic pathways resulting in abnormal calpain activation that affects synaptic plasticity and learning, as well as memory function [38 - 41]. Decreased phosphorylation and/or increased degradation of the transcription factor cAMP response element-binding protein (CREB) results in synaptic dysfunction and cognitive impairment. Calpain inhibition resulted in improvement in memory loss in an animal model of AD by re-establishing synaptic connections [42, 43]. Additionally Cdk 5 and calpain-associated neurodegeneration contributes to the pathophysiology of AD. This further strengthens the role of calpain in the pathology of this disease. Treatment with calpain inhibitor as well as others agents that result in calcium, Cdk and calpain regulation contribute to improvement of symptoms in AD [44 - 46]. Recently a selective calpain2 inhibitor showed enhanced learning and memory by modulating the extracellular receptor kinase (ERK) activation [47].

Amyotrophic Lateral Sclerosis (ALS)

Various mechanisms have been proposed to explain the loss of motor neurons in ALS. These mechanisms include abnormal calpain activation, oxidative damage, excitotoxicity from impaired clearing of glutamate, toxicity mediated by intracellular aggregates of mutant superoxide dismutase 1 (SOD1) and disruption of axonal transport caused by neurofilament disorganization. An estimated 10% of ALS cases are believed to be familial and approximately 20% of these are the result of missense mutations in the Cu/Zn SOD1 enzyme resulting in motor neuron degeneration [48 - 55]. Given the central role of calpain activation in ALS, treatment with calpain inhibitor is an important aspect of therapy. More evidence is emerging regarding the involvement of the Cdk family in neurodegenerative disorders including ALS [56]. Blocking Cdk 5 activity resulted in protection of cultured cortical and hippocampal neurons from fibrillary Aβ-mediated toxicity both *in vitro* and *in vivo* experiments. This indicates that controlled Cdk5 activity affects the degeneration process of motor neurons [28, 31, 56 - 58]. Thus calpain inhibition may be a target in controlling Cdk 5 activity-related motor neuron dysfunction.

Cochleovestibular Pathology

The neurodegeneration associated with aging, noise exposure and side effects of drugs can cause loss of structure and function with symptoms of hearing loss, tinnitus, vertigo, pain and neuropsychiatric disorders in the cochleovestibular system. Elevation of cytosolic $Ca^{2}+$ levels has been shown in damaged hair cells supporting the role of calpain activation in the pathophysiology of cochleovestibular injury [59 - 69]. In the normal cochlea the structural protein alpha-spectrin is present in hair cells, supporting cells and neurons. Alpha-spectrin is concentrated in hair cells in the cuticular plate as well as along the lateral cell membrane. The degradation of alpha-spectrin by calpain in both the cortical lattice and cuticular plates of the outer hair cells leads to disorganization of both cell shape and structure [70 - 72]. The level of alpha-spectrin degradation has been used as a surrogate marker for calpain action/inhibition. The neurochemical mechanisms of neuroprotection and apoptosis have been recommended for investigations of "ototoxicity" with calpain inhibitors. The role of calpain in the pathophysiology of cochleovestibular injury and its inhibition as a potential therapeutic intervention has been shown in different studies. Application of exogenous calpain inhibitors in the cochlea have been shown to protect hair cells from acoustic trauma, antibiotic ototoxicity and against hypoxia in both the cochlear hair cells and ganglion neurons [73 - 78]. Long term safety of the calpain inhibitor leupeptin was established in guinea pigs by investigation of baseline and post treatment effects on cochlear blood flow, auditory sensitivity, and cochlear histology [79, 80]. The effects of sustained-release delivery of leupeptin on the hearing of chinchillas produced no hearing loss at early time points, but resulted in some hearing loss at later time points in 40% of the animals. Application of leupeptin to the middle ear cavity reduced hearing loss as a result of exposure to impulse noise [81]. Although calpain inhibitors are not strictly selective, these findings strongly suggest that calpain plays a role in hair cell and primary neuron degeneration in the damaged cochlea. Recently the use of a dual agent that inhibits both calpain and lipid peroxidation resulted in a reduction in cochlear injury from trauma [77].

Epilepsy

Excitotoxicity is a hall mark of several disorders of the CNS, including epilepsy. The hippocampus has highly enriched glutamatergic synapses and activation of glutamate receptors during epileptic phenomena can lead to excitotoxicity-induced neuronal damage. Excitotoxicity is an overactivation of ionotropic and metabotropic glutamate receptors leading to an increase in cytosolic calcium concentration [82 - 86]. This triggers a cascade of cellular events resulting in calpain activation and tissue damage. Calpain is involved in the pathophysiology of seizure-dependent neurodegeneration and its inhibition is a target for therapeutic approaches. Furthermore, calpain is believed to have an early role in seizure-related neurodegeneration independent of caspase [17, 87]. Seizure activity leads to calpain activation and proteolysis of alpha-spectrin as a result of kainic acid (KA) injection in the hippocampus resulting in cell death in the hippocampus from excitotoxicity [86, 88 - 92]. Several experiments have shown that calpain inhibition was effective in ameliorating seizure burden, slowing the seizure offsets and long term potentiation [93 - 98]. Moreover, it has been shown that overexpression of calpain 1 in the temporal neocortex results in the same clinical pathology as in patients with intractable epilepsy [99].

Ischemic Stroke

Interruption of the blood circulation to the brain causes membrane depolarization and disrupts Ca^{2+} homeostasis in neurons. The excitotoxic ischemic injury following reduced blood flow increases intra-neuronal free calcium levels, leading to calpain activation.

Mechanisms involved in neuronal injury after ischemia include the formation/release of highly reactive free radicals and cytotoxic cytokines which directly participate in brain ischemia, or combine with calpain activation during brain ischemia [86, 100 - 107]. Calpain and other proteases play major role in the degradation of various cellular proteins that participate in apoptotic cell death in the lesion and the penumbra after brain ischemia. These same proteases play a role in delayed neuronal death in the ischemic penumbra [104, 108 - 111]. In addition, oxygen and glucose deprivation in brain slices caused calpain dependent conversion of the Cdk 5 activation, leading to an increase in p25 activity [112 - 114]. Overall, inappropriate imbalance between proteases and protease inhibitors in cerebral ischemia has led to extensive examination of calpain inhibitors as therapeutic targets for ischemic stroke. Using an animal model, multiple agents with calpain inhibiting properties have been tested [110, 115 - 119]. Administration of MDL 28,170 resulted in a dose-dependent reduction in infarct volume when administered 30 minutes after middle cerebral artery occlusion (MCAO). The protective effect of MDL 28,170 was lost after an 8-hour delay [120]. Rats treated with Cbz-Val-Phe-H showed significantly smaller infarct volumes. Effective reduction in infarction and edema, as well as a reduction in calcium activated proteolysis were observed after intravenous injections of cumulative doses of 30 mg/kg or 60 mg/kg of Cbz-Val-Phe-H [101, 121]. The calpain inhibitor Calpeptin has resulted in an improvement in neurological function and decreases in infarct volume and neuronal apoptosis of the CA1 sector of the hippocampus following reperfusion after focal cerebral ischemia in rats. These results further confirmed that calpain inhibition plays a role in neuroprotection from reperfusion injury following focal cerebral ischemia [122]. Experiment with conditional knock-out (CKO) of Cdk5 as well as pharmacological inhibition Cdk5 demonstrated prevention of neuronal death from focal cerebral ischemia by blocking excitotoxicity [113, 114, 123].

Huntington's Disease (HD)

Huntington's disease is an inherited neurodegenerative disorder that results from expansion of a CAG trinucleotide repeat encoding polyglutamine (polyGLYN). Calpain-mediated processing of mutant huntingtin (mhtt) is regarded as a key event in the pathogenesis of HD and the presence of calpain cleavage products has been observed in brains of HD patients. Fragments of mHtt containing a polyGLYN expansion are more cytotoxic than the full length mHtt. The degradation process can be blocked by calcium chelators. Mutant huntingtin is easily cleaved by calpain, resulting in two huntingtin fragments that easily enter the nucleus to form intranuclear inclusions [124 - 128]. Cleavage of huntingtin mainly occurs in dying cells and inhibition of huntingtin cleavage reduces huntingtin aggregates and toxicity, further supporting the role of calpain in the disease process and its inhibition in the potential treatment regimen of HD When primary neurons were exposed to glutamate or 3-nitropropionic acid (3-NP), degradation of wild-type huntingtin was observed and abnormal activation of calpain was found to contribute to degeneration of striatal neurons after exposure to 3-NP. Treatment with calpain inhibitors mediate protection against polyglutamine toxicity as well as 3-NP-induced neuronal damage [129 - 133]. These results suggest that calpain cleavage of huntingtin and calpain-mediated injury of striatal neurons plays a role in HD pathogenesis and calpain inhibition is a potential target for therapeutic intervention.

Similar to other neurodegenerative diseases, Cdk 5 plays a role in the pathophysiology of HD [134, 135].

Multiple Sclerosis (MS)

Calpain-mediated proteolysis as well as axonal injury subsequently leading to long term disability in MS is a potential target for therapeutic strategies. Elevated levels of calpain were found in the white matter of patients with MS and it was present in large quantities inside activated inflammatory cells surrounding the MS plaques [136 - 152]. There is a recent report that bidirectional cytotoxicity from neuron-microglia interaction is associated with activation of calpain [153, 154]. Although other proteases are also involved in myelin degradation as well as axonal injury, calpain appears to play a major role in these processes since neuronal protein degradation (alpha-spectrin and NFP) is significantly decreased when calpain is inhibited [155 - 159].

The exact mechanism of axonal injury is not fully understood, but several factors including abnormally activated calpain are believed to play a key role. Demyelination results in impairment or loss of conduction of electrical signals, progressively leading to compensatory increases in sodium channel ($Na_v1.6$ channels) expression to restore conduction. The resulting increased influx of sodium into the axons via the Na^+/Ca^{2+} exchanger (NCX) triggers increased Ca^{2+} release which activates a number of enzyme cascades including one that leads to increased calpain activation. This phenomenon is particularly important in the chronic phase of MS and experimental autoimmune encephalomyelitis (EAE). The disease severity and the degree of permanent disability correspond to the extent of axonal damage rather than myelin damage [160 - 171].

A reduction in axonal injury was achieved using flecainide or phenytoin via the inhibition of sodium channels. Calpain inhibition exhibited the same effect in EAE [158, 172, 173]. Similar calpain-related pathophysiology and treatment strategies with calpain inhibitors were observed in optic neuritis, a form of MS [156, 174 - 178].

Muscular Dystrophy (MD)

Proteolysis in muscle fibers leads to degeneration in different neuromuscular and muscular dystrophy diseases. Some of the disease entities include Duchenne and Becker muscular dystrophies (DMD/BMD), inflammatory myopathy, acute quadriplegic myopathy and distal myopathy. Dystrophin deficiency is believed to result in membrane lesions causing leakage of intracellular constituents and influx of calcium ions. This influx of calcium ions has been proposed to account for myofiber necrosis secondary to activation of calpain. Abnormal calcium accumulation in DMD myofibers as well as in murine MDX myofibers is a well-known phenomenon [179 - 185]. This fact suggests that proteases such as calpain may play a role in the pathology. Several calpain types are associated with the pathology of the muscular apparatus. Calpain 3 seems to play substantial role, as alterations in calpain 3 seems to predispose a person to the familial type of muscle girdle dystrophy [186, 187].

Further supporting the role of calpain in muscle injury, calpain inhibitors have been used to delay muscle degeneration and necrosis in animal models. In addition, transgenic mice that overexpressed calpastatin showed reductions in dystrophic pathology [179, 188 - 194].

Parkinson's Disease (PD)

Parkinson's disease is a progressive neurological disease characterized by loss of dopaminergic neurons in the substantia nigra pars compacta. The molecular mechanisms leading to neurodegeneration of dopamine neurons in PD are poorly understood, but calpain plays a significant role as calpain expression and activity is elevated in postmortem brains of patients with PD. Increased calpain expression was also observed in the mesencephalon of patients that suffer from PD. Calpain activation and alpha-synuclein (α-syn) deposits appear to be relevant components of the disease. The aggregation and accumulation of α-syn deposits, one hall mark of PD that leads to synaptic dysfunction and neuronal death, is proposed to play a central role in the pathophysiology of PD. It has been shown that overexpression of calpastatin reduced human α-syn processing and aggregation, suggesting calpain's role [195 - 225]. In 1-methyl-4-Phenylpyridinium ion (MPP+) treated granule neurons, calpain activation was determined showing an increase in calpain (74%) as measured by alpha-spectrin cleavage products. The results indicate that the cleavage is mediated by calpain. Another hint for the role of calpain in PD is that overexpression of calpastatin leads to a reduction in truncated and aggregated α-Syn as well as decreasing synaptic impairment in transgenic animal models of PD [226].

Another mechanism proposed in the pathophysiology of PD as well as other neurodegenerative diseases is the breakdown of Cdk5/p35 into CDK5/p25, leading to increases in its kinase activity and neurotoxicity [227]. MPP+ prompted an increase in Cdk 5 expression, as well as the cleavage of p35-p25, in a time-dependent manner. Increased Cdk 5/p25 expression has been shown in the brains of patients with PD [200, 228 - 232].

Administration of N-methyl-4-phenyl-1,2,3,6-tetrahydropyridine (MPTP) increases calpain mediated proteolysis in nigral dopamine neurons and causes behavioral changes resembling PD. Inhibition of calpain resulted in a reduction in behavioral and neuronal deficit in an MPTP model [233 - 235]. Studies have shown that treatment with calpain inhibitors (*e.g.*, calpeptin, MDL-28170) prevents neuronal death and restores function in rodent and cell culture models of PD [233]. Similarly, inhibition of calpain using animals overexpressing calpastatin, the endogenous calpain inhibitor, significantly attenuated the loss of nigral dopaminergic neurons in an MPTP animal model [226]. Our group has tested two calpain inhibitors in a small number of transgenic animal models of PD. Intraperitoneal administration of both calpain inhibitors, Gabadur and Neurodur for 30 days at 2mg/mouse/day in the PDGF α-Syn mouse model, is seen to have a dramatic effect on the deposition of α-Syn in examined brain tissue (hippocampus and cortex). Gabadur decreases α-Syn deposition by approximately 60%, while Neurodur decreases it by approximately 40% in both regions. Calpain activity is decreased by approximately 70% in the Gabadur group. The animals tolerated the therapy without any observable toxic effects (unpublished data).

Traumatic Brain (TBI) and Spinal Cord Injuries (SCI)

Injuries to the brain or spinal cord trigger a process that results in neuronal damage in phases. The initial proposed mechanism after focal or global contusion appears to be excitotoxicity resulting in increased glutamate release and sustained overactivation of the N-methyl-D-aspartate (NMDA) receptors. This results in increased Ca^{2+} overload immediately following CNS trauma, which then further leads to calpain activation [86, 236 - 240]. In the secondary or delayed phase, tissue damage results from ischemia, loss of ion homeostasis, excitotoxicity, and free-radical production. TBI mediated axonal injury causes secondary damage to the myelin sheath and the myelin membrane of adjacent structures [241 - 245].

A relative shift in μ-calpain activity from the cytosol to the total membrane fraction was observed from 3 to 24 h following injury, a time frame consistent with increased calpain autolysis and proteolytic activity. The effect of calpain activation on proteolysis of the neuronal cytoskeletal protein was evaluated using alpha-spectrin degradation products [240, 246 - 248]. Calpain expression in the cortex significantly changed during the time from TBI to death, and the most prominent expression was detected in the cortex 3 days after TBI. Immunoreactivity for alpha-spectrin breakdown products was detectable within 15 min after injury in cortical samples ipsilateral to the injury site. The levels of alpha-spectrin breakdown products increased in a biphasic manner, with a large increase between 15 min and 6 h after injury, followed by a smaller increase between 6 and 24 h after the insult. No further accumulation of alpha-spectrin breakdown products was observed between 24 and 48 h after injury [241 - 243, 249]. Thus, calpain inhibition is appealing for SCI and TBI treatment as it can lead to reduction in neuronal injury by ameliorating cytoskeletal degradation [250, 251]. Another mechanism that has been targeted in neurodegenerative diseases is the Cdk 5 pathway. Calpain inhibition has been shown to attenuate Cdk 5 activation and improve neurological function after spinal cord injury [252].

The role of calpain in TBI and or SCI was tested using various calpain inhibitors in transgenic animals that overexpressed the endogenous inhibitor calpastatin, as well as calpain1 knockout animal models [253 - 255]. Pharmacological calpain inhibition has been tested in different models of TBI/SCI [256, 257]. Controlled cortical impact (CCI) is a widely used model [258 - 260]. An experiment using lentiviral vectors (LV) encoding calpain 1 shRNA (CAPN1shRNA) in a Calpain 1 knockdown model demonstrated a significant improvement in locomotor function over 6 weeks after the initial injury when compared to LV control groups. In addition, calpain 1 protein levels were reduced by 54% 2 weeks after shRNA-mediated knockout when compared to the LV control group, while calpain 2 levels were unchanged. The results from this experiment support the hypothesis that calpain 1 activation plays a role in tissue damage and impaired locomotor function, and strengthens the potential of calpain inhibitors as therapeutic agents [254]. Further supporting the role of calpain in TBI/SCI, Calpastatin overexpression significantly attenuated calpain-mediated proteolysis of these selected substrates immediately after severe CCI [254, 255]. Pre-injury administration of MDL28170 resulted in improvement in axonal injury after TBI. Similarly, application of MDL28170 abated calpain I activation, thereby inhibiting apoptosis and neuronal loss, as well as activating microglia. The consequence of these mechanisms was a significant improvement in locomotor function one week after spinal cord hemisection [245, 256, 261]. Recently, protection of neuronal injury from TBI was shown using a selective calpain 2 inhibitor [262].

OVERVIEW OF CURRENT PROTEASE INHIBITORS

Several attempts have been made to identify, develop and use calpain inhibitors. The major difficulties in this matter have been calpain inhibitor specificity, water-solubility, cell membrane penetration and the ability to cross the blood-brain barrier (BBB). Over the years, some inhibitors have been developed that have better affinity and potency, but they still exhibit some of these limitations [22 - 25, 263 - 277].

The major protease inhibitors are broadly subdivided into 4 classes:

1. Peptidyl epoxides: irreversibly inhibit calpain and other cysteine proteases by forming a thioester bond with the active site cysteine. Its charged groups, however, prevent it from passing through the plasma membrane (*e.g.* E64).
2. Peptidyl aldehydes: form a reversible hemiacetal bond with the active site thiol. They suffer from poor solubility, poor membrane permeability and the inability to cross the BBB (*e.g.* leupeptin).
3. Peptidyl α ketomides: inhibit calpain reversibly and show improved cell and membrane permeability over the above mentioned groups (*e.g.* AK275 and AK295).
4. Non-peptide inhibitors: they target a site other than the active site and may show better specificity to calpain than other cysteine proteases. The inhibition mode is non-competitive and reversible. The binding of the inhibitor at an allosteric site may bring an alteration in the structure of calpain leading to an impaired confirmatory change and inactivation of the enzyme (*e.g.* PD150606 and PD151746).

Advances in biopharmaceutical methods and techniques have led to the development of improved characteristics of calpain inhibitors. A newer agent with improved cell penetration capacity is a synthetic *N*-acetylated 27-mer peptide derived from exon B of the human calpastatin inhibitory domain 1. This peptide was *N*-terminally extended with, or disulfide-linked to the *C*-terminal 7-mer fragment of penetratin, a vector for cell membrane translocation of bioactive compounds [269]. Another promising agent is a nanomolecular inhibitor that was created by applying chemical modifications, site-directed mutagenesis and molecular modeling, in order to covalently bind thalassospiramide's α,β-unsaturated carbonyl moiety to the thiol group of calpain's catalytic Cys115 residue [278]. A newer version of a calpain 1 inhibitor is the substrate-based azapeptide. This inhibitor was derived from a potent m-calpain substrate, TPLKSPPPSPR. The oligopeptide is modified by systematic replacements of amino acids at different substrate binding positions [265]. Two additional 3rd generation selective and potent calpain 1 inhibitors are NYC438 and NYC488. These agents are derived from a well-known epoxide-based generic calpain inhibitor: E64. These agents have shown promising results in an animal model of AD with less overall toxicity and longer half-life [279].

Moreover, targeting calpain action can be achieved with methods other than pharmacological inhibition. Newer strategies include genetic alterations of the enzyme or its natural inhibitor. Several researchers have conducted experiments using calpain knockout mice and animals overexpressing calpastatin. Both experimental approaches strengthen the role of calpain in various pathological conditions as well as the role its inhibition plays in treating diseases, as discussed in each individual diseases. Of note, some of the calpain inhibitors exert their effect via mechanisms other than calpain inhibition. For instance Calpeptin, a known calpain inhibitor, can exert its effect independent of calpain inhibition. Experiment using Calpeptin showed a direct inhibitory effect on mitochondrial ion channels affecting thrombin- and collagen-mediated platelet activation [280, 281]. Application of PD150606, a known non-peptide calpain inhibitor, ameliorated neuronal damage by irreversibly inhibiting calcium influx through alpha-amino-3-hydroxy-5-methyl-4-isoxazole propionic acid (AMPA) receptors [96].

TARGETED PROTEASE INHIBITION

Our laboratory has been working on developing targeted protease inhibitors with improved characteristics for optimal effect. We have developed three protease inhibitors with distinct features. Here, we describe the different protease inhibitors and their unique properties.

Gabadur (ALA 1.0)

Gabadur (ALA1.0) is synthesized by combining the modified anti-seizure/pain medication Pregabalin as a vehicle and leupeptin as calpain inhibitor. The concept was developed from the clinical observation of the efficacy of Gabapentin for a particular type of disabling subjective idiopathic tinnitus with early signs of neurodegeneration. Pregabalin is an analog of gamma-aminobutyric acid (GABA) and has been approved by FDA for use in neuropathic pain, adjunct therapy for partial seizure and as an anxiolytic agent [282]. The leucyl-argininal part exerts its effect on calpain that is abnormally activated due to the excitotoxicity caused by the seizure. Pregabalin is a α2-δ ligand of the voltage-gated calcium channel similar to GABA [283 - 285]. Pregabalin binding sites are upregulated in response to nerve damage, thus probably targeting the leucyl-argininal to the site of injury/insult [286, 287]. Gabadur's structure is (3-aminomethyl-4amio-5methylhexanoic acid)-suc-leul-argininal (Fig. **1**). The pregabalin part of Gabadur acts on the voltage-gated calcium channel, thereby rendering its potential effect on seizure activity [282, 285]. The combined effect is thought to minimize the amount of the individual drugs needed, reduce their side effects as well as provide additive advantage through synergistic therapy.

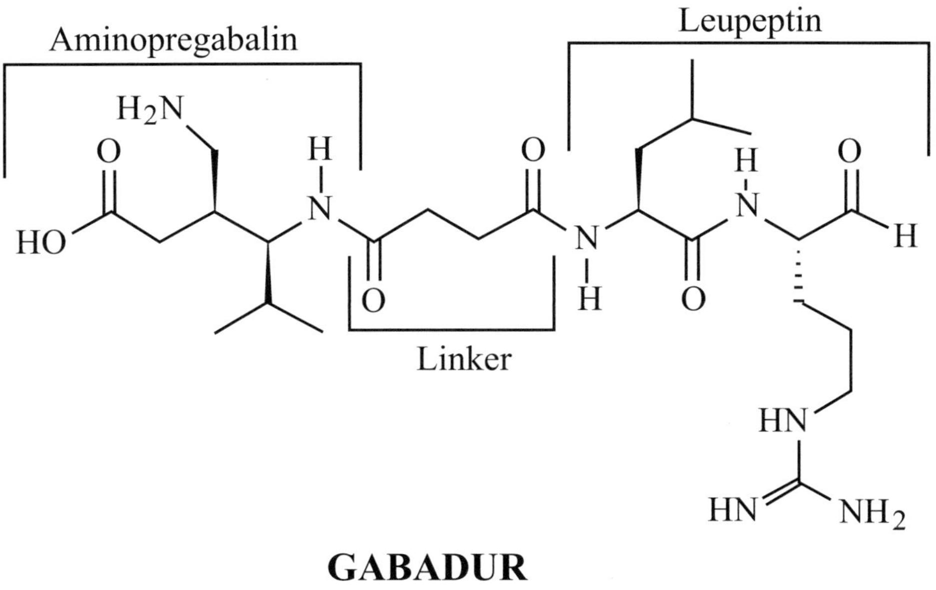

Fig. (1). Structure of Gabadur.

Myodur

It has already been described in literature that naturally occurring carnitine is distributed in muscle tissue [288, 289]. We thus conceived the concept of covalently attaching carnitine to the active end of the leupeptin molecule, leucyl-argininal, to allow selective muscle absorption. The structure of leupeptin, a well-known calpain inhibitor, and Myodur are identical at two positions, and it is the leucyl-argininal moiety that is directly involved in calpain inhibition.

Leupeptin contains an acetyl-leucinyl group attached to the N-terminal leucyl and Myodur contains an aminocarnitine group attached to the amino group via a succinyl linker (Fig. **2**). Myodur targets the high affinity carnitine transporter: organic cation transporter (OCTN2), which is localized in the heart, the kidney and in skeletal muscle. Organic cation transporter 2 co-transports sodium and L-carnitine with high affinity along with drugs such as quinidine and verapamil [290, 291]. This targeting principle results in enhanced potency and reduction in side effects when compared to leupeptin alone. Myodur can be delivered to muscle tissue approximately 115 times more effectively than leupeptin alone (preliminary result).

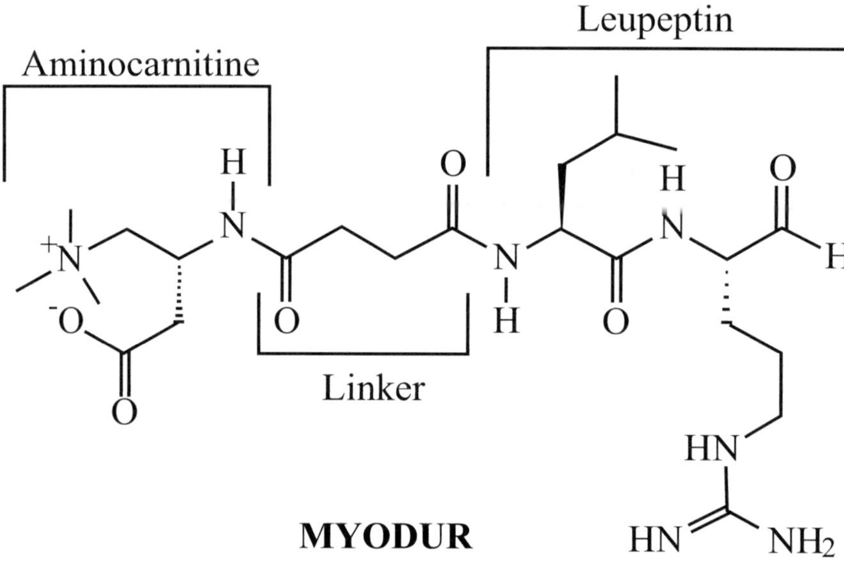

Fig. (2). Structure of Myodur.

Neurodur

Taurine (2-aminoethanesulfonic acid) is an essential β-amino acid that is dependent on a Na^+-dependent transport system to pass through cell membranes. Two distinct high affinity Na^+-dependent systems help transport Taurine. Taurine is synthesized in limited amounts in the brain and the vast majority of this essential amino acid must be transported across the BBB [292 - 294]. Due to structural similarity with taurine, cysteic acid (α-amino-β-sulfo-propionic acid) utilizes taurine transport to cross membranes [295 - 297]. Neurodur is synthesized by attaching the carboxyl group of cysteic acid to the leucyl-argininal of Leupeptin (Fig. **3**). This enables Neurodur to use taurine transporters to cross the BBB. Moreover, the carrier molecule taurine by itself has anti-inflammatory, calpain inhibitory and calpastatin upregulatory effects. This is an additional benefit of Neurodur. Limited experiments have shown the beneficial effect of taurine in closed head injury models *in vivo* [298 - 300]. We have shown the ability of Neurodur in suppressing inflammation, demyelination and protection of axonal injury in experimental autoimmune encephalomyelitis (EAE) both in acute and chronic forms [159, 172]. The synergistic effect of leupeptin and taurine make Neurodur a very appealing therapeutic agent in treating TBI patients.

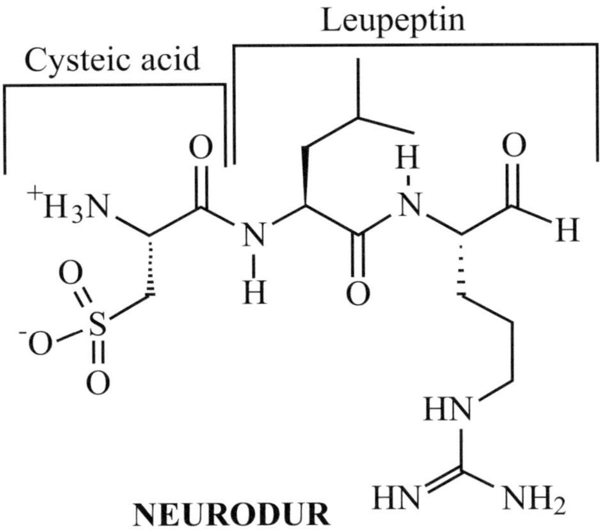

Fig. (3). Structure of Neurodur.

DISCUSSION

All forms of tissue breakdown are regulated by protein synthesis and protein degradation. When protein degradation exceeds the synthesis pathway, atrophy occurs in all forms of tissue wasting. This is most easily observed in muscle as it makes up approximately 40%-50% of the mass of an animal. Muscle wasting can also be the result of neuromuscular junction dysfunction or neuronal injury, in which proteases play a role [301 - 305]. Thus, one should consider the role of protease inhibition in the treatment of diseases with extensive tissue wasting. With the discovery of calpain and the role of calpain in different disease conditions, the focused attention on inhibition of this protease began [273, 306 - 308]. The initial studies using leupeptin, a thiol protease inhibitor discovered by the Umezawa group, showed promising results [309, 310]. The early studies using cultured muscles incubated with leupeptin showed a remarkable extension of the fiber lifespan and robustness of the fibers. These studies were sufficiently encouraging to enter into a series of *in vivo* animal model studies, including denervation atrophy, the MDX genetic mouse models of DMD and EAE, an animal model of MS [159, 172, 179, 189, 311 - 314]. Earlier studies from our laboratory using leupeptin showed both a delay in muscle degeneration and necrosis in MDX mice, as well as recovery of neuromuscular segments after peripheral nerve injury. An early study of denervated chicken pectoral muscle showed that the calpain inhibitor leupeptin, when injected intramuscularly into the denervated pectoral muscle decreased muscle atrophy by approximately 45 to 48% [315]. This *in vivo* demonstration of the therapeutic effectiveness of calpain inhibitor was extremely encouraging and led to an extensive *in vivo* study in monkeys using leupeptin to prevent denervation atrophy. Similar studies with leupeptin were carried out in an MDX mouse model of human DMD. In this study, although untreated muscle leads to loss in muscle fiber size, calpain inhibition can prevent the decrease in myofiber diameter in both the gastrocnemius and diaphragm of the MDX mouse after 60 days of treatment with leupeptin [179, 312, 314, 316]. Most interesting was the observation that calpain activity did not return to zero, but rather close to control values depending upon the doses used. This observation suggests that calpain inhibitors act in a manner to replace calpastatin, the endogenous inhibitor of calpain.

Another area of calpain involvement is MS. Leupeptin has been used for the treatment of EAE. Unfortunately leupeptin does not cross the BBB and needs to be directly injected in to the CNS or liposome-encapsulated in order to cross the BBB [317, 318]. The disadvantage of these ways of administering leupeptin is the invasiveness of the intrathecal application and the degradation of the liposome-encapsulated drug when administered orally.

It became apparent that attaching the protease inhibitor to a carrier for selective delivery would have significant advantages. Targeted inhibition allows dose reduction of the individual agent and results in fewer side effects. It also increases the amount of drug available at the desired site of action. The advantages of targeted protease inhibitors are numerous, including:

1. Delivery of the drug to the area of calpain over-activation by concentrating the amount of inhibitor in the area of interest and reducing the amount of calpain inhibition in different organs systems where calpain is physiologically active.

2. Reduction of the adverse effects of the drug and toxicity by using a smaller dose.
3. Increasing the window of opportunity in treating diseases, since calpain is involved in the late stages of disease.
4. Combining two agents that will provide additive/synergistic effect.

For instance given the roles of pregabalin and calpain inhibition in the treatment of seizure–related neurodegeneration, combining the two drugs provides an excellent double therapeutic intervention for the treatment of seizure disorders.

Our multiple sclerosis project showed suppression of inflammation and demyelination along with prevention of axonal injury using Neurodur. In a series of experiments, we have shown a dose-dependent inhibition of calpain and suppression of demyelination and inflammation. In another experiment using an animal model of retinal ischemia, we found that post-ischemic administration of 20 mg/kg of Neurodur provided a significant preservation of retinal cells [159, 172, 311].

Preliminary results from an animal model of Huntington's disease (3-nitropropionic acid-induced striatal damage) using Gabadur showed approximately 50% preservation of the striatal structure. Western blot analysis using alpha-spectrin antibody showed suppression of the full-length alpha-spectrin proteolysis in the Gabadur treated groups. Partial results from this experiment were presented at the Experimental Biology (EB) scientific meeting in April, 2009. The preliminary results from another project using an animal model of Parkinson's disease showed reduction of α-Syn by Neurodur (40%) and Gabadur (60%) (Unpublished data). This model gives the strongest indirect evidence that the protease inhibitors can cross the intact BBB as compared to other models where the disease process disrupts the BBB to some extent. Currently experiments are being conducted in animal models of noise induced sensorineural hearing tinnitus as well as traumatic brain injury using our targeted calpain inhibitors.

The previously described works illustrate how diverse the involvement of calpain is in a wide variety of disorders. Thus the genesis of the title and the use of the term "magic bullet". With calpain as a "target" we have designed a potential "magic bullet" inhibitor of calpain and have shown its effect in animal models of multiple neuromuscular and neurodegenerative disorders. Thus, it is not unrealistic to consider that Ehrlich's dream of a "magic bullet" to treat a class of diseases pharmacologically may be more a reality than previously imagined.

Lastly, it is important to note that calpains are ubiquitous enzymes and have important physiological functions. Treatment with calpain inhibitors may help treat pathologies that result from abnormally elevated calpain activation, but the inhibition may concurrently affect the normal function of calpain in other organ systems. This may lead to complications or worsening of the pathological condition for which the treatment was intended. One example of this is the role of calpain in platelet aggregation. Calpain in known to affect platelet aggregation and its inhibition may affect the coagulation cascade [281, 319 - 323]. In the setting of trauma and TBI, calpain activation is believed to ameliorate brain injury, but may also affect platelet aggregation and lead to bleeding complications. This fact and other potential complications have to be taken in to account when considering calpain inhibitors as a therapeutic agents.

CONCLUSION

Given the role of calpain in the molecular mechanisms of numerous disease states, including various neurodegenerative and neuromuscular diseases, and especially considering that their involvement in delayed tissue destruction allows an increased window of opportunity for treatment, calpain inhibitors either as a single agent or in combination with other pharmaceutical agents are appealing new therapeutic agents.

CONFLICT OF INTEREST

The authors declare no conflict of interest, financial or otherwise.

ACKNOWLEDGEMENTS

We thank Drs. Pashmforoosh and Shaw for reviewing and editing the Manuscript as well as the Michael J. Fox Foundation and the Martha Entenmann Tinnitus Research Center Inc. for their support. Moreover, we would like to thank Dr. Satendra for his support with the chemical structures of these varies drugs and his valuable scientific advice.

REFERENCES

[1] Perrin BJ, Huttenlocher A. Calpain. Int J Biochem Cell Biol 2002; 34(7): 722-5. [http://dx.doi.org/10.1016/S1357-2725(02)00009-2] [PMID: 11950589]

[2] Wu HY, Lynch DR. Calpain and synaptic function. Mol Neurobiol 2006; 33(3): 215-36. [http://dx.doi.org/10.1385/MN:33:3:215] [PMID: 16954597]

[3] Glading A, Lauffenburger DA, Wells A. Cutting to the chase: calpain proteases in cell motility. Trends Cell Biol 2002; 12(1): 46-54. [http://dx.doi.org/10.1016/S0962-8924(01)02179-1] [PMID: 11854009]

[4] Wells A, Huttenlocher A, Lauffenburger DA. Calpain proteases in cell adhesion and motility. Int Rev Cytol 2005; 245: 1-16. [http://dx.doi.org/10.1016/S0074-7696(05)45001-9] [PMID: 16125543]

[5] Jánossy J, Ubezio P, Apáti A, Magócsi M, Tompa P, Friedrich P. Calpain as a multi-site regulator of

cell cycle. Biochem Pharmacol 2004; 67(8): 1513-21.
[http://dx.doi.org/10.1016/j.bcp.2003.12.021] [PMID: 15041468]

[6] Zimmerman UJ, Boring L, Pak JH, Mukerjee N, Wang KK. The calpain small subunit gene is essential: its inactivation results in embryonic lethality. IUBMB Life 2000; 50(1): 63-8.
[http://dx.doi.org/10.1080/15216540050176610] [PMID: 11087123]

[7] Suzuki K, Saido TC, Hirai S. Modulation of cellular signals by calpain. Ann N Y Acad Sci 1992; 674: 218-27.
[http://dx.doi.org/10.1111/j.1749-6632.1992.tb27490.x] [PMID: 1337690]

[8] Suzuki K, Sorimachi H, Yoshizawa T, Kinbara K, Ishiura S. Calpain: novel family members, activation, and physiologic function. Biol Chem Hoppe Seyler 1995; 376(9): 523-9.
[PMID: 8561910]

[9] Zimmerman UJ, Schlaepfer WW. Two-stage autolysis of the catalytic subunit initiates activation of calpain I. Biochim Biophys Acta 1991; 1078(2): 192-8.
[http://dx.doi.org/10.1016/0167-4838(91)99009-H] [PMID: 2065086]

[10] Saido TC, Nagao S, Shiramine M, *et al.* Autolytic transition of mu-calpain upon activation as resolved by antibodies distinguishing between the pre- and post-autolysis forms. J Biochem 1992; 111(1): 81-6.
[http://dx.doi.org/10.1093/oxfordjournals.jbchem.a123723] [PMID: 1607367]

[11] Wendt A, Thompson VF, Goll DE. Interaction of calpastatin with calpain: a review. Biol Chem 2004; 385(6): 465-72.
[http://dx.doi.org/10.1515/BC.2004.054] [PMID: 15255177]

[12] Johnson GV, Guttmann RP. Calpains: intact and active? BioEssays 1997; 19(11): 1011-8.
[http://dx.doi.org/10.1002/bies.950191111] [PMID: 9394623]

[13] Hanna RA, Campbell RL, Davies PL. Calcium-bound structure of calpain and its mechanism of inhibition by calpastatin. Nature 2008; 456(7220): 409-12.
[http://dx.doi.org/10.1038/nature07451] [PMID: 19020623]

[14] Potz BA, Abid MR, Sellke FW. Role of calpain in pathogenesis of human disease processes. J Nat Sci 2016; 2(9): e218.
[PMID: 27747292]

[15] Wu HY, Tomizawa K, Oda Y, *et al.* Critical role of calpain-mediated cleavage of calcineurin in excitotoxic neurodegeneration. J Biol Chem 2004; 279(6): 4929-40.
[http://dx.doi.org/10.1074/jbc.M309767200] [PMID: 14627704]

[16] Vosler PS, Brennan CS, Chen J. Calpain-mediated signaling mechanisms in neuronal injury and neurodegeneration. Mol Neurobiol 2008; 38(1): 78-100.
[http://dx.doi.org/10.1007/s12035-008-8036-x] [PMID: 18686046]

[17] Vanderklish PW, Bahr BA. The pathogenic activation of calpain: a marker and mediator of cellular toxicity and disease states. Int J Exp Pathol 2000; 81(5): 323-39.
[http://dx.doi.org/10.1046/j.1365-2613.2000.00169.x] [PMID: 11168679]

[18] Camins A, Verdaguer E, Folch J, Pallàs M. Involvement of calpain activation in neurodegenerative processes. CNS Drug Rev 2006; 12(2): 135-48.
[http://dx.doi.org/10.1111/j.1527-3458.2006.00135.x] [PMID: 16958987]

[19] Zimmerman UJ, Schlaepfer WW. Activation of calpain I and calpain II: a comparative study using terbium as a fluorescent probe for calcium-binding sites. Arch Biochem Biophys 1988; 266(2): 462-9.
[http://dx.doi.org/10.1016/0003-9861(88)90278-0] [PMID: 2847653]

[20] Zimmerman UP, Schlaepfer WW. Multiple forms of Ca-activated protease from rat brain and muscle. J Biol Chem 1984; 259(5): 3210-8.
[PMID: 6321500]

[21] Zimmerman UJ, Schlaepfer WW. Calcium-activated neutral protease (CANP) in brain and other

tissues. Prog Neurobiol 1984; 23(1-2): 63-78.
[http://dx.doi.org/10.1016/0301-0082(84)90012-1] [PMID: 6097938]

[22] Siklos M, BenAissa M, Thatcher GR. Cysteine proteases as therapeutic targets: does selectivity matter? A systematic review of calpain and cathepsin inhibitors. Acta Pharm Sin B 2015; 5(6): 506-19.
[http://dx.doi.org/10.1016/j.apsb.2015.08.001] [PMID: 26713267]

[23] Donkor IO. Calpain inhibitors: a survey of compounds reported in the patent and scientific literature. Expert Opin Ther Pat 2011; 21(5): 601-36.
[http://dx.doi.org/10.1517/13543776.2011.568480] [PMID: 21434837]

[24] Donkor IO. An updated patent review of calpain inhibitors (2012 - 2014). Expert Opin Ther Pat 2015; 25(1): 17-31.
[PMID: 25399719]

[25] Pietsch M, Chua KC, Abell AD. Calpains: attractive targets for the development of synthetic inhibitors. Curr Top Med Chem 2010; 10(3): 270-93.
[http://dx.doi.org/10.2174/156802610790725489] [PMID: 20166953]

[26] Ikiz B, Przedborski S. A sequel to the tale of p25/Cdk5 in neurodegeneration. Neuron 2008; 60(5): 731-2.
[http://dx.doi.org/10.1016/j.neuron.2008.11.020] [PMID: 19081365]

[27] Patrick GN, Zukerberg L, Nikolic M, de la Monte S, Dikkes P, Tsai LH. Conversion of p35 to p25 deregulates Cdk5 activity and promotes neurodegeneration. Nature 1999; 402(6762): 615-22.
[http://dx.doi.org/10.1038/45159] [PMID: 10604467]

[28] Camins A, Verdaguer E, Folch J, Canudas AM, Pallàs M. The role of CDK5/P25 formation/inhibition in neurodegeneration. Drug News Perspect 2006; 19(8): 453-60.
[http://dx.doi.org/10.1358/dnp.2006.19.8.1043961] [PMID: 17160145]

[29] Hamdane M, Buée L. The complex p25/Cdk5 kinase in neurofibrillary degeneration and neuronal death: the missing link to cell cycle. Biotechnol J 2007; 2(8): 967-77.
[http://dx.doi.org/10.1002/biot.200700059] [PMID: 17571276]

[30] Kanungo J. Special Issue on "Cdk5 and Brain Disorders": Prologue. Brain Disord Ther 2012; Suppl 1.

[31] Kanungo J, Zheng YL, Amin ND, Pant HC. Targeting Cdk5 activity in neuronal degeneration and regeneration. Cell Mol Neurobiol 2009; 29(8): 1073-80.
[http://dx.doi.org/10.1007/s10571-009-9410-6] [PMID: 19455415]

[32] Lee MS, Kwon YT, Li M, Peng J, Friedlander RM, Tsai LH. Neurotoxicity induces cleavage of p35 to p25 by calpain. Nature 2000; 405(6784): 360-4.
[http://dx.doi.org/10.1038/35012636] [PMID: 10830966]

[33] Ahlijanian MK, Barrezueta NX, Williams RD, *et al.* Hyperphosphorylated tau and neurofilament and cytoskeletal disruptions in mice overexpressing human p25, an activator of cdk5. Proc Natl Acad Sci USA 2000; 97(6): 2910-5.
[http://dx.doi.org/10.1073/pnas.040577797] [PMID: 10706614]

[34] Mohamed T, Shakeri A, Rao PP. Amyloid cascade in Alzheimer's disease: Recent advances in medicinal chemistry. Eur J Med Chem 2016; 113: 258-72.
[http://dx.doi.org/10.1016/j.ejmech.2016.02.049] [PMID: 26945113]

[35] Shen J, Wu J. Nicotinic Cholinergic Mechanisms in Alzheimer's Disease. Int Rev Neurobiol 2015; 124: 275-92.
[http://dx.doi.org/10.1016/bs.irn.2015.08.002] [PMID: 26472533]

[36] Oz M, Lorke DE, Yang KH, Petroianu G. On the interaction of β-amyloid peptides and α7-nicotinic acetylcholine receptors in Alzheimer's disease. Curr Alzheimer Res 2013; 10(6): 618-30.
[http://dx.doi.org/10.2174/15672050113109990132] [PMID: 23627750]

[37] Grimaldi M, Marino SD, Florenzano F, *et al.* β-Amyloid-acetylcholine molecular interaction: new role

of cholinergic mediators in anti-Alzheimer therapy? Future Med Chem 2016; 8(11): 1179-89. [http://dx.doi.org/10.4155/fmc-2016-0006] [PMID: 27402297]

[38] Hasanbasic S, Jahic A, Karahmet E, Sejranic A, Prnjavorac B. The role of cysteine protease in alzheimer disease. Mater Sociomed 2016; 28(3): 235-8. [http://dx.doi.org/10.5455/msm.2016.28.235-238] [PMID: 27482169]

[39] Higuchi M, Iwata N, Matsuba Y, *et al.* Mechanistic involvement of the calpain-calpastatin system in Alzheimer neuropathology. FASEB J 2012; 26(3): 1204-17. [http://dx.doi.org/10.1096/fj.11-187740] [PMID: 22173972]

[40] Higuchi M, Iwata N, Saido TC. Understanding molecular mechanisms of proteolysis in Alzheimer's disease: progress toward therapeutic interventions. Biochim Biophys Acta 2005; 1751(1): 60-7. [http://dx.doi.org/10.1016/j.bbapap.2005.02.013] [PMID: 16054018]

[41] Liang B, Duan BY, Zhou XP, Gong JX, Luo ZG. Calpain activation promotes BACE1 expression, amyloid precursor protein processing, and amyloid plaque formation in a transgenic mouse model of Alzheimer disease. J Biol Chem 2010; 285(36): 27737-44. [http://dx.doi.org/10.1074/jbc.M110.117960] [PMID: 20595388]

[42] Seo J, Giusti-Rodríguez P, Zhou Y, *et al.* Activity-dependent p25 generation regulates synaptic plasticity and Aβ-induced cognitive impairment. Cell 2014; 157(2): 486-98. [http://dx.doi.org/10.1016/j.cell.2014.01.065] [PMID: 24725413]

[43] Trinchese F, Fa' M, Liu S, *et al.* Inhibition of calpains improves memory and synaptic transmission in a mouse model of Alzheimer disease. J Clin Invest 2008; 118(8): 2796-807. [http://dx.doi.org/10.1172/JCI34254] [PMID: 18596919]

[44] Utreras E, Maccioni R, González-Billault C. Cyclin-dependent kinase 5 activator p35 over-expression and amyloid beta synergism increase apoptosis in cultured neuronal cells. Neuroscience 2009; 161(4): 978-87. [http://dx.doi.org/10.1016/j.neuroscience.2009.04.002] [PMID: 19362124]

[45] Alvarez A, Toro R, Cáceres A, Maccioni RB. Inhibition of tau phosphorylating protein kinase cdk5 prevents beta-amyloid-induced neuronal death. FEBS Lett 1999; 459(3): 421-6. [http://dx.doi.org/10.1016/S0014-5793(99)01279-X] [PMID: 10526177]

[46] Park J, Kim B, Chae U, *et al.* Peroxiredoxin 5 decreases beta-amyloid-mediated cyclin-dependent kinase 5 activation through regulation of Ca(2+)-mediated calpain activation. Antioxid Redox Signal 2017; 27(11): 715-26. [http://dx.doi.org/10.1089/ars.2016.6810] [PMID: 28358580]

[47] Liu Y, Wang Y, Zhu G, Sun J, Bi X, Baudry M. A calpain-2 selective inhibitor enhances learning & memory by prolonging ERK activation. Neuropharmacology 2016; 105: 471-7. [http://dx.doi.org/10.1016/j.neuropharm.2016.02.022] [PMID: 26907807]

[48] Stifanese R, Averna M, De Tullio R, *et al.* Role of calpain-1 in the early phase of experimental ALS. Arch Biochem Biophys 2014; 562: 1-8. [http://dx.doi.org/10.1016/j.abb.2014.08.006] [PMID: 25151305]

[49] Gou-Fabregas M, Ramírez-Núñez O, Cacabelos D, *et al.* Calpain activation and CaMKIV reduction in spinal cords from hSOD1G93A mouse model. Mol Cell Neurosci 2014; 61: 219-25. [http://dx.doi.org/10.1016/j.mcn.2014.07.002] [PMID: 25063475]

[50] Watanabe S, Ilieva H, Tamada H, *et al.* Mitochondria-associated membrane collapse is a common pathomechanism in SIGMAR1- and SOD1-linked ALS. EMBO Mol Med 2016; 8(12): 1421-37. [http://dx.doi.org/10.15252/emmm.201606403] [PMID: 27821430]

[51] Yamashita T, Aizawa H, Teramoto S, Akamatsu M, Kwak S. Calpain-dependent disruption of nucleo-cytoplasmic transport in ALS motor neurons. Sci Rep 2017; 7: 39994. [http://dx.doi.org/10.1038/srep39994] [PMID: 28045133]

[52] Nguyen MD, Boudreau M, Kriz J, Couillard-Després S, Kaplan DR, Julien JP. Cell cycle regulators in

the neuronal death pathway of amyotrophic lateral sclerosis caused by mutant superoxide dismutase 1. J Neurosci 2003; 23(6): 2131-40.
[PMID: 12657672]

[53] Rosen DR, Siddique T, Patterson D, *et al.* Mutations in Cu/Zn superoxide dismutase gene are associated with familial amyotrophic lateral sclerosis. Nature 1993; 362(6415): 59-62.
[http://dx.doi.org/10.1038/362059a0] [PMID: 8446170]

[54] Tradewell ML, Durham HD. Calpastatin reduces toxicity of SOD1G93A in a culture model of amyotrophic lateral sclerosis. Neuroreport 2010; 21(15): 976-9.
[PMID: 20736867]

[55] Wootz H, Hansson I, Korhonen L, Lindholm D. XIAP decreases caspase-12 cleavage and calpain activity in spinal cord of ALS transgenic mice. Exp Cell Res 2006; 312(10): 1890-8.
[http://dx.doi.org/10.1016/j.yexcr.2006.02.021] [PMID: 16566922]

[56] Bajaj NP. Cyclin-dependent kinase-5 (CDK5) and amyotrophic lateral sclerosis. Amyotroph Lateral Scler Other Motor Neuron Disord 2000; 1(5): 319-27.
[http://dx.doi.org/10.1080/146608200300079563] [PMID: 11464850]

[57] Patzke H, Tsai LH. Cdk5 sinks into ALS. Trends Neurosci 2002; 25(1): 8-10.
[http://dx.doi.org/10.1016/S0166-2236(00)02000-2] [PMID: 11801324]

[58] Takahashi S, Kulkarni AB. Mutant superoxide dismutase 1 causes motor neuron degeneration independent of cyclin-dependent kinase 5 activation by p35 or p25. J Neurochem 2004; 88(5): 1295-304.
[http://dx.doi.org/10.1046/j.1471-4159.2003.02256.x] [PMID: 15009685]

[59] Shulman A. Noise, calpain, calpain inhibitors, and neuroprotection: a preliminary report of tinnitus control. Int Tinnitus J 1998; 4(2): 134-40.
[PMID: 10753402]

[60] Forge A. Outer hair cell loss and supporting cell expansion following chronic gentamicin treatment. Hear Res 1985; 19(2): 171-82.
[http://dx.doi.org/10.1016/0378-5955(85)90121-2] [PMID: 4055536]

[61] Forge A, Li L. Apoptotic death of hair cells in mammalian vestibular sensory epithelia. Hear Res 2000; 139(1-2): 97-115.
[http://dx.doi.org/10.1016/S0378-5955(99)00177-X] [PMID: 10601716]

[62] Jiang H, Sha SH, Forge A, Schacht J. Caspase-independent pathways of hair cell death induced by kanamycin *in vivo.* Cell Death Differ 2006; 13(1): 20-30.
[http://dx.doi.org/10.1038/sj.cdd.4401706] [PMID: 16021180]

[63] Taylor RR, Nevill G, Forge A. Rapid hair cell loss: a mouse model for cochlear lesions. J Assoc Res Otolaryngol 2008; 9(1): 44-64.
[http://dx.doi.org/10.1007/s10162-007-0105-8] [PMID: 18057986]

[64] Ding L, McFadden SL, Salvi RJ. Calpain immunoreactivity and morphological damage in chinchilla inner ears after carboplatin. J Assoc Res Otolaryngol 2002; 3(1): 68-79.
[http://dx.doi.org/10.1007/s101620020004] [PMID: 12083725]

[65] Ding ZJ, Chen X, Tang XX, *et al.* Apoptosis-inducing factor and calpain upregulation in glutamate-induced injury of rat spiral ganglion neurons. Mol Med Rep 2015; 12(2): 1685-92.
[http://dx.doi.org/10.3892/mmr.2015.3626] [PMID: 25891494]

[66] Dodson HC. Loss and survival of spiral ganglion neurons in the guinea pig after intracochlear perfusion with aminoglycosides. J Neurocytol 1997; 26(8): 541-56.
[http://dx.doi.org/10.1023/A:1015434524040] [PMID: 9350806]

[67] Chang L, Wang A. Calpain mediated cisplatin-induced ototoxicity in mice. Neural Regen Res 2013; 8(21): 1995-2002.
[PMID: 25206508]

[68] Lefebvre PP, Malgrange B, Lallemend F, Staecker H, Moonen G, Van De Water TR. Mechanisms of cell death in the injured auditory system: otoprotective strategies. Audiol Neurootol 2002; 7(3): 165-70.
[http://dx.doi.org/10.1159/000058304] [PMID: 12053139]

[69] Vago P, Humbert G, Lenoir M. Amikacin intoxication induces apoptosis and cell proliferation in rat organ of Corti. Neuroreport 1998; 9(3): 431-6.
[http://dx.doi.org/10.1097/00001756-199802160-00014] [PMID: 9512385]

[70] Holley MC, Ashmore JF. Spectrin, actin and the structure of the cortical lattice in mammalian cochlear outer hair cells. J Cell Sci 1990; 96(Pt 2): 283-91.
[PMID: 2211870]

[71] Holley MC, Ashmore JF. A cytoskeletal spring for the control of cell shape in outer hair cells isolated from the guinea pig cochlea. Eur Arch Otorhinolaryngol 1990; 247(1): 4-7.
[http://dx.doi.org/10.1007/BF00240939] [PMID: 2310549]

[72] Hafidi A, Despres G, Romand R. Cochlear innervation in the developing rat: an immunocytochemical study of neurofilament and spectrin proteins. J Comp Neurol 1990; 300(2): 153-61.
[http://dx.doi.org/10.1002/cne.903000202] [PMID: 2124223]

[73] Momiyama J, Hashimoto T, Matsubara A, Futai K, Namba A, Shinkawa H. Leupeptin, a calpain inhibitor, protects inner ear hair cells from aminoglycoside ototoxicity. Tohoku J Exp Med 2006; 209(2): 89-97.
[http://dx.doi.org/10.1620/tjem.209.89] [PMID: 16707850]

[74] Ding D, Stracher A, Salvi RJ. Leupeptin protects cochlear and vestibular hair cells from gentamicin ototoxicity. Hear Res 2002; 164(1-2): 115-26.
[http://dx.doi.org/10.1016/S0378-5955(01)00417-8] [PMID: 11950531]

[75] Salvi RJ, Shulman A, Stracher A, Ding D, Wang J. Protecting the inner ear from acoustic trauma. Int Tinnitus J 1998; 4(1): 11-5.
[PMID: 10753379]

[76] Abaamrane L, Raffin F, Schmerber S, Sendowski I. Intracochlear perfusion of leupeptin and z-VA--FMK: influence of antiapoptotic agents on gunshot-induced hearing loss. Eur Arch Otorhinolaryngol 2011; 268(7): 987-93.
[http://dx.doi.org/10.1007/s00405-011-1487-0] [PMID: 21246210]

[77] Wang J, Pignol B, Chabrier PE, *et al.* A novel dual inhibitor of calpains and lipid peroxidation (BN82270) rescues the cochlea from sound trauma. Neuropharmacology 2007; 52(6): 1426-37.
[http://dx.doi.org/10.1016/j.neuropharm.2007.02.007] [PMID: 17449343]

[78] Gavriel H, Shulman A, Stracher A, Sohmer H. Leupeptin reduces impulse noise induced hearing loss. J Occup Med Toxicol 2011; 6: 38.
[http://dx.doi.org/10.1186/1745-6673-6-38] [PMID: 22206578]

[79] Tang W, Seidman MD, Henig JP, Shulman A, Stracher A. The effects of leupeptin on cochlear blood flow, auditory sensitivity, and histology. Int Tinnitus J 2001; 7(1): 4-12.
[PMID: 14964948]

[80] Cheng AG, Huang T, Stracher A, *et al.* Calpain inhibitors protect auditory sensory cells from hypoxia and neurotrophin-withdrawal induced apoptosis. Brain Res 1999; 850(1-2): 234-43.
[http://dx.doi.org/10.1016/S0006-8993(99)01983-6] [PMID: 10629769]

[81] Hoffer ME, Finley JC, Killian P, *et al.* Sustained-release delivery of leupeptin in the chinchilla: hearing results. Int Tinnitus J 2003; 9(2): 76-8.
[PMID: 15106277]

[82] Choi DW. Excitotoxic cell death. J Neurobiol 1992; 23(9): 1261-76.
[http://dx.doi.org/10.1002/neu.480230915] [PMID: 1361523]

[83] Jarrard LE, Meldrum BS. Selective excitotoxic pathology in the rat hippocampus. Neuropathol Appl Neurobiol 1993; 19(5): 381-9. [http://dx.doi.org/10.1111/j.1365-2990.1993.tb00458.x] [PMID: 8278020]

[84] Meldrum BS. Excitotoxicity and selective neuronal loss in epilepsy. Brain Pathol 1993; 3(4): 405-12. [http://dx.doi.org/10.1111/j.1750-3639.1993.tb00768.x] [PMID: 8293196]

[85] Araújo IM, Xapelli S, Gil JM, *et al.* Proteolysis of NR2B by calpain in the hippocampus of epileptic rats. Neuroreport 2005; 16(4): 393-6. [http://dx.doi.org/10.1097/00001756-200503150-00017] [PMID: 15729144]

[86] Xu W, Wong TP, Chery N, Gaertner T, Wang YT, Baudry M. Calpain-mediated mGluR1alpha truncation: a key step in excitotoxicity. Neuron 2007; 53(3): 399-412. [http://dx.doi.org/10.1016/j.neuron.2006.12.020] [PMID: 17270736]

[87] Lankiewicz S, Marc Luetjens C, Truc Bui N, *et al.* Activation of calpain I converts excitotoxic neuron death into a caspase-independent cell death. J Biol Chem 2000; 275(22): 17064-71. [http://dx.doi.org/10.1074/jbc.275.22.17064] [PMID: 10828077]

[88] Bi X, Chang V, Siman R, Tocco G, Baudry M. Regional distribution and time-course of calpain activation following kainate-induced seizure activity in adult rat brain. Brain Res 1996; 726(1-2): 98-108. [http://dx.doi.org/10.1016/0006-8993(95)01360-1] [PMID: 8836550]

[89] Bi X, Chen J, Baudry M. Developmental changes in calpain activity, GluR1 receptors and in the effect of kainic acid treatment in rat brain. Neuroscience 1997; 81(4): 1123-35. [http://dx.doi.org/10.1016/S0306-4522(97)00218-2] [PMID: 9330373]

[90] Miettinen R, Kotti T, Tuunanen J, Toppinen A, Riekkinen P Sr, Halonen T. Hippocampal damage after injection of kainic acid into the rat entorhinal cortex. Brain Res 1998; 813(1): 9-17. [http://dx.doi.org/10.1016/S0006-8993(98)00915-9] [PMID: 9824657]

[91] Putkonen N, Kukkonen JP, Mudo G, *et al.* Involvement of cyclin-dependent kinase-5 in the kainic acid-mediated degeneration of glutamatergic synapses in the rat hippocampus. Eur J Neurosci 2011; 34(8): 1212-21. [http://dx.doi.org/10.1111/j.1460-9568.2011.07858.x] [PMID: 21978141]

[92] Sharma AK, Searfoss GH, Reams RY, *et al.* Kainic acid-induced F-344 rat model of mesial temporal lobe epilepsy: gene expression and canonical pathways. Toxicol Pathol 2009; 37(6): 776-89. [http://dx.doi.org/10.1177/0192623309344202] [PMID: 19700661]

[93] Fitzpatrick JS, Shahi K, Baudry M. Effect of seizure activity and calpain inhibitor I on LTP in juvenile hippocampal slices. Int J Dev Neurosci 1992; 10(4): 313-9. [http://dx.doi.org/10.1016/0736-5748(92)90020-Z] [PMID: 1384274]

[94] Higuchi M, Tomioka M, Takano J, *et al.* Distinct mechanistic roles of calpain and caspase activation in neurodegeneration as revealed in mice overexpressing their specific inhibitors. J Biol Chem 2005; 280(15): 15229-37. [http://dx.doi.org/10.1074/jbc.M500939200] [PMID: 15699033]

[95] Meade AJ, Meloni BP, Mastaglia FL, Watt PM, Knuckey NW. AP-1 inhibitory peptides attenuate *in vitro* cortical neuronal cell death induced by kainic acid. Brain Res 2010; 1360: 8-16. [http://dx.doi.org/10.1016/j.brainres.2010.09.007] [PMID: 20833150]

[96] Van den Bosch L, Van Damme P, Vleminckx V, *et al.* An alpha-mercaptoacrylic acid derivative (PD150606) inhibits selective motor neuron death via inhibition of kainate-induced Ca2+ influx and not via calpain inhibition. Neuropharmacology 2002; 42(5): 706-13. [http://dx.doi.org/10.1016/S0028-3908(02)00010-2] [PMID: 11985829]

[97] Ni H, Ren SY, Zhang LL, Sun Q, Tian T, Feng X. Expression profiles of hippocampal regenerative sprouting-related genes and their regulation by E-64d in a developmental rat model of penicillin-induced recurrent epilepticus. Toxicol Lett 2013; 217(2): 162-9.

[http://dx.doi.org/10.1016/j.toxlet.2012.12.010] [PMID: 23266720]

[98] Lam PM, Carlsen J, González MI. A calpain inhibitor ameliorates seizure burden in an experimental model of temporal lobe epilepsy. Neurobiol Dis 2017; 102: 1-10. [http://dx.doi.org/10.1016/j.nbd.2017.02.003] [PMID: 28237317]

[99] Feng ZH, Hao J, Ye L, *et al.* Overexpression of μ-calpain in the anterior temporal neocortex of patients with intractable epilepsy correlates with clinicopathological characteristics. Seizure 2011; 20(5): 395-401. [http://dx.doi.org/10.1016/j.seizure.2011.01.010] [PMID: 21315622]

[100] Araújo IM, Carreira BP, Carvalho CM, Carvalho AP. Calpains and delayed calcium deregulation in excitotoxicity. Neurochem Res 2010; 35(12): 1966-9. [http://dx.doi.org/10.1007/s11064-010-0323-z] [PMID: 21110090]

[101] Hong SC, Lanzino G, Goto Y, *et al.* Calcium-activated proteolysis in rat neocortex induced by transient focal ischemia. Brain Res 1994; 661(1-2): 43-50. [http://dx.doi.org/10.1016/0006-8993(94)91178-9] [PMID: 7834383]

[102] Lai TW, Zhang S, Wang YT. Excitotoxicity and stroke: identifying novel targets for neuroprotection. Prog Neurobiol 2014; 115: 157-88. [http://dx.doi.org/10.1016/j.pneurobio.2013.11.006] [PMID: 24361499]

[103] Liebetrau M, Staufer B, Auerswald EA, *et al.* Increased intracellular calpain detection in experimental focal cerebral ischemia. Neuroreport 1999; 10(3): 529-34. [http://dx.doi.org/10.1097/00001756-199902250-00016] [PMID: 10208584]

[104] Lipton P. Ischemic cell death in brain neurons. Physiol Rev 1999; 79(4): 1431-568. [PMID: 10508238]

[105] Neumar RW, Meng FH, Mills AM, *et al.* Calpain activity in the rat brain after transient forebrain ischemia. Exp Neurol 2001; 170(1): 27-35. [http://dx.doi.org/10.1006/exnr.2001.7708] [PMID: 11421581]

[106] Xu J, Kurup P, Zhang Y, *et al.* Extrasynaptic NMDA receptors couple preferentially to excitotoxicity via calpain-mediated cleavage of STEP. J Neurosci 2009; 29(29): 9330-43. [http://dx.doi.org/10.1523/JNEUROSCI.2212-09.2009] [PMID: 19625523]

[107] Curcio M, Salazar IL, Mele M, Canzoniero LM, Duarte CB. Calpains and neuronal damage in the ischemic brain: The swiss knife in synaptic injury. Prog Neurobiol 2016; 143: 1-35. [http://dx.doi.org/10.1016/j.pneurobio.2016.06.001] [PMID: 27283248]

[108] Rami A, Agarwal R, Botez G, Winckler J. mu-Calpain activation, DNA fragmentation, and synergistic effects of caspase and calpain inhibitors in protecting hippocampal neurons from ischemic damage. Brain Res 2000; 866(1-2): 299-312. [http://dx.doi.org/10.1016/S0006-8993(00)02301-5] [PMID: 10825507]

[109] White BC, Sullivan JM, DeGracia DJ, *et al.* Brain ischemia and reperfusion: molecular mechanisms of neuronal injury. J Neurol Sci 2000; 179(S 1-2): 1-33. [http://dx.doi.org/10.1016/S0022-510X(00)00386-5]

[110] Ray SK. Currently evaluated calpain and caspase inhibitors for neuroprotection in experimental brain ischemia. Curr Med Chem 2006; 13(28): 3425-40. [http://dx.doi.org/10.2174/092986706779010342] [PMID: 17168715]

[111] Yamashima T, Saido TC, Takita M, *et al.* Transient brain ischaemia provokes Ca2+, PIP2 and calpain responses prior to delayed neuronal death in monkeys. Eur J Neurosci 1996; 8(9): 1932-44. [http://dx.doi.org/10.1111/j.1460-9568.1996.tb01337.x] [PMID: 8921284]

[112] Tan VB, Zhang B, Lim KM, Tay TE. Explaining the inhibition of cyclin-dependent kinase 5 by peptides derived from p25 with molecular dynamics simulations and MM-PBSA. J Mol Model 2010; 16(1): 1-8. [http://dx.doi.org/10.1007/s00894-009-0514-1] [PMID: 19466465]

[113] Barros-Miñones L, Martín-de-Saavedra D, Perez-Alvarez S, *et al.* Inhibition of calpain-regulated p35/cdk5 plays a central role in sildenafil-induced protection against chemical hypoxia produced by malonate. Biochim Biophys Acta 2013; 1832(6): 705-17. [http://dx.doi.org/10.1016/j.bbadis.2013.02.002] [PMID: 23415811]

[114] Meyer DA, Torres-Altoro MI, Tan Z, *et al.* Ischemic stroke injury is mediated by aberrant Cdk5. J Neurosci 2014; 34(24): 8259-67. [http://dx.doi.org/10.1523/JNEUROSCI.4368-13.2014] [PMID: 24920629]

[115] Wei Xu , Miou Zhou , Baudry M. Neuroprotection by cell permeable TAT-mGluR1 peptide in ischemia: synergy between carrier and cargo sequences. Neuroscientist 2008; 14(5): 409-14. [http://dx.doi.org/10.1177/1073858407309762] [PMID: 18000067]

[116] Zhou M, Xu W, Liao G, Bi X, Baudry M. Neuroprotection against neonatal hypoxia/ischemia-induced cerebral cell death by prevention of calpain-mediated mGluR1alpha truncation. Exp Neurol 2009; 218(1): 75-82. [http://dx.doi.org/10.1016/j.expneurol.2009.04.006] [PMID: 19374898]

[117] Sun A, Cheng J. Novel targets for therapeutic intervention against ischemic brain injury. Clin Neuropharmacol 1999; 22(3): 164-71. [PMID: 10367181]

[118] Sun M, Gu Y, Zhao Y, Xu C. Protective functions of taurine against experimental stroke through depressing mitochondria-mediated cell death in rats. Amino Acids 2011; 40(5): 1419-29. [http://dx.doi.org/10.1007/s00726-010-0751-8] [PMID: 20862501]

[119] Sun M, Xu C. Neuroprotective mechanism of taurine due to up-regulating calpastatin and down-regulating calpain and caspase-3 during focal cerebral ischemia. Cell Mol Neurobiol 2008; 28(4): 593-611. [http://dx.doi.org/10.1007/s10571-007-9183-8] [PMID: 17712625]

[120] Markgraf CG, Velayo NL, Johnson MP, *et al.* Six-hour window of opportunity for calpain inhibition in focal cerebral ischemia in rats. Stroke 1998; 29(1): 152-8. [http://dx.doi.org/10.1161/01.STR.29.1.152] [PMID: 9445345]

[121] Hong SC, Goto Y, Lanzino G, Soleau S, Kassell NF, Lee KS. Neuroprotection with a calpain inhibitor in a model of focal cerebral ischemia. Stroke 1994; 25(3): 663-9. [http://dx.doi.org/10.1161/01.STR.25.3.663] [PMID: 8128523]

[122] Peng S, Kuang Z, Zhang Y, Xu H, Cheng Q. The protective effects and potential mechanism of Calpain inhibitor Calpeptin against focal cerebral ischemia-reperfusion injury in rats. Mol Biol Rep 2011; 38(2): 905-12. [http://dx.doi.org/10.1007/s11033-010-0183-2] [PMID: 20473717]

[123] Tan X, Chen Y, Li J, *et al.* The inhibition of Cdk5 activity after hypoxia/ischemia injury reduces infarct size and promotes functional recovery in neonatal rats. Neuroscience 2015; 290: 552-60. [http://dx.doi.org/10.1016/j.neuroscience.2015.01.054] [PMID: 25665755]

[124] Qin ZH, Gu ZL. Huntingtin processing in pathogenesis of Huntington disease. Acta Pharmacol Sin 2004; 25(10): 1243-9. [PMID: 15456523]

[125] Majumder P, Raychaudhuri S, Chattopadhyay B, Bhattacharyya NP. Increased caspase-2, calpain activations and decreased mitochondrial complex II activity in cells expressing exogenous huntingtin exon 1 containing CAG repeat in the pathogenic range. Cell Mol Neurobiol 2007; 27(8): 1127-45. [http://dx.doi.org/10.1007/s10571-007-9220-7] [PMID: 17902043]

[126] Landles C, Sathasivam K, Weiss A, *et al.* Proteolysis of mutant huntingtin produces an exon 1 fragment that accumulates as an aggregated protein in neuronal nuclei in Huntington disease. J Biol Chem 2010; 285(12): 8808-23. [http://dx.doi.org/10.1074/jbc.M109.075028] [PMID: 20086007]

[127] Cowan CM, Fan MM, Fan J, *et al.* Polyglutamine-modulated striatal calpain activity in YAC transgenic huntington disease mouse model: impact on NMDA receptor function and toxicity. J Neurosci 2008; 28(48): 12725-35.
[http://dx.doi.org/10.1523/JNEUROSCI.4619-08.2008] [PMID: 19036965]

[128] Gafni J, Ellerby LM. Calpain activation in Huntington's disease. J Neurosci 2002; 22(12): 4842-9.
[PMID: 12077181]

[129] Menzies FM, Garcia-Arencibia M, Imarisio S, *et al.* Calpain inhibition mediates autophagy-dependent protection against polyglutamine toxicity. Cell Death Differ 2015; 22(3): 433-44.
[http://dx.doi.org/10.1038/cdd.2014.151] [PMID: 25257175]

[130] Clemens LE, Weber JJ, Wlodkowski TT, *et al.* Olesoxime suppresses calpain activation and mutant huntingtin fragmentation in the BACHD rat. Brain 2015; 138(Pt 12): 3632-53.
[http://dx.doi.org/10.1093/brain/awv290] [PMID: 26490331]

[131] Weber JJ, Ortiz Rios MM, Riess O, Clemens LE, Nguyen HP. The calpain-suppressing effects of olesoxime in Huntington's disease. Rare Dis 2016; 4(1): e1153778.
[http://dx.doi.org/10.1080/21675511.2016.1153778] [PMID: 27141414]

[132] Bizat N, Galas MC, Jacquard C, *et al.* Neuroprotective effect of zVAD against the neurotoxin 3-nitropropionic acid involves inhibition of calpain. Neuropharmacology 2005; 49(5): 695-702.
[http://dx.doi.org/10.1016/j.neuropharm.2005.04.030] [PMID: 15998526]

[133] Bizat N, Hermel JM, Boyer F, *et al.* Calpain is a major cell death effector in selective striatal degeneration induced *in vivo* by 3-nitropropionate: implications for Huntington's disease. J Neurosci 2003; 23(12): 5020-30.
[PMID: 12832525]

[134] Paoletti P, Vila I, Rifé M, Lizcano JM, Alberch J, Ginés S. Dopaminergic and glutamatergic signaling crosstalk in Huntington's disease neurodegeneration: the role of p25/cyclin-dependent kinase 5. J Neurosci 2008; 28(40): 10090-101.
[http://dx.doi.org/10.1523/JNEUROSCI.3237-08.2008] [PMID: 18829967]

[135] Anne SL, Saudou F, Humbert S. Phosphorylation of huntingtin by cyclin-dependent kinase 5 is induced by DNA damage and regulates wild-type and mutant huntingtin toxicity in neurons. J Neurosci 2007; 27(27): 7318-28.
[http://dx.doi.org/10.1523/JNEUROSCI.1831-07.2007] [PMID: 17611284]

[136] Banik NL, Chakrabarti AK, Hogan EL. Distribution of calcium activated neutral proteinase (mM CANP) in myelin and cytosolic fractions in bovine brain white matter. Life Sci 1987; 41(9): 1089-95.
[http://dx.doi.org/10.1016/0024-3205(87)90626-6] [PMID: 3039281]

[137] Banik NL, Chou CH, Deibler GE, Krutzch HC, Hogan EL. Peptide bond specificity of calpain: proteolysis of human myelin basic protein. J Neurosci Res 1994; 37(4): 489-96.
[http://dx.doi.org/10.1002/jnr.490370408] [PMID: 7517457]

[138] Banik NL, McAlhaney WW, Hogan EL. Calcium-stimulated proteolysis in myelin: evidence for a Ca2+-activated neutral proteinase associated with purified myelin of rat CNS. J Neurochem 1985; 45(2): 581-8.
[http://dx.doi.org/10.1111/j.1471-4159.1985.tb04026.x] [PMID: 2409235]

[139] Banik NL, Shields DC. A putative role for calpain in demyelination associated with optic neuritis. Histol Histopathol 1999; 14(2): 649-56.
[PMID: 10212825]

[140] de Rosbo NK, Bernard CC. Multiple sclerosis brain immunoglobulins stimulate myelin basic protein degradation in human myelin: a new cause of demyelination. J Neurochem 1989; 53(2): 513-8.
[http://dx.doi.org/10.1111/j.1471-4159.1989.tb07363.x] [PMID: 2473168]

[141] Baud L, Fouqueray B, Bellocq A, Peltier J. Calpains participate in inflammatory reaction development. Med Sci (Paris) 2003; 19(1): 71-6.

[http://dx.doi.org/10.1051/medsci/200319171] [PMID: 12836194]

[142] Schaecher KE, Shields DC, Banik NL. Mechanism of myelin breakdown in experimental demyelination: a putative role for calpain. Neurochem Res 2001; 26(6): 731-7. [http://dx.doi.org/10.1023/A:1010903823668] [PMID: 11519732]

[143] Shields DC, Banik NL. Upregulation of calpain activity and expression in experimental allergic encephalomyelitis: a putative role for calpain in demyelination. Brain Res 1998; 794(1): 68-74. [http://dx.doi.org/10.1016/S0006-8993(98)00193-0] [PMID: 9630523]

[144] Shields DC, Banik NL. Pathophysiological role of calpain in experimental demyelination. J Neurosci Res 1999; 55(5): 533-41. [http://dx.doi.org/10.1002/(SICI)1097-4547(19990301)55:5<533::AID-JNR1>3.0.CO;2-8] [PMID: 10082076]

[145] Shields DC, Deibler GE, Banik NL. Calpain, a mediator of myelin breakdown in demyelinating diseases. Ann N Y Acad Sci 1997; 825: 128-30. [http://dx.doi.org/10.1111/j.1749-6632.1997.tb48422.x] [PMID: 9369981]

[146] Shields DC, Schaecher KE, Hogan EL, Banik NL. Calpain activity and expression increased in activated glial and inflammatory cells in penumbra of spinal cord injury lesion. J Neurosci Res 2000; 61(2): 146-50. [http://dx.doi.org/10.1002/1097-4547(20000715)61:2<146::AID-JNR5>3.0.CO;2-C] [PMID: 10878587]

[147] Shields DC, Schaecher KE, Saido TC, Banik NL. A putative mechanism of demyelination in multiple sclerosis by a proteolytic enzyme, calpain. Proc Natl Acad Sci USA 1999; 96(20): 11486-91. [http://dx.doi.org/10.1073/pnas.96.20.11486] [PMID: 10500203]

[148] Rosenberger TA. Targeting calpain-mediated proteolysis and peptide signaling as a strategy to reduce injury in multiple sclerosis. J Neurochem 2014; 130(2): 161-4. [http://dx.doi.org/10.1111/jnc.12732] [PMID: 24844646]

[149] Imam SA, Guyton MK, Haque A, *et al.* Increased calpain correlates with Th1 cytokine profile in PBMCs from MS patients. J Neuroimmunol 2007; 190(1-2): 139-45. [http://dx.doi.org/10.1016/j.jneuroim.2007.07.016] [PMID: 17765980]

[150] Das A, Guyton MK, Butler JT, Ray SK, Banik NL. Activation of calpain and caspase pathways in demyelination and neurodegeneration in animal model of multiple sclerosis. CNS Neurol Disord Drug Targets 2008; 7(3): 313-20. [http://dx.doi.org/10.2174/187152708784936699] [PMID: 18673215]

[151] Deshpande RV, Goust JM, Chakrabarti AK, Barbosa E, Hogan EL, Banik NL. Calpain expression in lymphoid cells. Increased mRNA and protein levels after cell activation. J Biol Chem 1995; 270(6): 2497-505. [http://dx.doi.org/10.1074/jbc.270.6.2497] [PMID: 7852311]

[152] Deshpande RV, Goust JM, Hogan EL, Banik NL. Calpain secreted by activated human lymphoid cells degrades myelin. J Neurosci Res 1995; 42(2): 259-65. [http://dx.doi.org/10.1002/jnr.490420214] [PMID: 8568927]

[153] Podbielska M, Banik NL, Kurowska E, Hogan EL. Myelin recovery in multiple sclerosis: the challenge of remyelination. Brain Sci 2013; 3(3): 1282-324. [http://dx.doi.org/10.3390/brainsci3031282] [PMID: 24961530]

[154] Podbielska M, Das A, Smith AW, *et al.* Neuron-microglia interaction induced bi-directional cytotoxicity associated with calpain activation. J Neurochem 2016; 139(3): 440-55. [http://dx.doi.org/10.1111/jnc.13774] [PMID: 27529445]

[155] Smith AW, Doonan BP, Tyor WR, Abou-Fayssal N, Haque A, Banik NL. Regulation of Th1/Th17 cytokines and IDO gene expression by inhibition of calpain in PBMCs from MS patients. J Neuroimmunol 2011; 232(1-2): 179-85.

[http://dx.doi.org/10.1016/j.jneuroim.2010.09.030] [PMID: 21075457]

[156] Smith AW, Rohrer B, Wheless L, *et al.* Calpain inhibition reduces structural and functional impairment of retinal ganglion cells in experimental optic neuritis. J Neurochem 2016; 139(2): 270-84. [http://dx.doi.org/10.1111/jnc.13770] [PMID: 27513991]

[157] Smith ME, Amaducci LA. Observations on the effects of protease inhibitors on the suppression of experimental allergic encephalomyelitis. Neurochem Res 1982; 7(5): 541-54. [http://dx.doi.org/10.1007/BF00965121] [PMID: 6750429]

[158] Trager N, Smith A, Wallace Iv G, *et al.* Effects of a novel orally administered calpain inhibitor SNJ-1945 on immunomodulation and neurodegeneration in a murine model of multiple sclerosis. J Neurochem 2014; 130(2): 268-79. [http://dx.doi.org/10.1111/jnc.12659] [PMID: 24447070]

[159] Hassen GW, Feliberti J, Kesner L, Stracher A, Mokhtarian F. A novel calpain inhibitor for the treatment of acute experimental autoimmune encephalomyelitis. J Neuroimmunol 2006; 180(1-2): 135-46. [http://dx.doi.org/10.1016/j.jneuroim.2006.08.005] [PMID: 17007940]

[160] Craner MJ, Newcombe J, Black JA, Hartle C, Cuzner ML, Waxman SG. Molecular changes in neurons in multiple sclerosis: altered axonal expression of Nav1.2 and Nav1.6 sodium channels and Na+/Ca2+ exchanger. Proc Natl Acad Sci USA 2004; 101(21): 8168-73. [http://dx.doi.org/10.1073/pnas.0402765101] [PMID: 15148385]

[161] Stys PK, Waxman SG, Ransom BR. Ionic mechanisms of anoxic injury in mammalian CNS white matter: role of Na+ channels and Na(+)-Ca2+ exchanger. J Neurosci 1992; 12(2): 430-9. [PMID: 1311030]

[162] Waxman SG. Demyelinating diseases--new pathological insights, new therapeutic targets. N Engl J Med 1998; 338(5): 323-5. [PMID: 9445415]

[163] Bjartmar C, Wujek JR, Trapp BD. Axonal loss in the pathology of MS: consequences for understanding the progressive phase of the disease. J Neurol Sci 2003; 206(2): 165-71. [http://dx.doi.org/10.1016/S0022-510X(02)00069-2] [PMID: 12559505]

[164] Wujek JR, Bjartmar C, Richer E, *et al.* Axon loss in the spinal cord determines permanent neurological disability in an animal model of multiple sclerosis. J Neuropathol Exp Neurol 2002; 61(1): 23-32. [http://dx.doi.org/10.1093/jnen/61.1.23] [PMID: 11829341]

[165] Bjartmar C, Kidd G, Mörk S, Rudick R, Trapp BD. Neurological disability correlates with spinal cord axonal loss and reduced N-acetyl aspartate in chronic multiple sclerosis patients. Ann Neurol 2000; 48(6): 893-901. [http://dx.doi.org/10.1002/1531-8249(200012)48:6<893::AID-ANA10>3.0.CO;2-B] [PMID: 11117546]

[166] Bjartmar C, Kinkel RP, Kidd G, Rudick RA, Trapp BD. Axonal loss in normal-appearing white matter in a patient with acute MS. Neurology 2001; 57(7): 1248-52. [http://dx.doi.org/10.1212/WNL.57.7.1248] [PMID: 11591844]

[167] Bjartmar C, Yin X, Trapp BD. Axonal pathology in myelin disorders. J Neurocytol 1999; 28(4-5): 383-95. [http://dx.doi.org/10.1023/A:1007010205037] [PMID: 10739578]

[168] Trapp BD, Peterson J, Ransohoff RM, Rudick R, Mörk S, Bö L. Axonal transection in the lesions of multiple sclerosis. N Engl J Med 1998; 338(5): 278-85. [http://dx.doi.org/10.1056/NEJM199801293380502] [PMID: 9445407]

[169] Trapp BD, Ransohoff R, Rudick R. Axonal pathology in multiple sclerosis: relationship to neurologic disability. Curr Opin Neurol 1999; 12(3): 295-302. [http://dx.doi.org/10.1097/00019052-199906000-00008] [PMID: 10499174]

[170] Petzold A. Neurofilament phosphoforms: surrogate markers for axonal injury, degeneration and loss. J Neurol Sci 2005; 233(1-2): 183-98.
[http://dx.doi.org/10.1016/j.jns.2005.03.015] [PMID: 15896809]

[171] Lindberg RL, De Groot CJ, Certa U, *et al.* Multiple sclerosis as a generalized CNS disease--comparative microarray analysis of normal appearing white matter and lesions in secondary progressive MS. J Neuroimmunol 2004; 152(1-2): 154-67.
[http://dx.doi.org/10.1016/j.jneuroim.2004.03.011] [PMID: 15223248]

[172] Hassen GW, Feliberti J, Kesner L, Stracher A, Mokhtarian F. Prevention of axonal injury using calpain inhibitor in chronic progressive experimental autoimmune encephalomyelitis. Brain Res 2008; 1236: 206-15.
[http://dx.doi.org/10.1016/j.brainres.2008.07.124] [PMID: 18725211]

[173] Bechtold DA, Kapoor R, Smith KJ. Axonal protection using flecainide in experimental autoimmune encephalomyelitis. Ann Neurol 2004; 55(5): 607-16.
[http://dx.doi.org/10.1002/ana.20045] [PMID: 15122700]

[174] Hoffmann DB, Williams SK, Bojcevski J, *et al.* Calcium influx and calpain activation mediate preclinical retinal neurodegeneration in autoimmune optic neuritis. J Neuropathol Exp Neurol 2013; 72(8): 745-57.
[http://dx.doi.org/10.1097/NEN.0b013e31829c7370] [PMID: 23860028]

[175] Das A, Guyton MK, Smith A, *et al.* Calpain inhibitor attenuated optic nerve damage in acute optic neuritis in rats. J Neurochem 2013; 124(1): 133-46.
[http://dx.doi.org/10.1111/jnc.12064] [PMID: 23106593]

[176] Guyton MK, Sribnick EA, Ray SK, Banik NL. A role for calpain in optic neuritis. Ann N Y Acad Sci 2005; 1053: 48-54.
[http://dx.doi.org/10.1196/annals.1344.005] [PMID: 16179508]

[177] Smith AW, Das A, Guyton MK, Ray SK, Rohrer B, Banik NL. Calpain inhibition attenuates apoptosis of retinal ganglion cells in acute optic neuritis. Invest Ophthalmol Vis Sci 2011; 52(7): 4935-41.
[http://dx.doi.org/10.1167/iovs.10-7027] [PMID: 21613375]

[178] Zhu B, Moore GR, Zwimpfer TJ, *et al.* Axonal cytoskeleton changes in experimental optic neuritis. Brain Res 1999; 824(2): 204-17.
[http://dx.doi.org/10.1016/S0006-8993(99)01191-9] [PMID: 10196450]

[179] Badalamente MA, Stracher A. Delay of muscle degeneration and necrosis in mdx mice by calpain inhibition. Muscle Nerve 2000; 23(1): 106-11.
[http://dx.doi.org/10.1002/(SICI)1097-4598(200001)23:1<106::AID-MUS14>3.0.CO;2-D] [PMID: 10590413]

[180] Gailly P, De Backer F, Van Schoor M, Gillis JM. In situ measurements of calpain activity in isolated muscle fibres from normal and dystrophin-lacking mdx mice. J Physiol 2007; 582(Pt 3): 1261-75.
[http://dx.doi.org/10.1113/jphysiol.2007.132191] [PMID: 17510188]

[181] Matsumura K, Campbell KP. Deficiency of dystrophin-associated proteins: a common mechanism leading to muscle cell necrosis in severe childhood muscular dystrophies. Neuromuscul Disord 1993; 3(2): 109-18.
[http://dx.doi.org/10.1016/0960-8966(93)90002-2] [PMID: 8358236]

[182] Matsumura K, Campbell KP. Dystrophin-glycoprotein complex: its role in the molecular pathogenesis of muscular dystrophies. Muscle Nerve 1994; 17(1): 2-15.
[http://dx.doi.org/10.1002/mus.880170103] [PMID: 8264699]

[183] Ohlendieck K, Matsumura K, Ionasescu VV, *et al.* Duchenne muscular dystrophy: deficiency of dystrophin-associated proteins in the sarcolemma. Neurology 1993; 43(4): 795-800.
[http://dx.doi.org/10.1212/WNL.43.4.795] [PMID: 8469343]

[184] Purintrapiban J, Wang MC, Forsberg NE. Degradation of sarcomeric and cytoskeletal proteins in

cultured skeletal muscle cells. Comp Biochem Physiol B Biochem Mol Biol 2003; 136(3): 393-401. [http://dx.doi.org/10.1016/S1096-4959(03)00201-X] [PMID: 14602148]

[185] Whitehead NP, Yeung EW, Allen DG. Muscle damage in mdx (dystrophic) mice: role of calcium and reactive oxygen species. Clin Exp Pharmacol Physiol 2006; 33(7): 657-62. [http://dx.doi.org/10.1111/j.1440-1681.2006.04394.x] [PMID: 16789936]

[186] Toral-Ojeda I, Aldanondo G, Lasa-Elgarresta J, *et al.* Calpain 3 deficiency affects SERCA expression and function in the skeletal muscle. Expert Rev Mol Med 2016; 18: e7. [http://dx.doi.org/10.1017/erm.2016.9] [PMID: 27055500]

[187] Renjini R, Gayathri N, Nalini A, Srinivas Bharath MM. Analysis of calpain-3 protein in muscle biopsies of different muscular dystrophies from India. Indian J Med Res 2012; 135(6): 878-86. [PMID: 22825607]

[188] Spencer MJ, Mellgren RL. Overexpression of a calpastatin transgene in mdx muscle reduces dystrophic pathology. Hum Mol Genet 2002; 11(21): 2645-55. [http://dx.doi.org/10.1093/hmg/11.21.2645] [PMID: 12354790]

[189] Badalamente MA, Hurst LC, Stracher A. Neuromuscular recovery after peripheral nerve repair: effects of an orally-administered peptide in a primate model. J Reconstr Microsurg 1995; 11(6): 429-37. [http://dx.doi.org/10.1055/s-2007-1006557] [PMID: 8583456]

[190] Briguet A, Erb M, Courdier-Fruh I, *et al.* Effect of calpain and proteasome inhibition on Ca^{2+}-dependent proteolysis and muscle histopathology in the mdx mouse. FASEB J 2008; 22(12): 4190-200. [http://dx.doi.org/10.1096/fj.07-099036] [PMID: 18728218]

[191] Hollinger K, Selsby JT. The physiological response of protease inhibition in dystrophic muscle. Acta Physiol (Oxf) 2013; 208(3): 234-44. [http://dx.doi.org/10.1111/apha.12114] [PMID: 23648220]

[192] Libby P, Goldberg AL. Leupeptin, a protease inhibitor, decreases protein degradation in normal and diseased muscles. Science 1978; 199(4328): 534-6. [http://dx.doi.org/10.1126/science.622552] [PMID: 622552]

[193] Ono Y, Iemura S, Novak SM, *et al.* PLEIAD/SIMC1/C5orf25, a novel autolysis regulator for a skeletal-muscle-specific calpain, CAPN3, scaffolds a CAPN3 substrate, CTBP1. J Mol Biol 2013; 425(16): 2955-72. [http://dx.doi.org/10.1016/j.jmb.2013.05.009] [PMID: 23707407]

[194] Wadosky KM, Li L, Rodríguez JE, *et al.* Regulation of the calpain and ubiquitin-proteasome systems in a canine model of muscular dystrophy. Muscle Nerve 2011; 44(4): 553-62. [http://dx.doi.org/10.1002/mus.22125] [PMID: 21826685]

[195] Al-Mansoori KM, Hasan MY, Al-Hayani A, El-Agnaf OM. The role of α-synuclein in neurodegenerative diseases: from molecular pathways in disease to therapeutic approaches. Curr Alzheimer Res 2013; 10(6): 559-68. [http://dx.doi.org/10.2174/15672050113100060002] [PMID: 23899170]

[196] Amschl D, Neddens J, Havas D, *et al.* Time course and progression of wild type α-synuclein accumulation in a transgenic mouse model. BMC Neurosci 2013; 14: 6. [http://dx.doi.org/10.1186/1471-2202-14-6] [PMID: 23302418]

[197] Baba M, Nakajo S, Tu PH, *et al.* Aggregation of alpha-synuclein in Lewy bodies of sporadic Parkinson's disease and dementia with Lewy bodies. Am J Pathol 1998; 152(4): 879-84. [PMID: 9546347]

[198] Beyer K, Ariza A. α-Synuclein posttranslational modification and alternative splicing as a trigger for neurodegeneration. Mol Neurobiol 2013; 47(2): 509-24. [http://dx.doi.org/10.1007/s12035-012-8330-5] [PMID: 22923347]

[199] Chung KK, Dawson VL, Dawson TM. New insights into Parkinson's disease. J Neurol 2003; 250

(Suppl. 3): III15-24.
[http://dx.doi.org/10.1007/s00415-003-1304-9] [PMID: 14579120]

[200] Czapski GA, Gąssowska M, Wilkaniec A, Cieślik M, Adamczyk A. Extracellular alpha-synuclein induces calpain-dependent overactivation of cyclin-dependent kinase 5 *in vitro*. FEBS Lett 2013; 587(18): 3135-41.
[http://dx.doi.org/10.1016/j.febslet.2013.07.053] [PMID: 23954626]

[201] Daher JP, Ying M, Banerjee R, *et al.* Conditional transgenic mice expressing C-terminally truncated human alpha-synuclein (alphaSyn119) exhibit reduced striatal dopamine without loss of nigrostriatal pathway dopaminergic neurons. Mol Neurodegener 2009; 4: 34.
[http://dx.doi.org/10.1186/1750-1326-4-34] [PMID: 19630976]

[202] Dauer W, Przedborski S. Parkinson's disease: mechanisms and models. Neuron 2003; 39(6): 889-909.
[http://dx.doi.org/10.1016/S0896-6273(03)00568-3] [PMID: 12971891]

[203] Dawson TM, Dawson VL. Molecular pathways of neurodegeneration in Parkinson's disease. Science 2003; 302(5646): 819-22.
[http://dx.doi.org/10.1126/science.1087753] [PMID: 14593166]

[204] Dev KK, Hofele K, Barbieri S, Buchman VL, van der Putten H. Part II: alpha-synuclein and its molecular pathophysiological role in neurodegenerative disease. Neuropharmacology 2003; 45(1): 14-44.
[http://dx.doi.org/10.1016/S0028-3908(03)00140-0] [PMID: 12814657]

[205] Drolet RE, Behrouz B, Lookingland KJ, Goudreau JL. Mice lacking alpha-synuclein have an attenuated loss of striatal dopamine following prolonged chronic MPTP administration. Neurotoxicology 2004; 25(5): 761-9.
[http://dx.doi.org/10.1016/j.neuro.2004.05.002] [PMID: 15288507]

[206] Dufty BM, Warner LR, Hou ST, *et al.* Calpain-cleavage of alpha-synuclein: connecting proteolytic processing to disease-linked aggregation. Am J Pathol 2007; 170(5): 1725-38.
[http://dx.doi.org/10.2353/ajpath.2007.061232] [PMID: 17456777]

[207] Eriksen JL, Dawson TM, Dickson DW, Petrucelli L. Caught in the act: alpha-synuclein is the culprit in Parkinson's disease. Neuron 2003; 40(3): 453-6.
[http://dx.doi.org/10.1016/S0896-6273(03)00684-6] [PMID: 14642269]

[208] Esteves AR, Arduíno DM, Swerdlow RH, Oliveira CR, Cardoso SM. Dysfunctional mitochondria uphold calpain activation: contribution to Parkinson's disease pathology. Neurobiol Dis 2010; 37(3): 723-30.
[http://dx.doi.org/10.1016/j.nbd.2009.12.011] [PMID: 20034566]

[209] Golbe LI. Alpha-synuclein and Parkinson's disease. Adv Neurol 2003; 91: 165-74.
[PMID: 12442675]

[210] Hashimoto M, Rockenstein E, Masliah E. Transgenic models of alpha-synuclein pathology: past, present, and future. Ann N Y Acad Sci 2003; 991: 171-88.
[http://dx.doi.org/10.1111/j.1749-6632.2003.tb07475.x] [PMID: 12846986]

[211] Kim SJ, Sung JY, Um JW, *et al.* Parkin cleaves intracellular alpha-synuclein inclusions *via* the activation of calpain. J Biol Chem 2003; 278(43): 41890-9.
[http://dx.doi.org/10.1074/jbc.M306017200] [PMID: 12917442]

[212] Kirik D, Rosenblad C, Burger C, *et al.* Parkinson-like neurodegeneration induced by targeted overexpression of alpha-synuclein in the nigrostriatal system. J Neurosci 2002; 22(7): 2780-91.
[PMID: 11923443]

[213] Li W, West N, Colla E, *et al.* Aggregation promoting C-terminal truncation of alpha-synuclein is a normal cellular process and is enhanced by the familial Parkinson's disease-linked mutations. Proc Natl Acad Sci USA 2005; 102(6): 2162-7.
[http://dx.doi.org/10.1073/pnas.0406976102] [PMID: 15684072]

[214] Liu CW, Giasson BI, Lewis KA, Lee VM, Demartino GN, Thomas PJ. A precipitating role for truncated alpha-synuclein and the proteasome in alpha-synuclein aggregation: implications for pathogenesis of Parkinson disease. J Biol Chem 2005; 280(24): 22670-8. [http://dx.doi.org/10.1074/jbc.M501508200] [PMID: 15840579]

[215] Ma QL, Chan P, Yoshii M, Uéda K. Alpha-synuclein aggregation and neurodegenerative diseases. J Alzheimers Dis 2003; 5(2): 139-48. [http://dx.doi.org/10.3233/JAD-2003-5208] [PMID: 12719631]

[216] Masliah E, Rockenstein E, Veinbergs I, *et al.* Dopaminergic loss and inclusion body formation in alpha-synuclein mice: implications for neurodegenerative disorders. Science 2000; 287(5456): 1265-9. [http://dx.doi.org/10.1126/science.287.5456.1265] [PMID: 10678833]

[217] Mishizen-Eberz AJ, Guttmann RP, Giasson BI, *et al.* Distinct cleavage patterns of normal and pathologic forms of alpha-synuclein by calpain I *in vitro*. J Neurochem 2003; 86(4): 836-47. [http://dx.doi.org/10.1046/j.1471-4159.2003.01878.x] [PMID: 12887682]

[218] Mouatt-Prigent A, Karlsson JO, Agid Y, Hirsch EC. Increased M-calpain expression in the mesencephalon of patients with Parkinson's disease but not in other neurodegenerative disorders involving the mesencephalon: a role in nerve cell death? Neuroscience 1996; 73(4): 979-87. [http://dx.doi.org/10.1016/0306-4522(96)00100-5] [PMID: 8809817]

[219] Mouatt-Prigent A, Karlsson JO, Yelnik J, Agid Y, Hirsch EC. Calpastatin immunoreactivity in the monkey and human brain of control subjects and patients with Parkinson's disease. J Comp Neurol 2000; 419(2): 175-92. [http://dx.doi.org/10.1002/(SICI)1096-9861(20000403)419:2<175::AID-CNE3>3.0.CO;2-2] [PMID: 10722997]

[220] Prasad K, Beach TG, Hedreen J, Richfield EK. Critical role of truncated α-synuclein and aggregates in Parkinson's disease and incidental Lewy body disease. Brain Pathol 2012; 22(6): 811-25. [http://dx.doi.org/10.1111/j.1750-3639.2012.00597.x] [PMID: 22452578]

[221] Rohn TT. Targeting alpha-synuclein for the treatment of Parkinson's disease. CNS Neurol Disord Drug Targets 2012; 11(2): 174-9. [http://dx.doi.org/10.2174/187152712800269678] [PMID: 22483285]

[222] Samantaray S, Knaryan VH, Shields DC, Banik NL. Critical role of calpain in spinal cord degeneration in Parkinson's disease. J Neurochem 2013; 127(6): 880-90. [http://dx.doi.org/10.1111/jnc.12374] [PMID: 23875735]

[223] Ulusoy A, Decressac M, Kirik D, Björklund A. Viral vector-mediated overexpression of α-synuclein as a progressive model of Parkinson's disease. Prog Brain Res 2010; 184: 89-111. [http://dx.doi.org/10.1016/S0079-6123(10)84005-1] [PMID: 20887871]

[224] Wakamatsu M, Ishii A, Iwata S, *et al.* Selective loss of nigral dopamine neurons induced by overexpression of truncated human alpha-synuclein in mice. Neurobiol Aging 2008; 29(4): 574-85. [http://dx.doi.org/10.1016/j.neurobiolaging.2006.11.017] [PMID: 17174013]

[225] Wan OW, Chung KK. The role of alpha-synuclein oligomerization and aggregation in cellular and animal models of Parkinson's disease. PLoS One 2012; 7(6): e38545. [http://dx.doi.org/10.1371/journal.pone.0038545] [PMID: 22701661]

[226] Diepenbroek M, Casadei N, Esmer H, *et al.* Overexpression of the calpain-specific inhibitor calpastatin reduces human alpha-Synuclein processing, aggregation and synaptic impairment in [A30P]αSyn transgenic mice. Hum Mol Genet 2014; 23(15): 3975-89. [http://dx.doi.org/10.1093/hmg/ddu112] [PMID: 24619358]

[227] Smith PD, Crocker SJ, Jackson-Lewis V, *et al.* Cyclin-dependent kinase 5 is a mediator of dopaminergic neuron loss in a mouse model of Parkinson's disease. Proc Natl Acad Sci USA 2003; 100(23): 13650-5. [http://dx.doi.org/10.1073/pnas.2232515100] [PMID: 14595022]

[228] Alvira D, Ferrer I, Gutierrez-Cuesta J, Garcia-Castro B, Pallàs M, Camins A. Activation of the calpain/cdk5/p25 pathway in the girus cinguli in Parkinson's disease. Parkinsonism Relat Disord 2008; 14(4): 309-13.
[http://dx.doi.org/10.1016/j.parkreldis.2007.09.005] [PMID: 17977053]

[229] Alvira D, Tajes M, Verdaguer E, *et al.* Inhibition of the cdk5/p25 fragment formation may explain the antiapoptotic effects of melatonin in an experimental model of Parkinson's disease. J Pineal Res 2006; 40(3): 251-8.
[http://dx.doi.org/10.1111/j.1600-079X.2005.00308.x] [PMID: 16499562]

[230] Crespo-Biel N, Camins A, Pelegrí C, Vilaplana J, Pallàs M, Canudas AM. 3-Nitropropionic acid activates calpain/cdk5 pathway in rat striatum. Neurosci Lett 2007; 421(1): 77-81.
[http://dx.doi.org/10.1016/j.neulet.2007.05.038] [PMID: 17566644]

[231] Qu D, Rashidian J, Mount MP, *et al.* Role of Cdk5-mediated phosphorylation of Prx2 in MPTP toxicity and Parkinson's disease. Neuron 2007; 55(1): 37-52.
[http://dx.doi.org/10.1016/j.neuron.2007.05.033] [PMID: 17610816]

[232] Wales SQ, Laing JM, Chen L, Aurelian L. ICP10PK inhibits calpain-dependent release of apoptosis-inducing factor and programmed cell death in response to the toxin MPP+. Gene Ther 2008; 15(20): 1397-409.
[http://dx.doi.org/10.1038/gt.2008.88] [PMID: 18496573]

[233] Crocker SJ, Smith PD, Jackson-Lewis V, *et al.* Inhibition of calpains prevents neuronal and behavioral deficits in an MPTP mouse model of Parkinson's disease. J Neurosci 2003; 23(10): 4081-91.
[PMID: 12764095]

[234] Crocker SJ, Liston P, Anisman H, *et al.* Attenuation of MPTP-induced neurotoxicity and behavioural impairment in NSE-XIAP transgenic mice. Neurobiol Dis 2003; 12(2): 150-61.
[http://dx.doi.org/10.1016/S0969-9961(02)00020-7] [PMID: 12667469]

[235] Hayley S, Crocker SJ, Smith PD, *et al.* Regulation of dopaminergic loss by Fas in a 1-methyl-4-phenyl-1,2,3,6-tetrahydropyridine model of Parkinson's disease. J Neurosci 2004; 24(8): 2045-53.
[http://dx.doi.org/10.1523/JNEUROSCI.4564-03.2004] [PMID: 14985447]

[236] Raghupathi R. Cell death mechanisms following traumatic brain injury. Brain Pathol 2004; 14(2): 215-22.
[http://dx.doi.org/10.1111/j.1750-3639.2004.tb00056.x] [PMID: 15193035]

[237] Liu S, Yin F, Zhang J, Qian Y. The role of calpains in traumatic brain injury. Brain Inj 2014; 28(2): 133-7.
[http://dx.doi.org/10.3109/02699052.2013.860479] [PMID: 24456052]

[238] Bralić M, Stemberga V. Calpain expression in the brain cortex after traumatic brain injury. Coll Antropol 2012; 36(4): 1319-23.
[PMID: 23390828]

[239] Kampfl A, Posmantur RM, Zhao X, Schmutzhard E, Clifton GL, Hayes RL. Mechanisms of calpain proteolysis following traumatic brain injury: implications for pathology and therapy: implications for pathology and therapy: a review and update. J Neurotrauma 1997; 14(3): 121-34.
[http://dx.doi.org/10.1089/neu.1997.14.121] [PMID: 9104930]

[240] Kampfl A, Posmantur R, Nixon R, *et al.* mu-calpain activation and calpain-mediated cytoskeletal proteolysis following traumatic brain injury. J Neurochem 1996; 67(4): 1575-83.
[http://dx.doi.org/10.1046/j.1471-4159.1996.67041575.x] [PMID: 8858942]

[241] Saatman KE, Abai B, Grosvenor A, Vorwerk CK, Smith DH, Meaney DF. Traumatic axonal injury results in biphasic calpain activation and retrograde transport impairment in mice. J Cereb Blood Flow Metab 2003; 23(1): 34-42.
[http://dx.doi.org/10.1097/01.WCB.0000035040.10031.B0] [PMID: 12500089]

[242] Saatman KE, Bozyczko-Coyne D, Marcy V, Siman R, McIntosh TK. Prolonged calpain-mediated

spectrin breakdown occurs regionally following experimental brain injury in the rat. J Neuropathol Exp Neurol 1996; 55(7): 850-60.
[http://dx.doi.org/10.1097/00005072-199607000-00010] [PMID: 8965100]

[243] Bartus RT, Chen EY, Lynch G, Kordower JH. Cortical ablation induces a spreading calcium-dependent, secondary pathogenesis which can be reduced by inhibiting calpain. Exp Neurol 1999; 155(2): 315-26.
[http://dx.doi.org/10.1006/exnr.1998.7001] [PMID: 10072307]

[244] Wingrave JM, Schaecher KE, Sribnick EA, *et al.* Early induction of secondary injury factors causing activation of calpain and mitochondria-mediated neuronal apoptosis following spinal cord injury in rats. J Neurosci Res 2003; 73(1): 95-104.
[http://dx.doi.org/10.1002/jnr.10607] [PMID: 12815713]

[245] Czeiter E, Büki A, Bukovics P, *et al.* Calpain inhibition reduces axolemmal leakage in traumatic axonal injury. Molecules 2009; 14(12): 5115-23.
[http://dx.doi.org/10.3390/molecules14125115] [PMID: 20032879]

[246] Brophy GM, Pineda JA, Papa L, *et al.* alphaII-Spectrin breakdown product cerebrospinal fluid exposure metrics suggest differences in cellular injury mechanisms after severe traumatic brain injury. J Neurotrauma 2009; 26(4): 471-9.
[http://dx.doi.org/10.1089/neu.2008.0657] [PMID: 19206997]

[247] Mondello S, Robicsek SA, Gabrielli A, *et al.* αII-spectrin breakdown products (SBDPs): diagnosis and outcome in severe traumatic brain injury patients. J Neurotrauma 2010; 27(7): 1203-13.
[http://dx.doi.org/10.1089/neu.2010.1278] [PMID: 20408766]

[248] Thompson SN, Gibson TR, Thompson BM, Deng Y, Hall ED. Relationship of calpain-mediated proteolysis to the expression of axonal and synaptic plasticity markers following traumatic brain injury in mice. Exp Neurol 2006; 201(1): 253-65.
[http://dx.doi.org/10.1016/j.expneurol.2006.04.013] [PMID: 16814284]

[249] McCracken E, Hunter AJ, Patel S, Graham DI, Dewar D. Calpain activation and cytoskeletal protein breakdown in the corpus callosum of head-injured patients. J Neurotrauma 1999; 16(9): 749-61.
[http://dx.doi.org/10.1089/neu.1999.16.749] [PMID: 10521135]

[250] Saatman KE, Creed J, Raghupathi R. Calpain as a therapeutic target in traumatic brain injury. Neurotherapeutics 2010; 7(1): 31-42.
[http://dx.doi.org/10.1016/j.nurt.2009.11.002] [PMID: 20129495]

[251] Thompson SN, Carrico KM, Mustafa AG, Bains M, Hall ED. A pharmacological analysis of the neuroprotective efficacy of the brain- and cell-permeable calpain inhibitor MDL-28170 in the mouse controlled cortical impact traumatic brain injury model. J Neurotrauma 2010; 27(12): 2233-43.
[http://dx.doi.org/10.1089/neu.2010.1474] [PMID: 20874056]

[252] Hung KS, Hwang SL, Liang CL, *et al.* Calpain inhibitor inhibits p35-p25-Cdk5 activation, decreases tau hyperphosphorylation, and improves neurological function after spinal cord hemisection in rats. J Neuropathol Exp Neurol 2005; 64(1): 15-26.
[http://dx.doi.org/10.1093/jnen/64.1.15] [PMID: 15715081]

[253] Yamada KH, Kozlowski DA, Seidl SE, *et al.* Targeted gene inactivation of calpain-1 suppresses cortical degeneration due to traumatic brain injury and neuronal apoptosis induced by oxidative stress. J Biol Chem 2012; 287(16): 13182-93.
[http://dx.doi.org/10.1074/jbc.M111.302612] [PMID: 22367208]

[254] Yu CG, Li Y, Raza K, Yu XX, Ghoshal S, Geddes JW. Calpain 1 knockdown improves tissue sparing and functional outcomes after spinal cord injury in rats. J Neurotrauma 2013; 30(6): 427-33.
[http://dx.doi.org/10.1089/neu.2012.2561] [PMID: 23102374]

[255] Schoch KM, von Reyn CR, Bian J, Telling GC, Meaney DF, Saatman KE. Brain injury-induced proteolysis is reduced in a novel calpastatin-overexpressing transgenic mouse. J Neurochem 2013; 125(6): 909-20.

[http://dx.doi.org/10.1111/jnc.12144] [PMID: 23305291]

[256] Yu CG, Joshi A, Geddes JW. Intraspinal MDL28170 microinjection improves functional and pathological outcome following spinal cord injury. J Neurotrauma 2008; 25(7): 833-40. [http://dx.doi.org/10.1089/neu.2007.0490] [PMID: 18627259]

[257] Saatman KE, Murai H, Bartus RT, *et al.* Calpain inhibitor AK295 attenuates motor and cognitive deficits following experimental brain injury in the rat. Proc Natl Acad Sci USA 1996; 93(8): 3428-33. [http://dx.doi.org/10.1073/pnas.93.8.3428] [PMID: 8622952]

[258] Osier ND, Dixon CE. The controlled cortical impact model: applications, considerations for researchers, and future directions. Front Neurol 2016; 7: 134. [http://dx.doi.org/10.3389/fneur.2016.00134] [PMID: 27582726]

[259] Osier ND, Korpon JR, Dixon CE. Controlled cortical impact model.brain neurotrauma: molecular, neuropsychological, and rehabilitation aspects edn. Boca Raton, FL 2015. [http://dx.doi.org/10.1201/b18126-20]

[260] Zhang Z, Huang Z, Dai H, Wei L, Sun S, Gao F. Therapeutic efficacy of E-64-d, a selective calpain inhibitor, in experimental acute spinal cord injury. BioMed Res Int 2015; 2015: 134242. [PMID: 26240815]

[261] Buki A, Farkas O, Doczi T, Povlishock JT. Preinjury administration of the calpain inhibitor MDL-28170 attenuates traumatically induced axonal injury. J Neurotrauma 2003; 20(3): 261-8. [http://dx.doi.org/10.1089/089771503321532842] [PMID: 12820680]

[262] Wang Y, Liu Y, Lopez D, *et al.* Protection against TBI-induced neuronal death with oost-treatment with a selective calpain-2 inhibitor in mice. J Neurotrauma 2017. [http://dx.doi.org/10.1089/neu.2017.5024] [PMID: 28594313]

[263] Ono Y, Saido TC, Sorimachi H. Calpain research for drug discovery: challenges and potential. Nat Rev Drug Discov 2016; 15(12): 854-76. [http://dx.doi.org/10.1038/nrd.2016.212] [PMID: 27833121]

[264] Abell AD, Jones MA, Coxon JM, *et al.* Molecular modeling, synthesis, and biological evaluation of macrocyclic calpain inhibitors. Angew Chem Int Ed Engl 2009; 48(8): 1455-8. [http://dx.doi.org/10.1002/anie.200805014] [PMID: 19145612]

[265] Bánóczi Z, Tantos Á, Farkas A, *et al.* New m-calpain substrate-based azapeptide inhibitors. J Pept Sci 2013; 19(6): 370-6. [http://dx.doi.org/10.1002/psc.2511] [PMID: 23613308]

[266] Cagmat EB, Guingab-Cagmat JD, Vakulenko AV, Hayes RL, Anagli J. Potential use of calpain inhibitors as brain injury therapy.brain neurotrauma: molecular, neuropsychological, and rehabilitation aspects edn. Boca Raton, FL 2015. [http://dx.doi.org/10.1201/b18126-47]

[267] Carragher NO. Calpain inhibition: a therapeutic strategy targeting multiple disease states. Curr Pharm Des 2006; 12(5): 615-38. [http://dx.doi.org/10.2174/138161206775474314] [PMID: 16472152]

[268] Crestanello JA. Calpain inhibitors: The aspirin of the 21st century? J Thorac Cardiovasc Surg 2017; 153(2): 358-9. [http://dx.doi.org/10.1016/j.jtcvs.2016.10.025] [PMID: 27865555]

[269] Fiorino F, Gil-Parrado S, Assfalg-Machleidt I, Machleidt W, Moroder L. A new cell-permeable calpain inhibitor. J Pept Sci 2007; 13(1): 70-3. [http://dx.doi.org/10.1002/psc.790] [PMID: 17019744]

[270] Kim HJ, Lee JY, Kim SM, *et al.* A new epicatechin gallate and calpain inhibitory activity from Orostachys japonicus. Fitoterapia 2009; 80(1): 73-6. [http://dx.doi.org/10.1016/j.fitote.2008.10.003] [PMID: 18977282]

[271] Mehdi S. Cell-penetrating inhibitors of calpain. Trends Biochem Sci 1991; 16(4): 150-3. [http://dx.doi.org/10.1016/0968-0004(91)90058-4] [PMID: 1877091]

[272] Neuhof C, Götte O, Trumbeckaite S, *et al.* A novel water-soluble and cell-permeable calpain inhibitor protects myocardial and mitochondrial function in postischemic reperfusion. Biol Chem 2003; 384(12): 1597-603. [http://dx.doi.org/10.1515/BC.2003.177] [PMID: 14719802]

[273] Saez ME, Ramirez-Lorca R, Moron FJ, Ruiz A. The therapeutic potential of the calpain family: new aspects. Drug Discov Today 2006; 11(19-20): 917-23. [http://dx.doi.org/10.1016/j.drudis.2006.08.009] [PMID: 16997142]

[274] Sanders ML, Donkor IO. A novel series of urea-based peptidomimetic calpain inhibitors. Bioorg Med Chem Lett 2006; 16(7): 1965-8. [http://dx.doi.org/10.1016/j.bmcl.2005.12.068] [PMID: 16412635]

[275] Stracher A. Calpain inhibitors as therapeutic agents in nerve and muscle degeneration. Ann N Y Acad Sci 1999; 884: 52-9. [http://dx.doi.org/10.1111/j.1749-6632.1999.tb08635.x] [PMID: 10842583]

[276] Wang KK, Yuen PW. Calpain inhibition: an overview of its therapeutic potential. Trends Pharmacol Sci 1994; 15(11): 412-9. [http://dx.doi.org/10.1016/0165-6147(94)90090-6] [PMID: 7855906]

[277] Zhang Y, Jung SY, Jin C, Kim ND, Gong P, Lee YS. Design and synthesis of 4-aryl-4-oxobutanoic acid amides as calpain inhibitors. Bioorg Med Chem Lett 2009; 19(2): 502-7. [http://dx.doi.org/10.1016/j.bmcl.2008.11.030] [PMID: 19041242]

[278] Lu L, Meehan MJ, Gu S, *et al.* Mechanism of action of thalassospiramides, a new class of calpain inhibitors. Sci Rep 2015; 5: 8783. [http://dx.doi.org/10.1038/srep08783] [PMID: 25740631]

[279] Fà M, Zhang H, Staniszewski A, *et al.* Novel selective calpain 1 inhibitors as potential therapeutics in alzheimer's disease. J Alzheimers Dis 2016; 49(3): 707-21. [http://dx.doi.org/10.3233/JAD-150618] [PMID: 26484927]

[280] Derksen M, Vorwerk C, Siemen D. Calpeptin, not calpain, directly inhibits an ion channel of the inner mitochondrial membrane. Protoplasma 2016; 253(3): 835-43. [http://dx.doi.org/10.1007/s00709-015-0846-x] [PMID: 26108743]

[281] Gwozdz AM, Leung R, Wang H, *et al.* Calpain inhibition by calpeptin does not prevent APLT activity reduction in PS-exposing platelets, but calpeptin has independent pro-apoptotic effects. Thromb Haemost 2010; 103(6): 1218-27. [http://dx.doi.org/10.1160/TH09-08-0557] [PMID: 20352156]

[282] Tassone DM, Boyce E, Guyer J, Nuzum D. Pregabalin: a novel gamma-aminobutyric acid analogue in the treatment of neuropathic pain, partial-onset seizures, and anxiety disorders. Clin Ther 2007; 29(1): 26-48. [http://dx.doi.org/10.1016/j.clinthera.2007.01.013] [PMID: 17379045]

[283] Horga de la Parte JF, Horga A. Pregabalin: new therapeutic contributions of calcium channel alpha2delta protein ligands on epilepsy and neuropathic pain. Rev Neurol 2006; 42(4): 223-37. [PMID: 16521062]

[284] Kelly KM. Gabapentin. Antiepileptic mechanism of action. Neuropsychobiology 1998; 38(3): 139-44. [http://dx.doi.org/10.1159/000026529] [PMID: 9778601]

[285] Stahl SM. Mechanism of action of alpha2delta ligands: voltage sensitive calcium channel (VSCC) modulators. J Clin Psychiatry 2004; 65(8): 1033-4. [http://dx.doi.org/10.4088/JCP.v65n0801] [PMID: 15323585]

[286] Field MJ, Cox PJ, Stott E, *et al.* Identification of the alpha2-delta-1 subunit of voltage-dependent

calcium channels as a molecular target for pain mediating the analgesic actions of pregabalin. Proc Natl Acad Sci USA 2006; 103(46): 17537-42.
[http://dx.doi.org/10.1073/pnas.0409066103] [PMID: 17088553]

[287] Melrose HL, Kinloch RA, Cox PJ, Field MJ, Collins D, Williams D. [3H] pregabalin binding is increased in ipsilateral dorsal horn following chronic constriction injury. Neurosci Lett 2007; 417(2): 187-92.
[http://dx.doi.org/10.1016/j.neulet.2007.02.068] [PMID: 17367933]

[288] Rebouche CJ. Kinetics, pharmacokinetics, and regulation of L-carnitine and acetyl-L-carnitine metabolism. Ann N Y Acad Sci 2004; 1033: 30-41.
[http://dx.doi.org/10.1196/annals.1320.003] [PMID: 15591001]

[289] Harris R.C., CVLFaDHSPccauimfoaiaEVJE. Plasma carnitine concentration and uptake into muscle following oral and intravenous administration 1995.

[290] Lahjouji K, Mitchell GA, Qureshi IA. Carnitine transport by organic cation transporters and systemic carnitine deficiency. Mol Genet Metab 2001; 73(4): 287-97.
[http://dx.doi.org/10.1006/mgme.2001.3207] [PMID: 11509010]

[291] Lamhonwah AM, Wong J, Tam C, Mai L, Tein I. Organic cation/carnitine transporter family expression patterns in adult murine heart. Pathol Res Pract 2009; 205(6): 395-402.
[http://dx.doi.org/10.1016/j.prp.2008.12.010] [PMID: 19233567]

[292] Huxtable RJ. Taurine. Past, present, and future. Adv Exp Med Biol 1996; 403: 641-50.
[http://dx.doi.org/10.1007/978-1-4899-0182-8_71] [PMID: 8915405]

[293] Kishi M, Ohkuma S, Kimori M, Kuriyama K. Characteristics of taurine transport system and its developmental pattern in mouse cerebral cortical neurons in primary culture. Biochim Biophys Acta 1988; 939(3): 615-23.
[http://dx.doi.org/10.1016/0005-2736(88)90109-5] [PMID: 2833312]

[294] Wu JY, Prentice H. Role of taurine in the central nervous system. J Biomed Sci 2010; 17 (Suppl. 1): S1.
[http://dx.doi.org/10.1186/1423-0127-17-S1-S1] [PMID: 20804583]

[295] Koyama Y, Baba A, Iwata H. Characteristics of Cl(-)-dependent L-[35S]cysteic acid transport into rat brain synaptic membrane vesicles. Neurochem Res 1990; 15(12): 1153-8.
[http://dx.doi.org/10.1007/BF01208574] [PMID: 2097511]

[296] Lähdesmäki P. Biosynthesis of taurine peptides in brain cytoplasmic fraction *in vitro*. Int J Neurosci 1987; 37(1-2): 79-84.
[http://dx.doi.org/10.3109/00207458708991804] [PMID: 3679692]

[297] Lähdesmäki P, Oja SS. On the mechanism of taurine transport at brain cell membranes. J Neurochem 1973; 20(5): 1411-7.
[http://dx.doi.org/10.1111/j.1471-4159.1973.tb00253.x] [PMID: 4716833]

[298] Gu Y, Zhao Y, Qian K, Sun M. Taurine attenuates hippocampal and corpus callosum damage, and enhances neurological recovery after closed head injury in rats. Neuroscience 2015; 291: 331-40.
[http://dx.doi.org/10.1016/j.neuroscience.2014.09.073] [PMID: 25290011]

[299] Sun M, Zhao Y, Gu Y, Zhang Y. Protective effects of taurine against closed head injury in rats. J Neurotrauma 2015; 32(1): 66-74.
[http://dx.doi.org/10.1089/neu.2012.2432] [PMID: 23327111]

[300] Su Y, Fan W, Ma Z, *et al.* Taurine improves functional and histological outcomes and reduces inflammation in traumatic brain injury. Neuroscience 2014; 266: 56-65.
[http://dx.doi.org/10.1016/j.neuroscience.2014.02.006] [PMID: 24530657]

[301] Koopman R. Dietary protein and exercise training in ageing. Proc Nutr Soc 2011; 70(1): 104-13.
[http://dx.doi.org/10.1017/S0029665110003927] [PMID: 21092364]

[302] Koopman R, van Loon LJ. Aging, exercise, and muscle protein metabolism. J Appl Physiol 2009; 106(6): 2040-8.
[http://dx.doi.org/10.1152/japplphysiol.91551.2008] [PMID: 19131471]

[303] Fry CS, Rasmussen BB. Skeletal muscle protein balance and metabolism in the elderly. Curr Aging Sci 2011; 4(3): 260-8.
[http://dx.doi.org/10.2174/1874609811104030260] [PMID: 21529326]

[304] Welle S, Thornton C, Jozefowicz R, Statt M. Myofibrillar protein synthesis in young and old men. Am J Physiol 1993; 264(5 Pt 1): E693-8.
[PMID: 8498491]

[305] Ryall JG, Schertzer JD, Lynch GS. Cellular and molecular mechanisms underlying age-related skeletal muscle wasting and weakness. Biogerontology 2008; 9(4): 213-28.
[http://dx.doi.org/10.1007/s10522-008-9131-0] [PMID: 18299960]

[306] Guroff G. A Neutral, Calcium-Activated Proteinase from the Soluble Fraction of Rat Brain. J Biol Chem 1964; 239: 149-55.
[PMID: 14114836]

[307] Huang Y, Wang KK. The calpain family and human disease. Trends Mol Med 2001; 7(8): 355-62.
[http://dx.doi.org/10.1016/S1471-4914(01)02049-4] [PMID: 11516996]

[308] Nixon RA. The calpains in aging and aging-related diseases. Ageing Res Rev 2003; 2(4): 407-18.
[http://dx.doi.org/10.1016/S1568-1637(03)00029-1] [PMID: 14522243]

[309] Aoyagi T, Miyata S, Nanbo M, Kojima F, Matsuzaki M. Biological activities of leupeptins. J Antibiot 1969; 22(11): 558-68.
[http://dx.doi.org/10.7164/antibiotics.22.558] [PMID: 4243683]

[310] Aoyagi T, Takeuchi T, Matsuzaki A, Kawamura K, Kondo S. Leupeptins, new protease inhibitors from Actinomycetes. J Antibiot 1969; 22(6): 283-6.
[http://dx.doi.org/10.7164/antibiotics.22.283] [PMID: 5810993]

[311] David J, Melamud A, Kesner L, *et al.* A novel calpain inhibitor for treatment of transient retinal ischemia in the rat. Neuroreport 2011; 22(13): 633-6.
[http://dx.doi.org/10.1097/WNR.0b013e32834959c5] [PMID: 21841454]

[312] Badalamente MA, Hurst LC, Stracher A. Recovery after delayed nerve repair: influence of a pharmacologic adjunct in a primate model. J Reconstr Microsurg 1992; 8(5): 391-7.
[http://dx.doi.org/10.1055/s-2007-1006724] [PMID: 1404069]

[313] Badalamente MA, Hurst LC, Stracher A. Localization and inhibition of calcium-activated neutral protease (CANP) in primate skeletal muscle and peripheral nerve. Exp Neurol 1987; 98(2): 357-69.
[http://dx.doi.org/10.1016/0014-4886(87)90248-2] [PMID: 2822459]

[314] Badalamente MA, Hurst LC, Stracher A. Neuromuscular recovery using calcium protease inhibition after median nerve repair in primates. Proc Natl Acad Sci USA 1989; 86(15): 5983-7.
[http://dx.doi.org/10.1073/pnas.86.15.5983] [PMID: 2548194]

[315] Stracher A, McGowan EB, Hedrych A, Shafiq SA. *In vivo* effect of protease inhibitors in denervation atrophy. Exp Neurol 1979; 66(3): 611-8.
[http://dx.doi.org/10.1016/0014-4886(79)90206-1] [PMID: 385335]

[316] Badalamente MA, Hurst LC, Stracher A. Calcium-induced degeneration of the cytoskeleton in monkey and human peripheral nerves. J Hand Surg [Br] 1986; 11(3): 337-40.
[http://dx.doi.org/10.1016/0266-7681(86)90153-1] [PMID: 3025318]

[317] Kieran D, Greensmith L. Inhibition of calpains, by treatment with leupeptin, improves motoneuron survival and muscle function in models of motoneuron degeneration. Neuroscience 2004; 125(2): 427-39.
[http://dx.doi.org/10.1016/j.neuroscience.2004.01.046] [PMID: 15062985]

[318] Osanai T, Nagai Y. Suppression of experimental allergic encephalomyelitis (EAE) with liposome-encapsulated protease inhibitor: therapy through the blood-brain barrier. Neurochem Res 1984; 9(10): 1407-16.
[http://dx.doi.org/10.1007/BF00964667] [PMID: 6514110]

[319] Croce K, Flaumenhaft R, Rivers M, *et al.* Inhibition of calpain blocks platelet secretion, aggregation, and spreading. J Biol Chem 1999; 274(51): 36321-7.
[http://dx.doi.org/10.1074/jbc.274.51.36321] [PMID: 10593923]

[320] Azam M, Andrabi SS, Sahr KE, Kamath L, Kuliopulos A, Chishti AH. Disruption of the mouse mu-calpain gene reveals an essential role in platelet function. Mol Cell Biol 2001; 21(6): 2213-20.
[http://dx.doi.org/10.1128/MCB.21.6.2213-2220.2001] [PMID: 11238954]

[321] Brown CS, Dean WL. Regulation of plasma membrane Ca^{2+}-ATPase in human platelets by calpain. Platelets 2007; 18(3): 207-11.
[http://dx.doi.org/10.1080/09537100600954037] [PMID: 17497432]

[322] Kuchay SM, Chishti AH. Calpain-mediated regulation of platelet signaling pathways. Curr Opin Hematol 2007; 14(3): 249-54.
[http://dx.doi.org/10.1097/MOH.0b013e3280ef68f8] [PMID: 17414215]

[323] Randriamboavonjy V, Fleming I. All cut up! The consequences of calpain activation on platelet function. Vascul Pharmacol 2012; 56(5-6): 210-5.
[http://dx.doi.org/10.1016/j.vph.2012.02.009] [PMID: 22386643]

Frontiers in CNS Drug Discovery, 2017, *Vol. 3*, 72-145

CHAPTER 3

Neurodegenerative and Neuropsychiatric Disorders: Present Clinical Drug Research and Future Perspectives

Sarika Garg[2,#], **Nikita Chordia**[1] and **Anil Kumar**[1,*]

[1] *School of Biotechnology, Devi Ahilya University, Takshashila Campus, Khandwa Road, INDORE-452001, India*

[2] *The University of Montreal Hospital Research Centre, CRCHUM R09.476, Tour Viger, 900 Rue St-Denis, Montreal H2X 0A9, Quebec, Canada*

[#] *Present address: Managing Editor and Founder, Canadian Journal of Biotechnology, 401-371 Rue Luciene-Milette, Saint Hubert J3Y 9H1, Canada*

Abstract: Neurodegenerative disorders are elucidated as genetic and intermittent diseases which are described by progressive nervous system dysfunctions. These disorders have often being correlated with the degeneration of nerve cells. Most prevalent diseases are Alzheimer's disease (AD) and related dementias, Encephalitis, Epilepsy, Parkinson's disease (PD), Multiple sclerosis, Amyotrophic lateral sclerosis, Huntington's disease, Schizophrenia and Prion diseases. All neurodegenerative diseases are disastrous and impact social as well as economic wellbeing. However, the majority of neuropatients are affected by AD, PD and together they cost the health care system almost billions of dollars per year. Besides, Schizophrenia is a severe mystery with no effective medical treatment. Therefore, AD, PD and Schizophrenia have been discussed at length in the present chapter. The AD is characterized by two neuropathological lesions, senile plaques composed of Aβ peptide and neurofibrillary tangles (NFTs) containing aggregated hyperphosphorylated Tau protein. The importance of Tau dysfunction in neurodegeneration is further supported by the enrichment of Tau genetic variants in cohorts of patients suffering from frontotemporal lobar degeneration disorder (FTLD). Memory loss, trouble sleeping, language problems, thinking and reasoning skills are the most common symptoms of AD. The PD is the second most common neurodegenerative disease which involves the breakdown and death of neurons in the brain. The core symptoms of PD are tremor, rigidity, bradykinesia and balance difficulties. Schizophrenia is a genetic brain disorder. Delusions, hallucinations, social withdrawal and disturbed thinking are some of its key symptoms. The genes causing these neurodegenerative disorders have been identified for more than two decades. Key researchers in this field have revealed numerous events at molecular and cellular levels, thus playing an important role in these fatal disorders. Many associated pathological events and therapeutic correlations

* **Corresponding authors Anil Kumar:** School of Biotechnology, Devi Ahilya University, Takshashila Campus, Khandwa Road, INDORE-452001, India; Tel:0091-731-2470373; Fax: 0091-731-2470372; E-mail: ak_sbt@yahoo.com

Atta-ur-Rahman & M. Iqbal Choudhary (Eds.)

are not clearly understood and therefore, there is no known cure for these chronic and progressive neurological disorders.

This chapter aims to address AD, PD and Schizophrenia researches that may divulge novel mechanisms and targets for therapeutic intervention. It collates the significant findings of various experts in studying these degenerative diseases and stimulates novel perception to the campaign against devastating neurodegenerative diseases.

Keywords: Alzheimer's disease, Bioinformatics, Clinical drugs, Neurodegeneration, Neurodevelopment, Parkinson's disease, Schizophrenia, Therapeutic approaches.

INTRODUCTION

Neurons are the building blocks of the nervous system, including the brain and the spinal cord. These are considered to be as special cells that process and transmit information through electrical and chemical signals. Normally, neurons do not replicate or replace themselves, so when they get injured or die they cannot be replaced by the body which may lead to neurodegenerative disease. Neurodegenerative diseases are considered to be irremediable and debilitating conditions that result in progressive degeneration and / or death of the nerve cells. Progressive loss of structure or function of neurons leads to neurodegeneration. It affects variety of functions, including movement, balance, talking, breathing, decision making and heart function. Many neurodegenerative diseases have a genetic basis and are caused by mutations in the genes. Unhealthy lifestyle, mainly tobacco smoking and alcohol consumption, also contributes to neurodegenerative diseases. There is no treatment that can cure neurodegenerative diseases, but may help to improve symptoms, relieve pain, and increase mobility [1]. Most prevalent neurodegenerative disorders especially in the middle and old aged groups are Alzheimer's disease and Parkinson's disease. Schizophrenia, a neurological disorder found in all aged humans is also much prevalent. Therefore, we have largely focused on the AD, PD and Schizophrenia in this chapter.

AD is a devastating neurodegenerative disorder. It is an irreversible, progressive and fatal brain disease. It is neither infectious nor contagious, but it is the single most common form of dementia, a term used to describe a general decline in all areas of the mental ability. The symptoms are deterioration in cognitive processes- memory, language, thinking and so on- with important repercussions on behaviour [2, 3]. About 50 per cent of the people with dementia suffer from AD, about 20 per cent from vascular dementia (caused by blockages in the supply of blood to the brain), and about 20 per cent from Lewy body dementia (characterized by tiny spherical deposits in the brain). The risk of getting AD increases as one gets older (beyond age 65) [4]. By age 85, about 35 out of 100 people have some form of dementia. AD is the ninth leading cause of death. It is estimated that more than 60 per cent of people with dementia live in developing countries, however, by 2040; it is expected to rise by 71 per cent.

PD is the second most common neurodegenerative disease. It is more prevalent in individuals older than 40. Only few PD cases are diagnosed with individuals younger than 40. Moreover, PD seems to occur more commonly in men than women. Motor and non-motor symptoms, the clinical features of the disease, are due to the death of dopaminergic neurons in the substantia nigra of the midbrain. The histological hallmark of the disease is the presence of fibrillary aggregates called Lewy bodies (LBs) in a proportion of surviving neurons. About 10 million people globally are living with PD. The disease is more prevalent in the United States of America where as many as 1 million people live with PD. Risk factors associated with this disease include family history, exposure to pesticides and metals, head injury and environmental chemicals like manganese. Despite decades of study, the ultimate cause of PD is still not much clear. Some experts believe that it is caused by the combination of genetic and environmental factors [5].Symptoms for PD can be divided into two categories: motor and non-motor symptoms. Motor symptoms include tremor or shaking, bradykinesia, postural instability, rigidity and shuffling gait. In addition to these symptoms, it is also characterized by some aging processes like blurred vision, decreased eye blink rate, speech impairment, masked facial expression, difficulty turning in bed and many more. Non-motor symptoms include behavioural and cognitive changes. These include altered personality, hallucinations, depression, anxiety, sleep disturbances, memory problems like memory retrieval, multi-tasking, problem in decision making and dementia [6].

There is no specific test to diagnose PD because of unavailability of an accurate biological marker. It is diagnosed based on the medical history and review of the signs and symptoms of the patient. Today, testing of disease can be done by using specialized brain scanning techniques that measure the amount of dopamine and brain metabolism [7]. Medical therapy for PD includes pharmacotherapy which compensates for dopamine deficit. The other therapy includes speech therapy, exercise, support groups, education and nutrition. Therapeutic approach depends on disease stage, troubling symptoms, patient's age, and the benefit/risk ratios of treatments. In addition, surgical therapies, *viz.* deep brain stimulation (DBS) and thalamotomy have been predicted as probable cure for the disease. Although there are no specific preventative measures known to prevent PD, there are reports that intake of high fibre food, fish, omega 3 rich oils, more fruits and vegetables in diet and avoidance of dairy products and meat protect the person from PD [8].

Schizophrenia is a chronic and severe neurodisorder that affects the person's thinking, feeling and behavior. People with schizophrenia have difficulty distinguishing between reality and fantasy. It is characterized by variety of symptoms like delusion, hallucinations, depression, emotionless, confusion, lack of motivation and disorganized speech. Its symptoms are sub-divided into positive and negative symptoms. Schizophrenia affects millions of people worldwide. The severity of the disease varies from person to person. The point prevalence is about five per thousand in global population. Schizophrenia can occur at any age but the mean onset age is 25 in males. It differs by 2 to 4 years in females [9]. The cause of schizophrenia includes several factors ranging from autoimmune, genetic and environmental. The risk factors include birth season, birth complications, parental age, urban residence, ethnicity and immune infections [10].

The antipsychotic drugs are primarily used for treating patients suffering from schizophrenia. Although these drugs do not cure illness, they help in reducing the symptoms. Chlorpromazine, aripiprazole, ziprasidone, zotepine and risperidone are few antipsychotics used for the treatment of schizophrenia [11]. Besides antipsychotics, pychosocial therapy and psychosurgery may be used to treat the patients. There is no specific test for the diagnosis of schizophrenia. It is diagnosed based on the symptoms of the patient. Lack of awareness is a common symptom of the disorder which leads to complicated treatment. There is no prevention of schizophrenia due to the lack of authentic markers for the later development of the disorder [12].

The etiological studies have focused on neuroimaging and genetic studies to support the neurodevelopmental hypothesis. Scientists have found out the neural abnormalities that lead to the aberrant neurodevelopment in schizophrenia. However, morphological changes in the brain and role of antipsychotic drugs in slowing down the disease support that schizophrenia is a neurodegenerative disease [13]. Here in this chapter, we have discussed both the theories of the schizophrenia.

HISTORY OF ALZHEIMER'S DISEASE

Alzheimer's disease is named after German psychiatrist and pathologist Dr. Alois Alzheimer. In 1907, he published an account of a 51-years old female patient named Auguste D from Frankfurt, who suffered from strong feelings of jealousy towards her husband, increased memory impairment, disorientation, hallucinations, and often loud and aggressive behavior [14]. After four and a half years of rapidly deteriorating mental illness, Auguste died in a completely demented state. Postmortem histological analysis of her brain using the Bielschowsky silver technique revealed dense bundles of unusual fibrils within nerve cells (neurofibrillary tangles or NFTs) and numerous focal lesions within the cerebral cortex, subsequently named as ”senile plaques” [15].

GENETICS OF ALZHEIMER'S DISEASE

Studies have supported the notion that 70 to 80% of the risk to develop AD is determined by genetic factors [16]. AD is not a single-gene disorder. Genetically, AD is a complex and heterogeneous disease involving mutations and polymorphisms in multiple genes on several chromosomes. The two basic types of AD are: the late sporadic AD (SAD) and the early familial AD (FAD). The SAD represents the vast majority of cases and aging is the important risk factor [17]. The apolipoprotein E (APOE) gene located on chromosome 19q13.2 has been confirmed unequivocally as a risk gene [18, 19]. Its ε4 allele increases the susceptibility to SAD whereas its ε2 allele confers protection against the late onset of AD [20]. Besides, cases arising sporadically and epidemiological studies indicated that about 30% of AD patients have a family history of disease and at least one first-degree relative is affected, however, only a few of them have a clear autosomal dominant inheritance [21]. The FAD starts before 60 and accounts for less than 1% of the total number of AD cases. It is associated with gene mutations on chromosomes 1, 14, and 21. Only 5% of the amyloid precursor protein (APP) mutations have been estimated for FAD. Most of the FAD cases are caused by mutations in two genes namely presenelin 1 (PSEN1) and presenelin 2 (PSEN2) [22, 23].More than 40 exonic and intronic mutations in MAPTgene present on chromosome 17q21.1 have been found in a familial dementia related to AD, and in the frontotemporal dementia with parkinsonism linked to chromosome 17 (FTDP-17) [24 - 26].

The actual causes of AD are not yet known with certainty. AD is a progressive neurodegenerative disorder characterized by two main types of protein aggregation [27, 28]; intracellular neurofibrillary tangles (NFTs) and extracellular senile plaques (SPs) [29 - 31]. The NFTs consist of paired helical filaments (PHF) resulting from the hyper-phosphorylation of the microtubule-binding protein Tau [32 - 36]. Senile plaques are principally composed of extracellular amyloid-ß (Aß) depositions [37 - 39]. The amyloid cascade hypothesis posits that Aß triggers Tau pathology [40], but details of this relationship are poorly understood. However, there has been surprisingly scant attention focused on Tau as a therapeutic target. Advances in generating animal models with Tau pathology are helping to erase this deficit [41] (Table **1**).

Table 1. Key discoveries in Tau protein research.

Year	Discovery	Reference
1906	Neurofibrillary tangles (NFTs) described by Alois Alzheimer	[41]
1960's	Paired helical filaments (PHF) form the structure of NFTs	[42, 43]
1975	Tau: A protein factor essential for microtubule assembly	[44]
1986	Tau is the major component of NFTs Abnormal p-Tau is the major protein subunit of PHF/NFTs Abnormal p-Tau inhibit Tau assembly in AD brain	[32, 45, 46] [47] [48]
1988	Cloning and sequence of Tau in the AD brain	[49, 50]
1994	First Tau knockout mouse Abnormal p-Tau is responsible of microtubule breakdown	[51] [52]
1995	AAY fibrils induce Tau phosphorylation Increased Tau levels in cerebrospinal fluid of AD patients First evidence of AAY and Tau interaction First transgenic mouse expressing the human Tau	[53] [54, 55] [53, 56] [57]
1997	Abnormal p-Tau sequester MAP1 and MAP2	[58]
1998	Tau mutations that cause a group of familial Tauopathies, frontotemporal dementia and parkinsonism linked to chromosome 17	[24, 25]
2001	Fibrillar AAY42 induces NFTs	[59]
2002	Tau is essential for the neurotoxicity induced by AAY	[60]
2003	AAY deposition precedes NFTs formation in 3xTg-AD	[61]
2004	Relation between Tau and inflammatory process	[62]
2005	NFTs formation does not lead to neuronal loss and neurodegeneration	[63]
2006	First transgenic rat expressing wild-type, truncated human Tau and producing NFT	[64]
2007	Genetic ablation of Tau blocks the AAY-and excitotoxin induced neuronal dysfunction	[65]

This table has been reproduced from the research paper of Medeiros *et al*., 2010 [41]

MICROTUBULE-ASSOCIATED PROTEIN TAU

Localization and Functions of Tau Protein

Tau protein belongs to the family of microtubule-associated proteins [44]. It is found in many animal species, *viz*. Caenorhabditis elegans [66, 67], Drosophila [68, 69], goldfish [70], bullfrog [71], rodents [72, 73], bovine [74, 75], goat [76], monkeys [76] and human [77, 78]. Tau is a low molecular weight component of cytoskeletal structures and it regulates the assembly of microtubules. The mRNAs encoding Tau protein are expressed predominantly in neurons, where Tau protein is localized mostly in axons of the CNS and PNS under normal physiological conditions [79, 80], whereas the neurofibrillary lesions in AD accumulate in the neuronal perikarya, axons, and dendrites. Lower expression of Tau mRNA and less abundant Tau protein have been observed in astrocytes as well as in oligodendrocytes [79, 80]. Tau mRNA and proteins can also be detected in several peripheral tissues such as heart, kidney, lung, muscle, pancreas, testis, as well as in fibroblasts [81 - 83].

Tau proteins play a major role in regulating neuronal microtubule assembly and stability [85 - 91]. Tau proteins promote the polymerization of tubulin into microtubules [44], and Tau bound to microtubules helps in stabilizing these structures in polymerized state [92]. Neurons have been treated with antisense oligonucleotides of Tau mRNA which blocked the expression of Tau protein. The treated neurons did not extend axon like processes. These results indicated that Tau protein is also involved in neuronal polarity [93, 94]. Mice lacking Tau protein showed decreased microtubule density and stability in some small-caliber axons [51], however, they showed motor impairments with age [95]. Tau is likely to play an essential role in the development of neurons and even glial cells, but it is also probable that other proteins such as MAP1A can be upregulated to partially compensate for the loss of Tau at least early in life [51, 95].

Expression of Multiple Tau Isoforms

In adult CNS, the single Tau gene on the long arm of chromosome 17 gives rise to six Tau isoforms by alternative mRNA splicing [49, 77, 78, 96] (Fig. **1**).

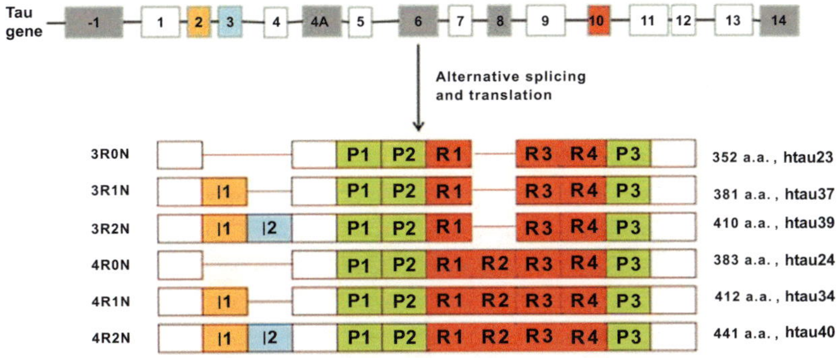

Fig. (1). Six human CNS Tau isoforms produced by alternative splicing of the Tau gene. The gene encoding Tau is a multi-exon gene that undergoes alternative post-transcriptional splicing of exons 2 (shown in orange), 3 (shown in blue) and 10 (shown in red) to yield six isoforms in the brain. The exons shown in dark grey are not found in translated human Tau. Exons 9-12 encode microtubule-binding repeat domains, and the exclusion or inclusion of exon 10 results in Tau with three (3R) or four (4R) microtubule-binding domains, respectively (shown as red boxes).

The six Tau isoforms differ in the presence of three (3R Tau) or four (4R Tau) microtubule binding repeats of 31 or 32 amino acids in the carboxy-terminal half, as well as in the presence of inserts of 29 or 58 amino acids or no insert at all in the amino terminal region [83, 84]. The tandem repeats in the carboxy-terminal half are encoded by exons 9, 10, 11, and 12, and the alternative splicing of exon 10 results in the generation of E10 + 4R Tau and E10 – 3R Tau mRNAs and their corresponding 4R and 3R Tau isoforms, respectively. This consecutive repeat region constitutes the microtubule binding domain of each Tau protein [97, 98]. The 4R Tau plays a much greater role in regulating the microtubule binding than 3R Tau [99]. The alternative splicing of the six brain Tau isoforms is developmentally regulated, and only the shortest Tau isoform with three repeats and no amino-terminal inserts (fetal Tau or 3R0N Tau) is present in fetal human brains [95]. The adult CNS contains the following Tau isoforms: Tau with one amino-terminal insert (1N Tau, 50%), Tau with no amino-terminal insert (0N, 40%) and Tau with two amino-terminal inserts (2N, 10%) in order of abundance. The ratio between 4R and 3R Tau isoforms has been found to be 1 [100]. Only three 4R Tau isoforms are known to be expressed in the adult rodent brain, while a 3R0N or fetal Tau isoform is expressed in the developing CNS of rodents [57].

Aggregation of Tau Protein

Tau is a highly soluble, natively unfolded protein, which shows little tendency for aggregation. Why it forms aggregates in AD and other neurodegenerative diseases remains unclear. The *in vitro* studies showed that Tau aggregation follows a nucleation-elongation pathway where an oligomeric nucleus is first formed by self-association of protein subunits, followed by addition of subunits to filament ends [101]. Tau aggregation is based on the partial structural transition from random coil to β-structure, which is regulated by two hexapeptide motifs [PHF6 (VQIVYK) and PHF6* (VQIINK)] within the repeat domains [102, 103]. Interruption of β-structure by introducing two prolines into the two hexapeptides suppresses Tau aggregation, while Tau mutant (e.g. ΔK280) which enhances β-propensity can promote Tau aggregation [104]. Although the mechanism for Tau aggregation is not well understood so far, it is known that it could be influenced by the post-translational modifications and degradation of Tau protein.

Phosphorylation of Tau Protein

It was demonstrated that phosphorylation of Tau negatively regulates its activity in promoting microtubule assembly [105]. Tau phosphorylation is regulated by various kinases and phosphatases (Fig. **2**). One or more protein kinases are subjected to act on each Tau phosphorylation site. Tau kinases can be divided into three classes: (i) protein kinases PDPKs (Proline-Directed Protein Kinases)-GSK3ß (Glycogen Synthase Kinase-3ß) [106], CDK5 (Cyclin-Dependent Kinase 5) [107] and MAPKs (Mitogen-Activated Protein Kinases) [108, 109] are protein kinases PDPKs which target several SP/TP motifs in the flanking regions of the repeats. (ii) protein kinases non PDPKs- PKA (Protein Kinase A), MARK (Microtubule Affinity Regulating Kinase) [110] and SADK (Synapses of Amphids Defective Family Kinases) [111] are protein kinases non PDPKs which target KXGS motifs in repeats. (iii) protein kinases specific for tyrosines- SFKs (Src Family Kinases) such as Src [112], Lck [113], Syk [114], Fyn [115, 116] and c-Abl Kinase [117] targets Tau tyrosine residues at Y18, Y29 and Y394.

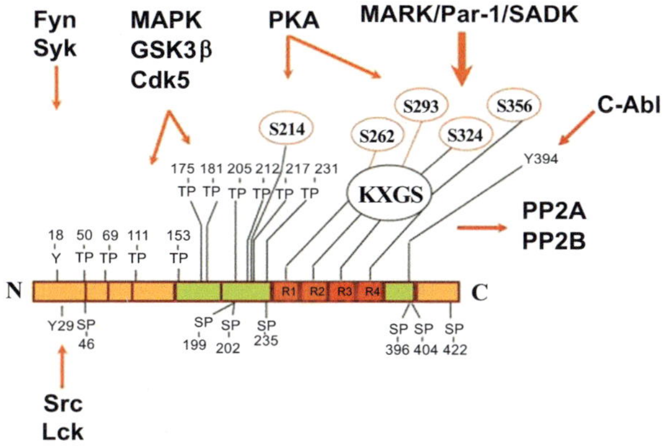

Fig. (2). Diagram of Tau phosphorylation sites. Different phosphorylation sites are targeted by many kinases in full length Tau (Ht40) isoform. Phosphorylation of SP/TP sites are targets of GSK3AY, CDK5 and MAPK. These phosphorylations have transitional effect on Tau-microtubule affinity. PKA, MARK and SADK phosphorylate KXGS motifs and S214. SFKs phosphorylate tyrosine residues at positions 18, 29 and 394. Tau can be readily dephosphorylated by phosphatases, PP2A and PP2B.

The phosphorylation at SP/TP motifs has only a weak influence on Tau-microtubule interactions [92, 118]. These phosphorylation sites are elevated in Alzheimer Tau [119].

The KXGS motifs in the repeat domain (S262, S293, S324, S356) can be phosphorylated by MARK, PKA, SADK, CamKII, and Par-1. PKA additionally phosphorylates S214 [120]. Tau phosphorylation in KXGS motifs results in decrease of Tau binding to microtubules [110, 121]. Moreover, phosphorylation of Tau at S262, T231, and S235 inhibits its binding to microtubules by ~35%, ~25%, and ~10%, respectively [122]. In AD brain, Tau is found to be hyperphosphorylated at almost all phosphorylation sites [123].

In 1985, Tau was shown to be phosphorylated on tyrosine *in vitro* by insulin receptor kinase [124]. The first study to demonstrate that Tau protein is phosphorylated on tyrosine residues in cells was published in 1998 by Gloria Lee and Co-workers [115]. Tyrosine residues of Tau protein have been shown to be phosphorylated by SFKs (Src Family Kinases) such as Src [112], Lck [113], Syk [114], Fyn [115, 116] and by c-Abl Kinase [117].

Tau is dephosphorylated by PP2A (Protein Phosphatase 2A) and PP2B (Protein Phosphatase 2B) [125, 126].

Proteolysis of Tau Protein

The microtubule associated protein Tau aggregates intracellularly in AD. Aggregation of Tau has also been reported in a number of other neurodegenerative diseases collectively called as tauopathies. It has been indicated that impaired proteolysis of Tau perturbs Tau turnover leading to its availability for aggregation [127]. Many studies showed Tau to be a substrate for large number of proteases, *viz.* trypsin, chymotrypsin, calpains, caspases, cathepsins, proteasomal proteases, and thrombin [128]. In spite of so many studies of proteases with Tau, still much is not known about proteases acting on Tau *in vivo*.

Clipping of Fuzzy Coat by Pronase

9.5 kD and 12.4 kD fragments have been isolated by digestion of paired helical filaments (PHFs) with pronase and amino acid sequencing analysis confirmed the derivation of these fragments from Tau [129].

PHFs are associated with a fuzzy outer coat which can be stripped off by a proteolytic digestion leaving the three- domain structure morphologically intact. PHFs are shown to be consisted of two structurally distinct parts. An external fuzzy region can be removed by pronase treatment to leave a pronase- resistant morphologically recognizable core. The mass per unit length was estimated to be 79 $kDa.nm^{-1}$ before pronase digestion and 65 $kDa.nm^{-1}$ after pronase digestion as determined using scanning transmission electron microscopy. The fuzzy region carries all the epitopes recognized by two different antisera against Tau. Immunoblotting studies revealed that a 9.5 kD central fragment of Tau protein forms a part of the pronase resistant core structure [50].

Chymotrypsin to Separate Projection Domain in Tau

The C-terminal half of Tau contains several (three or four) internal repeats which are responsible for the binding to microtubules [73, 75]. Tau is homologous to other MAPs in C-terminal region [130]. Tau protein is known to stabilize microtubules. However, phosphorylation reduces the stabilizing effect suggesting a regulatory function [131]. Steiner *et al.* [132] tried to separate the microtubule binding and non-binding regions of Tau protein. They incubated Taxol-stabilized microtubules with Tau and briefly digested with chymotrypsin. They found two fragments of Tau after digestion with chymotrypsin; one projection fragment was present in the supernatant after pelleting the microtubules. They confirmed the cleavage of Tau at Tyr186 by using amino acids sequencing. The fragment associated with the microtubules had residues from 187 to 430 confirming binding of C-terminal region of Tau with the microtubules.

Thrombin Cleavage of Tau

Thrombin is a serine protease involved in blood coagulation. It is generated by proteolytic cleavage of its precursor, prothrombin, which is made primarily in the liver and circulates in plasma. Expression of prothrombin mRNA has been found in the central nervous system [133-135]. Thrombin is normally present in the brain's neurons, where it cleaves Tau. It is necessary for thrombin to cleave Tau in order to prevent clumping of the microtubules for normal neuron function. It has been speculated that increased levels of thrombin could be directly involved in AD neuropathology [136, 137].

Thrombin is a brain protease which cleaves Tau. Tau breakdown was studied in the cytosolic fractions extracted from five normal human brains and complete inhibition of Tau breakdown in the fraction was reported using thrombin specific inhibitors, D-phenylalanyl-L-prolylarginyl chloromethyl ketone (PPACK). Inhibition of Tau breakdown from rat brain by PPACK has also been reported. The *in vitro* proteolysis of human recombinant Tau and Sarkosyl-insoluble Tau from a PHF preparation was carried out using thrombin. Thrombin initially cleaved recombinant Tau at the Arg155-Gly156 bond. Thereafter, it cleaved C-terminal Tau fragment bidirectionally at multiple Arg/Lys-Xaa bonds. Phosphorylated recombinant Tau and PHF-Tau are reported to be more resistant to thrombin proteolysis than non-phosphorylated recombinant Tau and dephosphorylated PHF-Tau. On the basis of these findings, a possible role for thrombin in proteolysis of Tau under physiological and/ or pathological conditions has been suggested [138].

The formation of a stable 25 kD fragment as a result of cleavage of Tau by thrombin in *in vitro* was reported. The fragment was derived from the C-terminal end of Tau as revealed by the immunoblotting and amino acid sequencing. The cleaved Tau has a reduced capacity to promote microtubule assembly compared with the full length Tau [139].

Cleavage of Tau by Caspases

Caspases belong to the cysteine- aspartate family of proteases which are critically involved in apoptosis. These enzymes have been broadly divided into initiator and executioner caspases. Caspases 2, 8, 9 and 10 are categorized as 'initiator caspases' because of their apical position in apoptotic protease cascades, and caspases 3, 6 and 7 are designated as 'executioner caspases' because they function as relatively downstream effectors of apoptosis, and cleave proteins that maintain the integrity of the nucleus and the plasma membrane, resulting in morphological manifestations of apoptosis. Many caspases have been shown to get activated in apoptotic neurons in AD and plays a critical role in Aβ induced neuronal apoptosis [140 - 142]. It has been postulated that caspases contribute to the proteolytic truncation of Tau observed in the neurofibrillar pathologies of AD.

Caspases 1, 3, 6, 7 and 8 are shown to cleave wild type Tau (WT Tau) into a major proteolytic product of nearly 5 kD smaller than WT Tau. Using 35S-labeled WT human Tau and recombinant caspases, analysis of proteolytic product(s) has been done using SDS-polyacrylamide gel electrophoresis. Tau has been reported to be cleaved by caspases at Asp421 in its C terminus. Cleavage of Tau at Asp421 by caspases is confirmed by using mutant Tau (D421E) which could not be cleaved by caspases. This cleavage was further confirmed with the help of specific monoclonal antibody TauC3, a specific antibody that recognizes Tau truncated at Asp421 site. Caspase cleavage of Tau has been shown to promote filament assembly more rapidly than WT Tau. Tau has also been shown to be specifically cleaved at Asp421 in neurons treated with amyloidogenic Aβ peptide and in the characteristic fibrillar pathologies in AD [143].

The studies showed that Tau is cleaved at Asp421 by caspase 3 [144, 145].A study reported cleavage of Tau at Asp421 by caspase 3 and caspase 7, both executioner caspases. Cleavage products are analyzed using sodium dodecyl sulfate polyacrylamide gel electrophoresis. Cleavage at Asp421 has been confirmed by primary amino acid sequencing of the smaller fragment. The molecular weights of the cleaved products have been determined by using electrospray mass spectrometry and found to be 45,900 Da and 1,997.99 Da for the larger fragment and smaller C-terminal fragment, respectively. A rabbit polyclonal antibody (α-ΔTau) directed against the caspase cleaved carboxy-terminus of Tau has been generated and its specificity is confirmed by western blot. Generated polyclonal antibody recognized the Asp421-cleaved fragment generated by caspase 3 or 7 but not full-length Tau [146].

It has been reported that caspase cleaved Tau (ΔTau) facilitates nucleation-dependent filament formation and readily adopts a conformational change recognized by the early pathological Tau marker MC1. The ΔTau can be phosphorylated by glycogen synthase kinase-3β and subsequently recognized by the NFT antibody PHF-1. In transgenic mice and AD brains, ΔTau associates with both early and late markers of NFTs. Additionally, ΔTau colocalizes with Aβ1–42 and is induced by Aβ1–42 *in vitro*. Aβ accumulation triggers caspase activation, leading to caspase-cleavage of Tau, and this is an early event that may precede hyperphosphorylation in the evolution of AD tangle pathology [146].

The role of caspases in the cleavage of important cellular proteins has been predicted. It has also been interpreted that full execution of apoptosis is not important for driving neuron dysfunction and pathology observed in AD. The role of caspase 9 in the AD brain using a caspase cleavage site directed antibody, directed towards the N-terminus of the auto activation cleavage site of caspase 9, has been investigated. Active caspase 9 is reported to colocalize with active caspase 8 and caspase 3 cleavage products of fodrin within neurons exhibiting NFT morphology. Caspase cleavage of Tau also occurs in the AD brain [147]. Lu *et al.* [148] also demonstrated the presence of activated caspase 9 in the AD brain by Western blot analysis. Canu *et al.* [149] showed the presence of a caspase cleavage site towards the amino terminal end of Tau. They showed the formation of 67000 Da and 28000 Da molecular weight fragments of Tau after caspase digestion analyzed by immunolabeling technique using Tau-CCP antibody.

Abraha *et al.* [150] showed that the C terminus of Tau inhibits its assembly into polymeric filaments *in vitro*. It is known that in apoptotic human neurons in primary cultures, caspase 6 is activated [150, 151]. Furthermore, when recombinant active caspase 6 is directly microinjected into the cytosol, there is induced human neuronal cell death [152]. Caspase 6 increases in the aging brain cortex and there is decrease in the learning paradigm [153]. Guo *et al.* [154] showed the presence of active caspase 6 in AD and age matched control short postmortem interval brains with neoepitope antibodies to the p20 subunit of human active caspase 6 and to caspase 6 cleaved Tau at Asp402. With the help of specific antibodies, they showed that caspase 6 is activated in human fetal and adult neuronal apoptosis and could contribute significantly to neuritic degeneration in AD. Albrecht *et al.* [155] also showed Tau cleavage by caspase 6 at Asp402 as detected by immunostaining. However, Horowitz *et al.* [156] showed that caspase 6 cleaves Tau *in vitro* at Asp13. They confirmed their results using mass spectrometric analysis. They suggested a role for caspase 6 and N-terminal truncation of Tau during neurofibrillary tangle evolution and the progression of AD.

Role of Calpains in Tau Cleavage

Calpains belong to a highly conserved family of calcium-dependent cysteine proteases that have been implicated in a variety of physiological processes. There are two ubiquitously expressed calpains, termed as μ-calpain (calpain-1) and m-calpain (calpain-2). The names, μ-calpain and m-calpain were coined for the μM and mM thresholds of calcium necessary for *in vitro* autolytic activation, respectively. Calpains are regulated by the ubiquitously expressed endogenous inhibitor, calpastatin. Calpains have been found at high concentrations in brain with neuronal localization [157, 158].

Tau can be cleaved by calpains and the process can be impeded by phosphorylation [159, 160]. Tau can be cleaved by calpains at nine putative calpain cleavage sites on the basis of P2-P1 rule [158]. Calpain cleavage of Tau generates a 17 kD fragment (A125-R230) spanning several PXXP motifs thereby displaying a potential of scrounging SH3-containing proteins [161, 162]. This 17 kD Tau fragment has been thought to intercede Aβ toxicity in neurons [163], but the role of the fragment in toxicity is a subject of debate.

Tau Cleavage by Cathepsin D

Cathepsins belong to cysteine family of proteases. A few cathepsins have also been reported to belong to serine and aspartate families of proteases. Cathepsins have been found to be localized in lysosomes and are monomeric in nature. Brain tissues display abundant cathepsin D levels [164 - 166]. Active cathepsin D and cathepsin B have been found in senile plaques in brains affected with AD [167]. It has been demonstrated that Tau is a substrate of cathepsin D [168, 169].

Kenessey *et al.* [170] studied degradation of different isoforms of human recombinant Tau and fetal Tau by cathepsin D using immunoblotting technique. The analyses revealed that amino and carboxy termini of Tau were cleaved before other regions. They demonstrated the cleavage of recombinant Tau between Phe8-Glu9, Met419-Val 420, Thr427-Leu428-Ala429, and Leu436-Ala437 as analyzed by amino acid sequencing and mass spectroscopy. They also showed additional cleavage sites dependent on pH. They observed additional sites between amino acids 34-161 and 267-358 at pH 3.5 whereas between amino acids 200-257 at pH 7.0. They suggested that cathepsin D cleavage of Tau could generate Tau fragments with intact microtubule binding domains which could have a role in the pathogenesis of paired helical filaments in AD.

AMYLOID-Β (AΒ)

A primary neuropathological hallmark of AD brains is the accumulation of β-amyloid peptide (Aβ) in amyloid (diffuse and later neuritic) plaques and, to a lesser extent, blood vessels. Aβ was first identified in 1984 as the main component of amyloid plaques [38]. The neurotoxic Aβ peptides are derived by the proteolytic processing of the amyloid precursor protein (APP) by certain proteases called beta- and gamma- secretases, generating three forms of Aβ corresponding to Aβ (1-40), Aβ (1-42), and Aβ (1-43). In the normal brain, most APP is processed in a way that prevents the formation of potentially amyloidogenic fragments. This non-amyloidogenic secretory pathway is predominant over the amyloidogenic pathway and involves the obligate cleavage of APP by a so-called alpha-secretase [171]. The C83 and C99 are the APP fragments generated by alpha-secretase and beta-secretase, respectively. These

APP fragments are substrates to gamma-secretase, which performs proteolysis in the middle of the transmembrane domain to liberate the 3 kD peptide from C83 and 4 kD peptide from C99 [172, 173] (Fig. **3**). Hence, beta-secretase initiated Aβ-generation is a prerequisite for "amyloidogenic" gamma-secretase activity. Gamma-secretase activity is largely due to the action of presenilins which are membrane bound aspartyl proteases. There are two homologous presenilins, PS1 and PS2. Initially, presenilins were linked to familial AD [22]. Mutations in the presenilin molecule itself play a pivotal role in early-onset AD [174]. Their role in sporadic AD is less clear. The dominant role of PS1 and PS2 in general amyloid formation is known from observations in PS1 knockout mice, which have drastically reduced Aβ generation [175]. Moreover, PS1/PS2 double knockout mice show no Aβ generation at all [176]. However, PS1 and PS2 alone do not explain gamma-secretase activity. There are number of factors which form complex with presenilins and are able to limit PS activity [173].

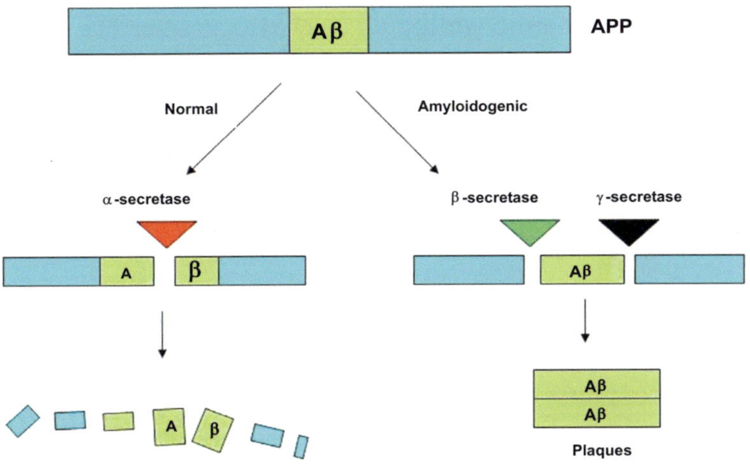

Fig. (3). A line diagram showing APP Processing by secretases. Under neuropathological conditions (amyloidogenic), APP is attacked by β- and γ-secretases forming different forms of Aβ plaques. In normal brain, α-secretase acts on APP forming C83 and C99 fragments.

Amyloid Cascade Hypothesis

John Hardy and David Allsop in 1991 proposed the amyloid cascade hypothesis. This hypothesis suggested that in AD pathogenesis, an initiating event is APP mismetabolism leading to the aggregation of Aβ. Further pathological events include the formation of neuritic plaques, NFTs and disruption of synaptic connections, which lead to a reduction in neurotransmitters, death of tangle bearing neurons and dementia [40]. One implication of this hypothesis is that plaques precede tangles.

Mechanism of Aβ Induced Cytotoxicity

Large amount of Aβ is neurotoxic to cells [177]. However, the precise mechanism of Aβ-induced cytotoxicity remains unknown. There are several ways via which Aβ may exert its neurotoxic effects. It has been shown that Aβ stimulates NO production through Ca^{2+} entry triggered by activated N-methyl-D-aspartate-gated channels [178]. Other reports have shown disruption of mitochondrial function via binding of the Aβ-binding alcohol dehydrogenase (ABAD) protein [179], induction of apoptotic genes through inhibition of Wnt [180], activation of microglia cells leading to the expression of pro-inflammatory genes, an increase in reactive oxygen species, and eventual neuronal toxicity and death [181]. Also Aβ inhibits glutamate uptake and causes extracellular glutamate increase [182].

THERAPEUTIC STRATEGIES FOR AD

The incidence of age-related neurodegenerative diseases such as AD continues to impact social as well as economic wellbeing. AD affects over 1% of the Canadian population and it currently costs the Health Care System (HCS) almost $20 billion per year. There is no cure for AD and the best 'therapy' resides in early intervention and delaying the onset of the disease. Here, therapeutic strategies will be discussed to provide insights for treatments of AD.

Tau Based Treatment Strategies

Tau is a highly soluble microtubule-associated protein that plays a critical role in microtubule stabilization. Tau hyperphosphorylation leads to the detachment of the protein from microtubules thus disrupting the structure of the neuronal cytoskeleton. Tau phosphorylation and aggregation leads to the formation of neurofibrillary tangles which is toxic to neurons. Thus, Tau based treatments intent to inhibit the phosphorylation and/or aggregation of the protein. Additionally, Tau clearance, microtubule-stabilizing drugs and immunotherapy could be used as a treatment strategy in AD.

Tau Phosphorylation Inhibition

Protein kinases are a group of critical enzymes responsible for Tau hyper-phosphorylation. Several kinases such as GSK3β, CDK5, p38, JNK, ERK1, ERK2, Fyn are reported to be expressed in increased amounts in the areas proximal to neurofibrillary tangles [183]. Much research work has been done towards the development of kinase inhibitors as a possible treatment strategy for AD.

Most important protein kinase involved in Tau phosphorylation is glycogen synthase kinase 3 beta (GSK3β); thus, GSK3β inhibitors are in the most advanced stages of clinical development for AD. In preclinical studies, Tideglusib, an irreversible inhibitor of GSK3β, has been reported to have favorable effects on reversing amyloid accumulation in brain tissue, preventing cell loss and reducing spatial memory deficits [184]. However, in the follow-up phase trial, Tideglusib administration to patients with mild-to-moderate AD did not show statistically significant behavioral therapeutic benefits leading to the discontinuation of the inhibitor [185].

Cyclin dependent kinase 5 (CDK5) belongs to the family of serine/threonine cyclin-dependent kinases and is associated with Tau hyperphosphorylation and neuronal cell death [186]. Thus, CDK5 selective inhibitors might also be potential drug targets. At present, Roscovitine and Flavopiridol have exhibited neuro-protective properties both in *in vitro* and *in vivo* models of excitotoxicity, and neurodegeneration [187].

The JNK3 is another important kinase reported to be present in the similar levels as that of Aβ (1-42) in the brain [188]. Moreover, JNK3 is upregulated in the CSF and is associated with the memory loss making it a promising target for future therapies [189]. SP600125, a JNK inhibitor, has been reported to reduce neurodegeneration in an APP/PS1 transgenic mouse model of AD [190].

Tau Aggregation Inhibition

Tau aggregation contributes to neurotoxicity in AD brain. Recently, methylene blue and its derivatives have displayed some promising results in inhibiting Tau aggregates. Rember, the first generation methylene blue derivative, successfully stabilized AD progression in a 50 weeks clinical trial. Later, the next generation purified derivative of methylene blue, TRx 0237 was developed and reported to inhibit Tau protein aggregation [191]. Several clinical trials are in the pipeline to evaluate the potential benefit of this drug in AD.

Microtubule Stabilizing Drugs

Microtubule stabilizing drugs may compensate for the loss of function of abnormally phosphorylated and aggregated Tau that cannot bind to and stabilize microtubules. Paclitaxel is the most common microtubule stabilizing drug. However, due to its incapability of crossing the blood brain barrier, its utility is limited in AD [192]. TPI-287 is another drug that stabilizes the microtubules by binding to tubulin. It is under a clinical trial which will determine its safety and tolerability in mild-to-moderate AD. Epothilone D is also a microtubule stabilizing drug and has been reported to display beneficial effects on axonal transport, axonal dystrophy, Tau neuropathology and neuronal loss. However, the drug failed to show promising results in a clinical trial and was therefore discontinued [193].

Immunotherapy

The Tau immunotherapy has been reported to play a pivotal role in reducing Tau aggregates and in clearing Tau oligomers and insoluble aggregates without any adverse effects [194]. AADvac-1, an active immunotherapy which consists of a synthetic peptide derived from the Tau sequence, displayed good preclinical safety profile for the treatment period of up to 6 months in rats, rabbits, and dogs [183].

Aβ Based Treatment Strategies

The Aβ centered theory for AD posits that the sequential cleavage of amyloid precursor protein (APP) by β-secretase and γ-secretase gives rise to the toxic β-amyloid (Aβ) and the deposition of Aβ is a central event in AD. Alternatively, APP can be processed by α-secretase under physiological conditions to produce a soluble sAPPα fragment and a carboxy-terminal 83-amino acid (C83) fragment [195]. Therefore, to crackdown the production of Aβ, focus is on the three enzymes involved in processing APP.

β-Secretase and γ-Secretase Inhibitors

The Aβ is generated by the cleavage of APP by β-secretase followed by γ-secretase. Therefore, to lower the production of Aβ, β-secretase and γ-secretase are good drug targets for the generation of inhibitors. However, besides APP, both the enzymes have several other substrates involved in physiological functions making the development of inhibitors a big challenge. For example, neuregulin-1 is a substrate of β-secretase and is involved in CNS axons myelination and synaptic plasticity [196]. Similarly, Notch protein, having role in cell proliferation, development, and communication, is a substrate of γ-secretase [197]. Thus, wide range of substrates increases the risk of side effects making it a major issue of concern.

Nonetheless, several β-secretase inhibitors such as E2609, MK-8931, and LY2886721 are tested and have shown the potency in reducing Aβ production drastically in the cerebrospinal fluid (CSF) in humans [198 - 200]. However, none of the inhibitors are available in the market as yet.

γ-secretase inhibitor, Semagacestat (LY450139), has been reported to decrease levels of Aβ in blood and in CSF in humans [201]. However, its clinical study results recorded the worsening of cognition with a bunch of other side effects including weight loss, increased probability of skin cancer and infection. Similarly, Avagacestat, another γ-secretase inhibitor was discontinued due to the lack of effectiveness [202].

Considering the deleterious side effects of both the enzymes inhibitors, efforts have been made in developing selective γ-secretase modulators in a way to avoid the side effects associated with enzyme inhibitors. This project began with the consideration that several nonsteroidal anti-inflammatory drugs (NSAIDs) such as ibuprofen, sulindac, indomethacin, and flurbiprofen decrease Aβ levels *in vitro* and *in vivo* [203]. Unfortunately, ibuprofen and flurbiprofen failed to perform in their respective clinical trials [203, 204]. The CHF5074, a NSAID similar to that of flurbiprofen, has been reported to inhibit Aβ *in vitro* [205].

Increase α-Secretase Levels

As α-secretase processing of APP impedes the Aβ production, increase of α-secretase activity is considered as a potential therapeutic target for AD. Interestingly, studies have shown that the α-secretase activity is increased by the drugs in use for the treatment of AD via the associated signaling cascades and it has been considered as the best therapeutic approach so far [206]. For example, Selegiline, an inhibitor used to slow down the progression of AD, has been reported to increase the α-secretase activity via a protein trafficking mechanism [207].

Etazolate (EHT 0202), a GABA receptor modulator, has been shown to protect rat cortical neurons against Aβ induced toxicity [208] and is in phase II clinical trials. Also, bryostatin, a powerful PKC modulator, is known to increase the sAPPα and is currently undergoing Phase II trials for use in AD [209].

Aggregation Inhibitors

The assemblage of Aβ peptides into oligomers and aggregates give rise to amyloid plaques and it is considered to be a major pathologic event in AD. Therefore, blocking the amyloid aggregation using small molecules is a promising strategy for the treatment of AD.

The inhibitor, 3-amino-1-propaneosulfonic acid (3-APS, Alzhemed, tramiprosate) has been designed to prevent the amyloid fibril formation by interfering with the interaction of Aβ with glycosaminoglycans. It reached the phase III clinical trials but failed to make it through and as a result has been suspended in Europe [184].

Colostrinin reached phase II clinical trial after showing promising results in mice models. Aβ aggregation is inhibited and cognitive performance is reportedly improved in mice models in the presence of Colostrinin. However, the drug failed to maintain its beneficial effects in phase II trial [210].

Aβ aggregation has also been shown to be inhibited with metal chelating 8-hydroxiquinolines (8-HQ) compounds, clioquinol and PBT2 [211]. Unfortunately, these molecules failed to perform in the phases II and III of clinical development.

Immunotherapy

Immunotherapy strategy intends to reduce the amyloid load in AD. The first-generation vaccine (AN1792) is consisted of a full length Aβ peptide and has been reported to have severe adverse effects including cerebral inflammation and aseptic meningoencephalitis [212] leading to its phase II trial discontinuation.

Afterwards, second-generation vaccines have also been designed using a shorter Aβ peptide to avoid the side effects faced with first-generation vaccines. CAD 106, the first second-generation vaccine, completed the phase II clinical trial without causing adverse reactions. The ACC-001, another second-generation vaccine has been reported to complete two-phase II trials and is currently undergoing an additional phase II trial [187].

Another approach of immunotherapy consists of the intravenous administration of anti- Aβ antibodies to the patient. This method is reported to reduce cerebral amyloid load and improve cognition in transgenic animals without having reduced the amyloid plaque numbers. Bapineuzumab, a humanized monoclonal antibody against Aβ (1-6) displayed significant reduction in brain amyloid plaques and phosphorylated Tau in CSF. However, it failed in phase III clinical trials due to the lack of effectiveness [213]. Solanezumab, a humanized monoclonal antibody against Aβ (12-28) improved cognition in mild AD [213]. At present, it is in phase III clinical trials.

Acetylcholinesterase Inhibitors

Acetylcholinesterase (AChE) remains a highly viable target for the symptomatic improvement in AD. AChE is involved in the termination of impulse transmission by rapid hydrolysis of the neurotransmitter acetylcholine in numerous cholinergic pathways in the central and peripheral nervous systems. Acetylcholinesterase inhibitors (AChEI) inhibit acetylcholinesterase enzyme and prevent it from breaking down acetylcholine, thereby increasing both the level and duration of action of the neurotransmitter acetylcholine [214]. Physostigmine was the first ChEI investigated for the treatment of AD. It is present in the seeds of

Physostigma venenosum as a parasympathomimetic plant alkaloid. Tacrine was the first drug approved for the treatment of AD in 1993. Donepezil was approved in 1996 for the treatment of mild-to-moderate AD. The other old AChEIs include rivastigmine, galantamine and metrifonate. Huperzine A and B, Nelumbo nucifera, Himatanthus lancifolius, Galangin, and Cardanol Derivatives are naturally derived AChEIs. Phenserine, tolserine, esolerine and tesofensine are new AChEI [215].The successful clinical trials led to the marketing of donepezil, rivastigmine and galantamine. Besides, many other compounds with AChEI properties have been developed and tested mainly in Phase I-II clinical trials in the last twenty years [216]. However, in spite of so much research work since long time, no effective treatment exists for the disease.

POLYPHARMACOLOGY

AD is one of the most complicated progressive neurodegeneration diseases that involve many genes, proteins, and their complex interactions. No effective medicines or treatments are available yet to stop or reverse the progression of the disease due to its polygenic nature [217]. Therefore, polypharmacology can be used to design the drugs for AD that act on multiple targets or disease pathways. The diverse cerebral mechanisms implicated in central nervous system (CNS) diseases together with the heterogeneous and overlapping nature of phenotypes indicated that the multitarget strategies may be appropriate for improved treatment of the complex brain diseases. It is shown that multipotent ligands targeting AChE/MAO-A/MAO-B and also D1-R/D2-R/5-HT2A -R/H3-R are promising novel drug candidates with improved efficacy and beneficial neuroleptic and procognitive activities in the treatment of Alzheimer's and related neurodegenerative diseases [218].

MICROBIOME

Recent genome-wide association studies (GWAS) indicated that a significant portion of AD-relevant gene signals are not located within gene coding regions suggesting the contribution of epigenetic or environmental factors to AD risk. Most of the changes seen in AD such as inflammation, brain cell atrophy, immunological aberrations, amyloidogenesis, altered gene expression and cognitive deficits are also seen as a consequence of microbial infection [219]. Humans contain a complex and dynamic community of microbes called the microbiome that forms a “metaorganism” with symbiotic or commensal benefit to the host. Emerging studies indicated that the human microbiome may contribute to the regulation of multiple neuro-chemical and neuro-metabolic pathways through a complex series of highly interactive and symbiotic host-microbiome signaling systems that mechanistically interconnect the gastrointestinal (GI) tract, skin, liver, and other organs with the central nervous system (CNS) [220]. The GI tract microbiome has been estimated to encode about 4×10^6 genes. Over 99% of gastrointestinal tract microbiota are anaerobic bacteria, with fungi, protozoa, archaebacteria and other microorganisms making up the remainder. There is currently much interest in the ability of gastrointestinal tract bacteria to influence host innate-immune, neuroinflammatory, neuromodulatory and neurotransmission-functions. Besides gastrointestinal tract microbes, there is also a potential contribution of pathogenic microbes, altered microbiome signaling and other disease-inducing agents to the development of AD [219].

INFECTIVE AGENTS

Various infectious agents and viruses in particular, have been proposed as potential causes of AD. Infection with several important pathogens could constitute risk factors for cognitive impairment, dementia, and AD. Infections with herpes simplex virus type 1, picornavirus, Borna disease virus, *Chlamydia pneumoniae*, *Helicobacter pylori*, and spirochete have been reported to contribute to the pathophysiology of AD [221]. Herpes simplex virus type 1 (HSV-1) is one of the stronger candidates because it is neurotropic, ubiquitous and able to establish lifelong latency in the host. Evidence for the role of HSV-1 in AD is still contradictory but its presence in the regions of the brain affected by AD is reported. The fact that HSV-1 is also present in elderly patients without the disease suggested that the virus is not an independent cause of the condition [222]. Contini *et al.* (2010) reported the role of *Chlamydophila pneumoniae* in the pathogenesis of mental or neurobehavioral disorders like Alzheimer and schizophrenia [223]. Association between Alzheimer and infectious agents like cytomegalovirus (CMV), herpes simplex virus type 1 (HSV-1), Borrelia burgdorferi, *Chlamydophila pneumoniae* and *Helicobacter pylori* has been reported using enzyme linked immunosorbent assay in 128 AD patients. Inflammation in brain vessels has also been reported to play a vital role in both vascular dementia and AD [224].

DATABASES FOR ALZHEIMER'S DISEASE

AlzGene Database

It is a publicly and continuously updated database of AD that comprehensively catalogs all the genetic association studies. It is available at http://www.alzgene.org. It is a collection of published Alzheimer's disease genetic association studies, random effects of meta-analyses for polymorphisms with genotype data in at least three case-control samples. Currently, AlzGene contains 695 genes taken from 1395 studies, 2973 polymorphisms and 320 meta-analyses. It can be searched using genes, protein, polymorphism, study or any keyword [225].

Alz Biomarker

Alz Biomarker contains data on the biomarkers of AD. Biomarker measurements from the cerebrospinal fluid and blood are curated from the primary literature and meta-analyzed. The database was developed by Henrik Zetterberg and colleagues at the University of Gothenburg. It is available at http://www.alzforum.org/alzbiomarker. The first version contains 25 biomarkers from 243 research papers and 34 meta-analyses [226].

AlzRisk

The AlzRisk database provides a comprehensive and publicly available collection of epidemiologic reports that evaluate environmental (i.e., non-genetic) risk factors for AD. It is regularly updated and available online at http://www.alzrisk.org/. The database can be searched by a variety of dropdown menus or by specific keywords. For each risk factor, a table or tables of all peer-reviewed studies published in English, the distribution of the risk factor (the "exposure"), the analytic methods, the effect size and statistical significance of the observed association and where appropriate a link to meta-analyses of the catalogued studies is also included [227].

NIAGADS

It is a national genetics repository created by National Institute on Aging Genetics of Alzheimer's Disease. It is created to facilitate access by qualified investigators to genotypic data for the study of genetics of late-onset AD. It can be accessed online at https://www.niagads.org/. As of January 2017, NIAGADS houses 34 datasets with almost 50k subjects and over 30 billion genotypes. With a streamlined application and submission process, NIAGADS is an enriched resource for AD researchers to utilize [228].

HISTORY OF PARKINSON'S DISEASE

Parkinson's disease is known since ancient times. It was being called as Kampavata in the ancient Indian medical system of Ayurveda. In 175 AD, physician Galen described the symptoms as the shaking palsy. In 1817, an English physician, James Parkinson recognized the medical condition and published a paper entitled "An Essay on the Shaking Palsy". It was based on six cases that he had observed during his practice and neighbourhood. He wrote this essay to encourage others to study the disease. After sixty years, a French neurologist, Jean Martin Charcot truly recognised the importance of Parkinson's work and he named the disease in the name of Parkinson [229].

In 1940, the frequency of Parkinsonism was reviewed by Kinnier Wilson where he reported the abundant cases of post-encephalitic type. In 1952, Garland made a survey for the prevalence of PD and concluded that Parkinson had a prevalence rate of 60 per 100,000. A study was carried out on Parkinsonism in patients aged 50 or more in Sweden and its prevalence was reported to be 1.6 per 1,000 [230].

In 1960, Ehringer and Hornykiewicz reported chemical difference in the Parkinson's patients. It was found that there was low level of dopamine in these patients that led to the degeneration of nerve cells in the part of brain called the substantia nigra. This discovery led to the identification of first effective medical treatment called Levodopa to treat the symptoms. Since 1960s, researches are being conducted at a faster rate, however, till now, no cure could be found for the disease. Only progress made is that now symptoms may be controlled and severity may be decreased [231].

SYMPTOMS OF PARKINSON'S DISEASE

Symptoms of PD vary from one person to another and the symptoms change as the disease progresses from its onset. Most of the time, the early symptoms are unnoticed. Disease causes two types of symptoms, *viz.* motor and non-motor symptoms. Motor symptoms are associated with the movement of the body. The motor symptoms are grouped by the acronym TRAP (Tremor, Rigidity, Akinesia (or bradykinesia) and Postural instability) [232].

Tremor is characterized by an involuntary or rhythmic movement of one or more body parts. In PD, different types of tremors are noticed according to the circumstances under which they occur, the body part involved and the frequency at which the tremor occurs. Tremor occurs only in 70 percent patients and varies in different cases. The most common tremor is resting tremor that appears when a person's muscles are relaxed or at rest and it again emerges when a person adopts a pose or move. It is called as re-emergent tremor. Other types of tremors include kinetic tremor having higher and non-harmonical frequency. Tremor is linked to the altered activity of two circuits: basal ganglia that trigger tremor and the cerebello-thalamo-cortical circuit that produces the tremor [233]. Tremor is marker of the benign PD. There are indications that patients with tremor symptoms have slow disease progression [234]. Tremor in Parkinson is generally provoked by stress or excitement.

Rigidity can be defined as the inability of muscles to relax normally. In general, muscles stretch when move and relax at rest. The inability of muscles to relax causes stiffness in the body. Rigidity is present in about 99% cases of Parkinson. Rigidity is characterized by the loss of arm swing with walking, fatigue, loss of facial expression and variety of muscle pain syndrome. Rigidity is commonly experienced in legs, neck and shoulder.

The basic symptom of Bradykinesia, also called Akinesia, is slowness of movement. Bradykinesia causes difficulty in repetitive movements and everyday functions such as brushing teeth, buttoning a shirt, cutting fruits and vegetables, *etc*. Bradykinesia is used synonymous with the word Akinesia and Hypokinesia. Akinesia is loss of spontaneous movement like facial expression or it is freezing of movement that leads to prolonged time taken in initiating a movement. Hypokinesia refers to a smaller movement as desired [235].

Postural instability or balance impairment is the loss of balance or tendency to be unstable when standing upright. This occurs because a person loses some of the reflexes that are required to keep the body in proper posture. This symptom generally appears in the early stage and becomes more disabling in the later stage of the disease. Due to postural instability, person falls while standing, turning or raising from chair. Some people might fall backwards and this problem is called as retropulsion. For postural instability, person can be treated using physical therapy or balancing exercises that reduce the risk of fall [236].

Besides this motor symptom, patients with PD also show non–motor symptoms like nausea, constipation, loss of smell and taste, vomiting, excessive saliva, changes in weight, insomnia, excessive daytime sleepiness, excessive sweating, depression, anxiety, hypotension, drolling, slow thinking, confusion, double vision, delusion, sexual dysfunction and hallucinations. Non-motor symptoms appear in the premotor phase of the disease and become complicated in the advanced phase. These symptoms are often undiagnosed and therefore are untreated. These non-motor symptoms cause significant burden on the quality of life of the patient and are the cause of hospitalization. Therefore, identification of these symptoms is essential in order to get them treated [236].

CAUSES OF PARKINSON'S DISEASE

In PD, many neurons gradually break down or die. These neurons produce the neuro-transmitter, dopamine, and therefore the dopamine level drops. Low level of dopamine leads to the abnormal brain activity that develops many symptoms of PD. The actual cause of Parkinson is still unknown but there are some genetic and environmental factors. Many experts think that Parkinson is caused by the combination of genetic and environmental factors and may vary in person to person.

Genetic Factors

Parkinson is generally a non-genetic disorder and therefore is not inherited. About 10 to 15% cases of the Parkinson are reported with the relatives having PD. About 4 to 9% cases are reported where parents had PD. Therefore, people with Parkinson parent(s) are more prone to this disorder compared to others whose parents do not suffer from PD. Researchers have identified several gene mutations that can directly cause the disease. These genes include PRKN (parkin), SNCA (α-synuclein gene), LRRK2 (leucine-rich repeat kinase 2), GBA (Glucocerebrosidase) and many more (Table **2**). In most of the cases, it has been observed that people with mutation in any of these genes develop Parkinson [237, 238].

Table 2. Genes and their mutations involved in Parkinson's Disease.

Gene	Mutations
SNCA	A30P, E46K, A53T, Genomic duplications/triplications
LRRK2	~50 missense variants, ~16 of them pathogenic, including the common G2019S
Parkin	>200 mutations (point mutations, exonic rearrangements)
PINK1	>40 point mutations, rare large deletions
DJ-1	>10 point mutations and large deletions
ATP13A2	>5 point mutations
FBXO7	Three point mutations
PLA2G6	Two missense mutations
Omi/HTRA2	Two missense variants
GIGYF2	Seven missense variants
UCHL1	One mutation in a single PD sibling pair

SNCA (α-Synuclein Gene)

The SNCA gene has six exons and it encodes for a cytosolic protein, α-synuclein, which has 140 amino acids in its polypeptide chain. It is the first gene that was reported to be mutated in Parkinson. This protein is abundant in the brain and is also found in the heart and muscles. In brain, α-synuclein is found in the presynaptic terminal which interacts with the fats and proteins and regulates the release of dopamine. Generally, SNCA gene mutation appears before the age of 50. Three different mutations are reported in SNCA gene which cause PD. Mutations reported are Ala53Thr, Ala30Pro, and Glu46Lys. Besides these mutations, duplication and triplication of SNCA gene are reported [239]. The α-synuclein genesis enriched in α- helical structure, however, when mutated it forms stable β sheet that induces the formation of toxic oligomers, protofibrils and fibrils. In turn, Lewy bodies are produced which suppress the toxic damaged α-synuclein [238].

LRKK2 (Leucine-Rich Repeat Kinase 2) Gene

Leucine-rich repeat kinase 2 gene is comparatively a larger gene that consisted of 51 exons and encodes for a protein of 2527 amino acids long chain, called as dardarin (LRKK2 protein). This protein is enriched in leucine repeats in the amino terminal region of the protein, a kinase domain in the carboxyl terminal region, and many other conserved domains in between. There are more than 50 mutations reported in this LRRK2 gene, and out of them 16 have been found to be pathogenic which are clustered in the 10 exons of carboxy-terminal region of the protein. The most common mutations are: Arg114Cys, Arg1441Gly, Arg1441His, Arg1628Pro, Tyr1699Cys, Gly2019Ser, Ile2020Thr, and Gly2385Arg [240]. How mutation(s) in LRKK2 gene causes PD is still unclear as the LRKK2 protein is much larger in size with many domains capable of interaction with many other proteins. However, a common mutation, Gly2019Ser affects the kinase activity. LRRK2 mutations result in inhibition of kinase activity which subsequently induces a progressive reduction in neurite length [241].

Parkin

Parkin gene is the second gene which was reported to be mutated in PD. Human Parkin gene contains 12 exons and encodes for a protein of 465 amino acids called as Parkin protein (Parkinson juvenile disease protein 2). This Parkin protein exhibits ubiquitin E3 ligase enzyme activity. Parkin protein plays an important role in the ubiquitin-proteasome system and acts as a regulator of protein breakdown [242]. Mutations in Parkin were first identified in 1998. About 887 exonic mutations have been described comprising 147 different changes. Mutations in parkin gene ranges from single base pair substitutions to small deletions and splice site mutations. Due to the loss of Parkin function, its catalytic activity decreases which subsequently leads to nitrosative stress (nitric oxide – NO), dopaminergic stress and oxidative stress (reactive oxygen species – ROS) [243]. As a result of mutation in Parkin protein, there is loss of E3 ligase enzyme activity and due to which there is accumulation of AIMP2 protein (Aminoacyl-tRNA synthetase interacting multifunctional protein type 2) and FBP-1 (Far upstream element binding protein 1) that are polyubiquitinated via lysine-48 chains and get accumulated that leads to the neurodegeneration. It has also been reported that parkin is essential for cellular mitochondrial integrity. Parkin mutation leads to the accumulation of misfolded, aggregated proteins and degenerated mitochondria (Fig. **4**).

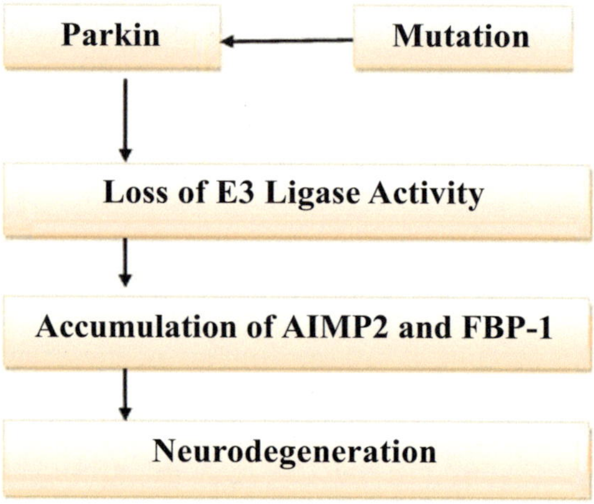

Fig. (4). Flowchart depicting the mutation in Parkin gene leads to neurodegeneration.

PINK1

Mutation(s) in PINK1 (Phosphatase and tensin homologue induced kinase1) gene may also cause PD. This gene contains 8 exons spanning in a length of 1.8 Kb [244]. The protein has been reported to have 581 amino acids long polypeptide chain with a conserved serine-threonine kinase domain. It exhibits kinase activity catalyzing phosphorylation of the mitochondrial proteins TRAP1 (Tumor necrosis factor receptor-associated protein 1) and Htr2a/OMI [5-hydroxytryptamine (serotonin) receptor 2a]. The PINK1 also associates with Hsp90 (heat shock protein 90)/Cdc37 (cell division cycle 37) chaperones [245]. Kumazawa *et al.* [246] carried mutation studies with hundreds of PD patients from many different countries. They identified 07 different novel mutations in PINK1 gene of these patients and out of which two were homozygous mutations (Asp297Met and Trp437Arg) and 05 were single heterozygous mutations (Ala78Val, Pro196Gln, Met342Val, Trp437Arg, Asn542Ser). Different researchers studied mutations in PINK1 gene, their relation with PD and reported ~50 mutation in PINK1 gene related to PD [247]. Loss or over expression of function of PINK1 effects apoptosis, abnormal mitochondrial morphology, impaired dopamine release and motor deficits.

DJ-1

DJ-1 gene has been reported to be consisted of seven exons and codes for 189 long amino acid protein which performs various functions, *viz.* transcriptional regulation, antioxidative stress reaction, cellular transformation, RNA binding, androgen-receptor signaling, spermatogenesis, fertilization and chaperone, protease, and mitochondrial regulation. Its activity is regulated by its oxidative status, especially of cysteine 106 [248, 249].Mutations in DJ-1 have been reported at various positions including Met26Ile, Glu64Asp, Arg98Gln, Ala104Thr and Asp149Ala and Leu166Pro [250]. The differently mutated DJ-1 proteins have been shown not to get folded properly resulting in reduction of the thermodynamic stability of the protein. The reduction in the thermodynamic stability of the protein results in the reduction of neuroprotective function and antioxidant activity of the protein [251].

Environmental Factors

Environmental factors include all other causes that are not of genetic in origin. Some scientists reported that Parkinson can be caused by the person's genetic makeup along with his activity and environment exposure. Some factors increase the risk of the disease, however many other factors may lower the risk. Similarly, some people have inherited the genetic makeup that makes them more susceptible to the disease. Scientists started to find the non- genetic factors by comparing the patients of Parkinson that make a person more susceptible to the disease. However, finding these factors is quite difficult since they did not provide the cause of Parkinson. It is important to perform statistical studies with the laboratory studies. A number of environmental risk factors have been reported such as rural environment, well water use, farming, use of herbicide/pesticide, exposure of toxins and many more.

Residence

The geographical distribution of Parkinson is not uniform and seems to be based on the environmental conditions. Area of residence may increase the risk of PD based on the exposure. Some reports indicated that urban areas have more incidence of Parkinson due to the exposure of industrial emissions of metals like copper and manganese [252]. However, in the rural areas, exposure to farm area and herbicides/pesticides leads to the higher risk of Parkinson [253]. In contrast, Gorell and co-workers in 1998 reported that there is no effect of rural living on incidence of Parkinson [254].

Occupation

Certain occupations, *viz.* welding and farming have been associated with higher risk of Parkinson. In contrast, some scientists reported that risk for Parkinson is not affected by the occupational factors [255]. Park *et al.* [256] reported that Parkinson is affected by the occupations like agriculture, hunting, forestry, whereas, Hertzman *et al.* [257] suggested that persons working in industries or mills are more prone to PD. On the other hand, Chen *et al.* [258] reported lower rate of Parkinson in people working in shifts and doing rigorous physical work.

Metal Exposure

Occupational exposure to specific metals specifically copper, manganese, lead, mercury, iron, aluminium and zinc increases the risk for PD. Elevated levels of these metals are found in the substantia nigra of Parkinson's patient. In PD, α-synuclein aggregates to form fibrils. It was observed that several di- and trivalent metal ions like copper(II), iron(III), cobalt(III), and manganese(II) increased the rate of synuclein fibril formation [259].

Pesticides/Toxin Exposure

Environmental toxins, specifically pesticides, implicate the risk factors for Parkinson. Some commonly used pesticides exhibited neurotoxicity and their exposure triggered the mechanism that can cause PD. Different pesticides exert different mechanisms for the pathogenesis of Parkinson. MPTP (1-methyl-4-phenyl-1,2,3,6-tetrahydropyridine) is lipid soluble which crosses BBB (Blood brain barrier) and enters into the brain cells. It has been shown that MPTP itself is not toxic but its oxidized form MPP+ (1-methyl-4-phenylpyridinium) is toxic. MPP+ accumulates in mitochondria, where it inhibits NADH dehydrogenase complex (complex I). This impairs oxidative phosphorylation in the brain [260]. Rotenone, a naturally occurring hydrophobic insecticide, is permeable to biological membranes. Rotenone withers dopaminergic neurons via free radical production [261]. Paraquat, a herbicide with high pulmonary toxicity, is a charged molecule which does not cross BBB. Like rotenone, paraquat also perturbs dopamine metabolism. Rotenone appears to affect all fluxes associated with dopamine compartmentalization, whereas paraquat perturbs fluxes associated with dopamine and its breakdown metabolites [262].

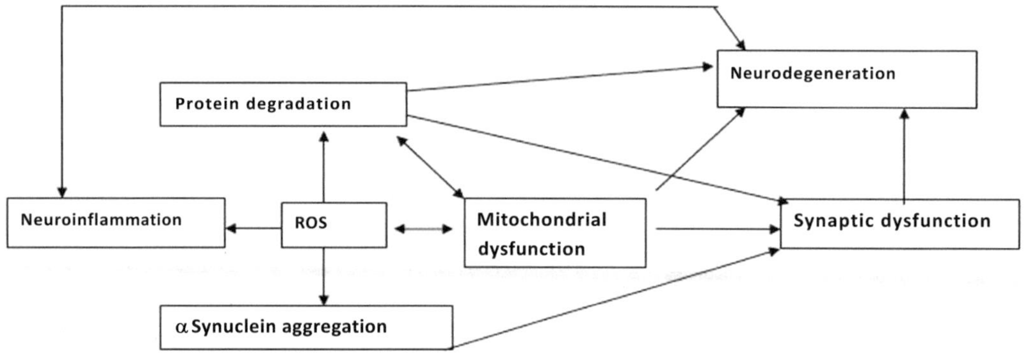

Fig. (5). Interaction of various pathways leading to neurodegeneration.

PATHWAY/MECHANISM

Parkinson is a progressive disease which is caused primarily due to the death of dopaminergic neurons of substantia nigra. It results in various inter linked activities like mitochondrial dysfunction, α-synuclein aggregation, impaired protein degradation and neuroinflammation [263] (Fig. **5**). As discussed above, these altered activities are due to various genetic and environmental factors.

Mitochondrial Dysfunction

Mitochondrial dysfunction plays a central role in the pathogenesis of Parkinson. Mitochondria are involved in many activities like energy metabolism, stress response, control apoptosis, and regulation of calcium homeostasis. A number of proteins, *viz.* Parkin, PINK1 and LRKK2 associated with the mitochondria are found to be involved in Parkinson. Mitochondrial protection against oxidative stress is mediated by kinase activity of PINK1 targeting Parkin, TRAP1 and HTRA2. Deficiency of PINK1 disturbs the mitochondrial respiration and calcium balance. This increases ROS (Reactive oxygen Species) that lowers the MOMP (mitochondrial outer membrane permeabilization) which in turn increases the susceptibility for cell death. Mitochondrial functions in the presence of oxidative environment are maintained by DJ-1 protein. Mitochondrial trafficking may also get impaired by Parkin, α-synuclein and LRRK2 as they modulate microtubule stability or by formation of α-synuclein aggregates [264] (Fig. **6**).

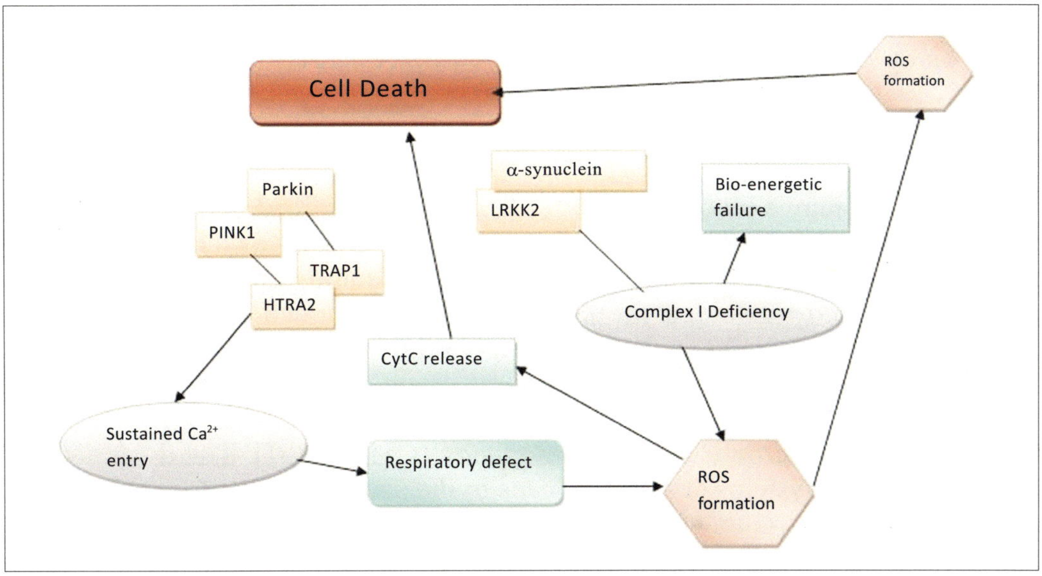

Fig. (6). A number of genes involved in mitochondrial dysfunction.

α-Synuclein Aggregation

α-synuclein is a highly conserved pre-synaptic protein that can adopt a number of different conformations depending on conditions and cofactors. It has been identified as the major component of Lewy bodies and Lewy neurites, proteinaceous deposits that are proteinaceous mark of Parkinson [265]. Mutated, misfolded or overexpressed α-synuclein is involved in a number of pathways associated with degeneration of dopaminergic neurons. This impairs synaptic function and mitochondrial turnover, morphology and respiration. Mutant α-synuclein induces chronic endoplasmic stress that may lead to neurodegeneration. α-synuclein over-expression reduces the lysosomal activity which may lead to α-synuclein aggregation [266] (Fig. 7).

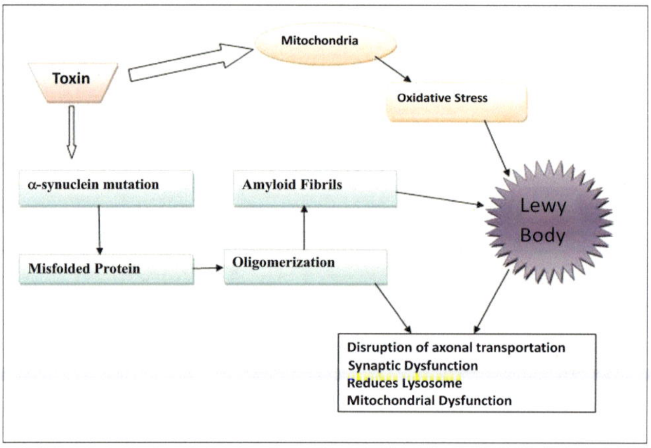

Fig. (7). α-synuclein aggregation.

Impaired protein degradation

Degradation system is involved in the clearance of misfolded or damaged proteins and dysfunctional organelles. This can be done via two pathways, *viz.* ubiquitin-proteasome system (UPS) and the autophagy-lysosome pathway. In UPS, short lived proteins and misfolded proteins in ER are degraded. The protein is first conjugated with a polyubiquitin tag through a three-step enzymatic cascade, and then degraded by the 20S or 26S proteasome complex. In autophagy, proteins are transported to lysosome for degradation. This can be done through macro-autophagy and chaperone mediated autophagy (CMA) [267]. The dysfunction of these degradation systems at synapse leads to the accumulation of α-synuclein and defective mitochondria that interfere with the proper synaptic function. This leads to the formation of toxic assemblies, oxidative stress and impairs energy function [268].

Neuroinflammation

Studies suggested that neuroinflammation and microglia activation play important role in the pathogenesis of PD. The glial cells maintain homeostasis that promotes neuronal survival. Microglia have a specialized immune surveillance role to invade pathogens by secreting factors, *viz.* cytokines, chemokines, reactive oxygen and nitrogen species, prostaglandins and growth factors. Some of these factors have neuroprotective role and help in brain repair processes while others enhance oxidative stress and trigger apoptotic pathways in neurons. Therefore, pro- and anti-inflammatory responses must be in balance to prevent the potential detrimental effects on neuronal populations [269]. Parkinson's stress factors disturb the balance of glial protective and detrimental effects. Microglial can detect misfoldedα-synuclein and increase the neurotoxicity. Deficiency of Parkin and DJ-1 also promote microglial activation that disturbs the balance of neurons and glial cells [263].

DIAGNOSIS OF PARKINSON'S DISEASE

There is no standard test for the diagnosis of PD. Generally, diagnosis is done on the basis of clinical information provided by the patient followed by some neurological tests like MRI (Magnetic resonance imaging) and Transcranial Sonography. These tests are performed to know the structural changes in the mid-brain. Structural changes in Parkinson patient include detection of nigra with 7 tesla MRI, diffusion weighted MRI, and transcranial sonography that helps in the diagnosis [270].

Traditional structural imaging results are ambiguous. Advances in MRI have shown significant results like functional imaging using dopaminergic tracers with either PET (Positron emission tomography) or SPECT (Single-photon emission computed tomography). PET and SPECT can detect the abnormal dopamine function [271].

TREATMENT FOR PARKINSON'S DISEASE

As per present day knowledge, there is no standard treatment known for the cure of the disease. However, treatment is done to control the symptoms based on type of the symptoms in the patient. Advanced Parkinson may be treated with surgery. In addition to medication and surgery, lifestyle changes, physical therapy, aerobic exercises may help in the treatment. Treatment of Parkinson can be divided into pharmacological and non-pharmacological treatments.

Pharmacological Treatment

Pharmacological treatment can be symptomatic therapy and neuroprotective therapy. In symptomatic therapy, efforts are done to control the symptoms of the disease. However, this therapy does not slow down the progression of the condition.

Levodopa

The use of levodopa to ameliorate the symptoms of Parkinson is highly effective. It is used as dopamine replacement therapy since many years. Levodopa is an amino acid that is decarboxylated to form dopamine. It is transported by the neutral amino acid transport system across the blood brain barrier into the brain. Treatment is started with lower dose of levodopa to avoid its acute symptoms like nausea, vomiting, and postural hypotension. However, there has been a concern that levodopa could enhance the oxidative stress and may promote the degeneration of residual dopamine neurons [272].

Dopamine Agonists

Dopamine agonists mimic the effect of dopamine in brain and directly simulate dopamine receptor by binding with the post-synaptic dopamine receptors. Dopamine agonists in use are bromocriptine, pergolide, pramipexole, ropinirole, apomorphine and rotigotine. Dopamine agonists may interact with either D1 or D2 dopamine receptor or both. Studies suggested that concurrent D1 and D2 receptors stimulation may be necessary for full expression of postsynaptic receptor-mediated effects of dopamine and dopamine agonists in the basal ganglia [273].

Monoamine Oxidase Type B Inhibitors

MAOB (Monoamine oxidase type B) inhibitors prevent the breakdown of dopamine by monoamine oxidase (MAO). The MAO increases the level of oxidative stress that may initiate the neurodegeneration and selective inhibition of MAO helps in lowering stress. There are two isoforms of MAO inhibitors –MAO-A and MAO-B. MAO-B inhibitors like selegiline and rasagiline are found to be useful in the treatment of PD [274].

Catechol-O-Methyltransferase (COMT) Inhibitors

Besides decarboxylases, levodopa can be metabolized by catechol--methyltransferase. COMT inhibitors improve levodopa availability to the brain by preventing their breakdown. Two most commonly used COMT inhibitors are entacapone and tolcapone. Entacapone inhibits the peripheral metabolism of levodopa by COMT and increases its availability to the brain. It has been observed that COMT inhibitors increase dopaminergic side effects due to increased levodopa availability to the brain [275].

Anticholinergics

Anticholinergics drugs are the first drugs that were used for the treatment of tremor in Parkinson. These include benztropine, ethopropazine, biperiden, procyclidine, trihexyphenidyl, diphenhydramine and orphenadrine. Parkinson causes imbalances between the dopaminergic and cholinergic neurological pathways. Anticholinergics drugs correct this imbalance by reducing the degree of neurotransmission mediated by neostriatal acetylcholine [276].

Amantadine

Amantadine is an anti-viral agent, however, it has been found useful in PD also. Parkinson affects the brain coordinates that move the muscles and leads to slow and abnormal nerve message to muscle. There are symptoms like slow movement, tremor and muscle stiffness. Amantadine helps in improving the motion and makes a person able to exercise. Amantadine hydrochloride is a tricyclic amine and has several mechanisms of action. It enhances the release of dopamine by directly acting on pre-synaptic membrane. Post-synaptically, it acts directly on the dopamine receptor and up regulates D2 receptors. Amantadine also has anti-glutamatergic, anti-muscarinic and immuno-modulatory properties [277].

Apomorphine

Apomorphine is a dopamine-receptor agonist. It acts on the same receptor as dopamine. It acts like dopamine and is able to treat on-off condition of Parkinson. In on-off condition, a person feels easy in movement in first minute and in another minute, it is difficult to move for the same person. Apomorphine works in the off condition. Its effect lasts for hours as it is given by injection subcutaneously [278].

Neuroprotective Therapy

Neuroprotective therapy is based on the concept that dopaminergic neurons can be protected from degeneration. Neuroprotective therapy can be given at the early stage of the disease or to those who are at genetic risk. Neuroprotective therapy includes the neurotrophic factor, growth factor and other drugs like pramipexole and ropinirole which can slow down the disease progression [279].

Neurotrophic Factor/Growth Factor

Neurotrophic factors are the secreted proteins that maintain and protect neurons in the developing and adult brain. Neurotrophic factors include BDNF (Brain-derived neurotrophic factor), GDNF (glial cell line-derived neurotrophic factor), Neurturin, MANF (mesencephalic astrocyte-derived neurotrophic factor), GDF (growth/differentiation factor) and cerebral dopaminergic neurotrophic factor (CDNF). Results of neurotrophic factors therapy are encouraging in clinical trials and proved to be most applicable in the early stages of the disease to provide neuroprotection. Much research still remains to be conducted in the area of neurotrophic factor therapy for Parkinson [280].

Nonpharmacological Treatment

Parkinson is a chronic disorder that requires pharmacological therapy as well as non-pharmacological treatments. Although pharmacological treatments are the main pillar of the treatment but non-pharmacological treatments help in facing the issues that are not treated with medications. Non-pharmacological treatments include therapies like exercise and physiotherapy, speech therapy, occupational therapy, language therapy, dance therapy, proper nursing, nutrition, *etc*.

Nursing

Nursing care for each of the symptoms of Parkinson improves the patient's quality of life. This can be done if trained nurse is appointed who takes care of the proper medication to maximize the drug effectiveness. Parkinson is a complex disease with variety of symptoms like tremor, rigidity, postural imbalance and many more that vary from case to case. Therefore, different kind of nursing is required for different patients [281].

Rehabilitation

Rehabilitation is specialized healthcare to improve the person's motion, strength and perception. Rehabilitation includes various therapies that are given according to the patient requirement. For example, physical therapy is given for impairment and disability in motion, fall prevention and flexibility.

Nutrition

Evidence suggests that nutrition plays an important role in the progression of PD. Biochemical studies have recently found out that there are some food components that can evoke the neuroprotection and some others trigger the neuroprotection. A balanced diet rich in variety of food like fruits, vegetables and small servings of tea, caffeine, omega-3 fatty acids and wine provide neuroprotection. A poor diet may lead to oxidative stress and affect mitochondrial energy function [282].

Surgical Treatment

Depletion of dopamine induces many changes in the motor circuit that affects many day to day activities. Medication can help in the early stages of the disease, but advanced stages are unresponsive to medication and this condition leads to the surgical/ transplantation. Surgical therapies for Parkinson are challenging but are not impossible [283]. Various kind of surgery can be done based on the patient's medical report. This includes [284]:

- **Thalamotomy:** It targets the ventral intermediate nucleus of the thalamus in the brain. It reduces the tremor and has little effect on the other Parkinson's symptoms.
- **DBS (Deep Brain Simulation):** It blocks the electrical signal from the targeted areas. It uses an electrical device called neurostimulator to deliver electrical stimulation to targeted areas in the brain. It shows significant reduction in rigidity, bradykinesia and gait disturbances.
- **Pallidotomy:** It targets the globus pallidus which is overactive in PD that leads to decrease activity of brain.
- **Subthalamic Nucleotomy**: Subthalamic nucleus is overactive in PD. So, subthalamus is removed from the brain.

DATABASES FOR PARKINSON'S DISEASE

PDbase

PDbase is a PD database having data about Parkinson related genes and genetic variation. The database in constructed by using substantia nigra normal tissues and EST (Expressed sequence tags) in Parkinson. PDbase is available freely at: http://bioportal.kobic.re.kr/PDbase/. This database contains experimentally confirmed annotation of substantia nigra EST's and genes information like gene regulating elements, gene expression and its pathway, genetic variation, protein-protein interaction and mitochondrial protein. Database can be accessed via its web interface providing alphabetically arranged genes list or by querying with the gene name. Currently PDbase contains 2,698 genes and their biological information [285].

PDmutDB

The PD Mutation Database (PDmutDB) archives all Parkinson related mutations reported in the literature or directly submitted to the database. The PDmutDB is available at http://www.molgen.vib-ua.be/PDmutDB. It provides information on the genes encoding α-synuclein (SNCA), Leucine-rich repeat kinase 2 (LRRK2), Parkin, PTEN-induced putative kinase 1 (PINK1) and DJ-1. It also holds information on 535 different DNA variations and 2084 families. The PDmutDB website was re-launched in 2009 as a locus-specific database [286].

PDGene

PDgene database comprehensively collects all Parkinson related gene and its genetic association studies. It is freely available at http://www.pdgene.org/. Database is created by screening ~27,000 research articles and individual-level data from three publicly available genome-wide association studies (GWAS). Currently PDGene contains data on 7,782,514 genetic variants from 13708 Parkinson cases and 95,282 control cases. Database can be searched with official gene names, SNP identifiers and chromosomal locations [287].

ParkDB

ParkDB is a database of gene expression data of PD. It can be queried at http://www2.cancer.ucl.ac.uk/Parkinson_Db2/. The ParkDB contains a complete set of re-analyzed, curated and annotated microarray datasets. This database helps the scientist in identifying the expression signature of the disease. ParkDB can be queried via gene query, experiment query, tissue query and comparison query. It is continuously updated via data from ArrayExpress, GEO and Stanford microarray databases. It also provides combination of features that can be used to compare relationship between Parkinson related human brain genes with multiple model organisms [288].

MDPD

MDPD (Mutation Database for Parkinson Disease) is integrated genetic information on mutations associated with PD. It is publicly available at http://datam.i2r.a-star.edu.sg/mdpd/. MDPD extract data from 576 publications and contains 2,391 entries on 202 genes. Every gene is reported with its summary containing information on variation impact, mutation position, mutation type, studied population and reference collection. Database can be queried by searching or browsing the gene id from gene list and from many other options like chromosome location. It also provides variation report, summary and statistical information [289].

HISTORY OF SCHIZOPHRENIA

Schizophrenia was first identified as a discrete mental illness in 1887 by Emil

Kraepelin. He gave the term dementia praecox to define the disorder. The term 'Schizophrenia' was first coined by the Eugen Bleuler in 1908, and its symptoms are noticeable from the ancient times. Earlier, symptoms were being considered as devil punishment or assault from god and were being treated with various treatments like exposing the patient to certain music or by drilling hole in the patient's skull to release the evil spirits. Ethnographic studies suggested that schizophrenia is present in all the existing culture by the presence of hole in the skull of Stone Age [290].

In 19th Century, psychiatrists noted different kinds of symptoms in young patients and no connection between symptoms was observed. It was considered that there is a link of mental illness with disease in mind. In 1851, Falvet described the disease as cyclical madness and named it as 'Folie Circulaire'. After twenty years in 1871, Hecker described it as silly undisciplined mind and gave the term 'Hebephrenia'. In 1874, Kahlbaum referred both catatonic and paranoid disorders of the mind. Thereafter, in 1878, Emil Kraepelin combined all these dementia into a single disease and gave the term dementia praecox or dementia of early onset. He gave this term to distinguish the disease with other dementia like Alzheimer's disease which occurs in the later stages of the life and he focused on the young adults with dementia. In 1911, Bleuler gave the term 'Schizophrenia' and he was the first to describe the symptoms as positive and negative. The word schizophrenia is a Greek word where schizo means split and phrene means mind to describe the fragmented thinking of the people in this disorder [291].

SCHIZOPHRENIA: NEURODEVELOPMENT OR NEURO-DEGENERATIVE DISORDER?

Schizophrenia is a severe mental disorder that affects the person thinking, feeling and behavior. A person with schizophrenia lost the touch with reality. The onset of schizophrenia usually occurs at 15 to 25 years of age in men and 25 to 35 years of age in women. The progress is so slow that sufferer does not even know that he/she has the disease from such a long time. It is estimated that schizophrenia decreases the average life span by 20%. It is also associated with a number of anatomical and physiological abnormalities outside of the brain. It accelerates the aging by fostering the physiological changes throughout the body as compared to normal aging [292].

Schizophrenia not only affects an individual, but its impact is also visible on the patient's family, friends, relatives and the society. There is wide range of impact including financial, social, work and family related stresses. It has been reported that person(s) who are living with schizophrenic patient had poorer self-reported physical health [293]. Schizophrenia is a challenging disorder but a person can lead a happy life with proper care and treatment. Schizophrenic person can live independently with proper medication and therapy.

There are several misconceptions on schizophrenia. It is considered to be a multiple personality disorder and patient has a split personality. This misconception arises from the literal meaning of the word schizophrenia means "split" given by Bleuer [294]. There is also a controversy on the etiology of the schizophrenia as neurodegenerative or neurodevelopment disorder. Both the causes are supported by theories and models given by various experts.

Neurodevelopment Theory

The neurodevelopmental hypothesis of schizophrenia is based on the symptom that it is related to abnormal brain development. It is considered on the basis of the data derived from clinical studies at different life phase, conception and birth, infancy and childhood up to the onset of the illness, after illness onset and post-mortem [295].

Pre- and Perinatal Complications (Obstetric Complication)

By investigating the linkage of pregnancy and birth records to psychiatric records, it has been reported that people with any obstetric complications are at twice the risk for schizophrenia than people without obstetric complications. The following three main categories of obstetric complications have been reported:

- complications of pregnancy (bleeding, pre-eclampsia, diabetes, and rhesus incompatibility)
- abnormal fetal growth and development (low birth weight, congenital malformations, and small head circumference)
- complications of delivery (asphyxia, uterine atony and emergency cesarean section)

Obstetrical events in schizophrenia have been considered as having a direct causative effect; however, one cannot deny that these may be markers of some other causal process as obstetric complications are multifactorial in origin [296]. For example, low birth weight and small head circumference reflect retarded fetal growth and any factor affecting the fetus adversely retards its growth. Many unspecific causes can perturb the brain and its development at different points in time and increase the risk for psychosis to emerge later. These observations about non-specificity makes the possibility that schizophrenia may not be an illness but is an abnormal pattern of neural responses that can be determined at an early stage of development [297].

Childhood Evidence

Abnormal brain development and maturation seems to begin prenatally but may continue throughout childhood. Abnormalities include delays in attainment of speech, problems in social adjustment and poorer academic and cognitive performance. Children at high risk for schizophrenia have more developmental problems. They have abnormalities in neurological and motor development from infancy which continue through school-age and adolescence [298]. Many factors can predict the later development of schizophrenia like poor relationship with the parents, low IQ and disruptive social behaviour [299]. The most consistently found neurocognitive deficit among schizophrenic children is attentional deficit [300]. Some studies on brain imaging found that the left amygdala–hippocampal complex is significantly smaller among schizophrenic children.

Adolescence Evidence

The neurodevelopmental hypothesis of schizophrenia suggested that a brain abrasion is present early in life. Many evidences support that there are consistent abnormalities in cognitive and behavioral development before the onset of psychosis [301]. Thompson and co-workers in 2001 reported that schizophrenic person has failure of normal maturation in neurological test performance during adolescence. During the development of schizophrenia in early adolescent, a dynamic wave of gray matter loss occurs, starting in parietal association cortices and proceeding frontally to envelop dorsolateral prefrontal cortex and temporal cortices including the superior temporal gyri [302].

Postmortem Evidence

Post-mortem studies of many schizophrenic patients revealed the structural changes in the brain. The major brain morphological abnormalities observed in schizophrenic patients are the loss of cortical gray matter, the reduced volume of the amygdala, the hippocampus, the frontal and temporal lobes and ventricular enlargement. Neurochemically, there is alterations in several transmitter systems including dopamine, glutamate, serotonin, and γ-aminobutyric acid (GABA) [303].

Some alterations in some specific molecular signals involved in cell formation and organization are found that lead to altered structure and function of the brain. For example, during post-mortem, shortage of tissue reelin expression has been observed in patients with schizophrenia. This protein guides certain neuron clusters to the appropriate place in the brain and is released at intense levels during neuron migration. Additionally, a reduced appearance of polysialic acid (PSA) has been observed on the neural cell adhesion molecules (NCAM) in patients with schizophrenia. This molecule is involved in axonal growth, the synaptogenesis of interneurons and the formation of inhibitor circuits related to the condition [304].

The model of altered neurodevelopment suggested that evolution of schizophrenia is diachronic. The individual is born with certain genetic factors that interact with certain environmental factors and prevent the brain from developing normally. Additionally, the person may be affected by the external and internal factors that trigger the onset of the condition. According to this theory, biological alterations and other characteristics of the illness would be present in the patient before the onset of the characteristic symptoms of this pathology but they would not be present until a certain level of development is reached upon interacting with certain external factors [304].

Neurodegeneration Theory

Alterations in brain morphology of the schizophrenic patients have led to the neurodevelopment hypothesis of schizophrenia. There are changes in some biochemical pathways resulting in neuronal death. The evidences of schizophrenia to be neurodegenerative disease include:

- Resemblance of schizophrenia to other neurodegenerative diseases like specific populations of neurons are affected and disconnectivity of midbrain, thalamic, limbic and cortical circuits occur.
- Progressive nature of schizophrenia as it is unclear when the illness actually begins.
- The emergence of cognitive dysfunction in schizophrenia.
- Decreased I3-aminobutyric acid interneuron-mediated inhibition of pyramidal neurons in the cingulated cortex.
- N-methyl-D-aspartate receptor hypofunction and glutamate excitotoxicity.
- N-acetylaspartate–glutamate oxidative stress damage [305].

SYMPTOMS OF SCHIZOPHRENIA

There are many characteristic symptoms of schizophrenia like delusions, hallucinations, disorganized speech, differential movement, confusion, disorganized behavior and many more. The signs and symptoms of schizophrenia vary from person to person both in pattern and severity. Not every person with schizophrenia will have all the symptoms and the symptoms of schizophrenia may also change from time to time. In 1991, Andreasen divided the symptoms of schizophrenia into two groups as positive and negative. The classification was first proposed by Crow in 1980, as type I (positive) and type II (negative) based on the phenomenology [306].

Positive Symptoms

Positive symptoms are disturbances that are "added" to the person's personality. It represents a change in behavior or thoughts. People with positive symptoms may lose touch with some aspects of reality. Positive symptoms may come and go frequently in some people and for others they may stay for a longer time. Sometimes these may be severe and sometimes hardly noticeable. The severity of positive symptoms may vary from case to case. Positive symptoms include the following:

Hallucination

Hallucinations are sounds or other sensations experienced as real when they exist only in the person's mind. Hallucinations can involve any of the five senses but auditory hallucinations and visual hallucinations are most common in schizophrenia. Hallucinations tend to be worse when the person is alone.

Delusion

Delusions are false beliefs that are not based on reality. Delusions are extremely common in schizophrenia occurring in more than 90% of cases. Common schizophrenic delusions include: Delusions of persecution, Delusions of grandeur, Delusions of reference and Delusions of control.

Disorganized Thinking (Speech)

People with schizophrenia are not able to organize their thoughts. They have trouble in concentrating and maintaining a train of thought. They may not be able to respond to queries, they answer with an unrelated answer. They start sentences with one topic and end somewhere completely different, speak incoherently, or say illogical things. It seems like they are zoning out or distracted. When they talk, their words can come out all jumbled and make no sense.

Disorganized Behavior

It includes difficulty in goal-directed behavior that leads to difficulties in daily living activities, unpredictable agitation or silliness, social disinhibition or behaviors that are bizarre. People may behave inappropriately or become extremely agitated and shout or swear for no reason.

Negative Symptoms

Negative symptoms are absence of normal behaviors that are found in healthy individuals. These are the capabilities which are "lost" from the person's personality. These symptoms are harder to recognize especially in teenagers because these can be mistaken with depression or other conditions. These symptoms include the following:

- Social withdrawal
- Lack of drive or initiative
- Emotional unresponsiveness
- Reduced speaking
- Lack of motivation/ enthusiasm

RISK FACTORS/CAUSES OF SCHIZOPHRENIA

The causes of schizophrenia are not yet understood. Scientists think that schizophrenia may develop from a combination of brain chemistry and genetic and environmental factors. Schizophrenia is caused by a combination of factors rather than a single one.

Genetic Factors

Positive family history is one of the factors of schizophrenia. Life time risk for general population is below 1% for schizophrenia but person with first order relative has nearly 6.5% risk for schizophrenia [307]. Genetic studies suggested that many genes are involved in schizophrenia. There are strong evidences that genes namely Dysbindin (DTNBP1) and Neuregulin1 (NRG1) are involved in schizophrenia. Other genes involved are Disrupted in Schizophrenia 1 (DISC1), D-amino-acid oxidase (DAO), D-amino-acid oxidase activator (DAOA) and Regulator of G-protein Signalling 4 (RGS4) [308].

Environmental Factors

Schizophrenia is not only a genetic disorder as evidenced by the fact that risk of schizophrenia for the identical co-twin of an affected individual is only about 40%. In recent years, environmental factors contributing to risk have been identified and are divided into three categories [309]. The probable reasons in each category have been summarized in Table **3**:

Table 3. Environmental factors contributing to schizophrenia.

Early Life	**Childhood**	**Later Life**
Obstetric complication	Adverse child rearing	Drug abuse
Season of birth	Child abuse	Migration/ethnicity
Prenatal/postnatal infection	Head injury	Urbanization
Maternal malnutrition		Social adversity

(Table 3) contd.....

Early Life	Childhood	Later Life
Maternal stress		Life events

Early Life

As described above, the neurodevelopmental theory of schizophrenia relies on the risk factors before and shortly after birth which leads to abnormal formation of the nervous system. These risk factors mainly include obstetric complications, Prenatal/postnatal infections, maternal malnutrition, maternal stress, season of birth and infection. Obstetric complications include:

i. Complications of pregnancy (bleeding, preeclampsia, diabetes, rhesus compatibility).
ii. Abnormal fetal growth and development (low birth weight, congenital malformations, small head circumference).
iii. Complications of delivery (asphyxia, uterine atony, emergency cesarean section) [310].

People who are born during winter or early spring are more likely to develop schizophrenia in later life than those born at other times of the year [311]. Gestational infectious particularly viruses such as influenza, rubella, cytomegalovirus, and herpes simplex are known to be associated with abnormalities in central nervous system (CNS) development [312]. Other factors such as maternal stress, maternal malnutrition, maternal diabetes, smoking, and rhesus incompatibility have also been considered as risk factors for schizophrenia [313 - 315].

Childhood

A number of environmental risk factors are the risk factors for schizophrenia. These include adverse child rearing, child abuse, atypical mother-infant interaction, early parental loss and poor mothering [316 - 318]. Head injury is also found to be associated with schizophrenia [319].

Later Life

Early life event supports the neurodevelopment model of the schizophrenia; however, later environmental factors supported the social and psychological mechanisms of illness. Later life event first considered was the drug abuse. Early and larger use of methamphetamine has been reported to be associated with schizophrenia [320]. D'Souza in 2000 reported that cannabis misuse can be a contributing cause for schizophrenia [321]. An increased prevalence of schizophrenia in urban compared to rural settings is one of the most consistent findings in schizophrenia research [322]. In addition, association between migration and schizophrenia has been known for 70 years. Recently Selten and Cantor-Graae have carried out a meta-analysis indicating that risk of schizophrenia got significantly increased among immigrants compared to native inhabitants [323]. Many scientists considered the role of social isolation and social disadvantage in increasing risk of schizophrenia. The factors may include social support, self-esteem, unemployment and poor physical health [324]. Finally, the occurrence of life events has been found to be associated with the onset and later symptoms of schizophrenia [325].

ALTERED PATHOLOGY IN SCHIZOPHRENIA

Schizophrenia has long been associated with an imbalance in dopamine (DA) neurotransmission. However, the dopamine hypothesis of schizophrenia cannot explain all the symptoms associated with this disorder. Therefore, recent studies focussed on other neurotransmitters like glutamate, GABA, acetylcholine and serotonin whose alterations are also involved in the pathology of schizophrenia [326].

Dopamine Hypothesis

Dopamine is produced in the substantia nigra and ventral tegmental regions of the brain and dopamine alterations are related to schizophrenia. The "initial dopamine hypothesis" states that hyperactive dopamine transmission results in schizophrenic symptoms [327]. The "revised dopamine hypothesis" proposes hyperactive dopamine transmission in the mesolimbic areas and hypoactive dopamine transmission in the prefrontal cortex in schizophrenia patients occur. Besides, dopamine dysregulation is also observed in other brain regions including the amygdala and prefrontal cortex which are important for emotional processing [328].

Dopamine receptors are G-protein-coupled receptors and can be divided into D1, D2, D3, and D4-receptors. In schizophrenia patients, D1 receptors are decreased in prefrontal cortex and increased in the parieto-temporal cortex [329]. Increased D2 receptors are found in the frontal cortex and decreased D2 receptors in the thalamus and anterior cingulate cortex in schizophrenia patients [330, 331]. Increased D3 and D4 receptors are reported in the limbic and cortical areas [332].

The Glutamate Hypothesis

L-Glutamic acid (as glutamate) is a major excitatory amino acid in the nervous system. Nearly half of the neurons in the brain, including all neurons that project from the cerebral cortex, are believed to use glutamate as their neurotransmitter.

Glutamate plays a major role in brain development, affecting neuronal migration, neuronal differentiation, axon genesis, and neuronal survival [333]. The glutamate hypothesis of schizophrenia assumes that the function of N-methyl-D-aspartate (NMDA) receptor is compromised in the patients of schizophrenia disease. NMDA receptors are a major subtype of glutamate receptors and mediate slow excitatory postsynaptic potentials (EPSPs). The idea of a glutamatergic abnormality in schizophrenia was first proposed by Kim and colleagues in 1980 based on their findings of low cerebrospinal fluid (CSF) glutamate levels in patients with schizophrenia [334]. Evidences that suggested disruptions in any of the numerous mechanisms influencing the function of NMDA receptors are [335]:

- Postmortem studies showed changes in glutamate receptor binding, transcription, and subunit protein expression in the prefrontal cortex, thalamus, and hippocampus of schizophrenia patients [336].
- Abnormalities in the neurotransmission in the postmortem studies of individuals with schizophrenia. Levels of amino acids N-acethylaspartate (NAA) and N-acethylaspartylglutamate (NAAG), and the activity of the enzyme that cleaves NAA to NAAG and glutamate are altered in the CSF [337].
- Imaging studies for the NMDA receptor (^{123}I) CNS-1261 reported reduced NMDA receptor binding in the hippocampus [338].

GABAergic Origin Hypothesis

Gamma-Aminobutyric Acid (GABA) is the endogenous neurotransmitter and synthesised in 20-30% of all CNS neurons. The GABAergic system is principally involved in the balance of excitation and inhibition in the brain [339]. Almost all neurons either express GABA receptors or release GABA or are innervated by neurons which do so. For these reasons, it is expected that most brain functions involve GABAergic transmission [340]. Therefore, role of GABA is crucial in normal information processing and it acts to keep the processes of CNS under control. Postmortem studies suggested changes in the structure of GABA receptor and its binding affinity. Communication between glutamatergic pyramidal and GABAergic local circuit neurons is altered that leads in a loss of inhibitory tone with consequent disinhibition of excitatory pyramidal cells leading to increased excitatory output to other areas of the brain. Due to loss of inhibitory tone in schizophrenia, interaction between dopamine and GABA may be compromised. Therefore, decreased GABAergic function may lead to increased dopaminergic activity [341].

Acetylcholine Hypothesis

Acetylcholine (Ach) has been recognized as a neurotransmitter and plays a crucial role in a variety of CNS and PNS functions, including motor function, sensory perception, cognitive processing, attention, sleep, nociception, motivation, memory, arousal, reward, mood, psychosis and neuroplasticity. The muscarinic and the nicotinic system are the two distinct families of the ACh system. The coordination of different cognitive and affective functions requires proper signaling through both muscarinic and nicotinic acetylcholine receptors (mAChRs and nAChRs). Disruptions in mAChR and nAChR signaling have been implicated in the symptoms observed in schizophrenic patients [342, 343]. Several post-mortem studies have indicated a significant decrease in muscarinic receptor density in different brain regions that are considered to be of crucial importance in the pathophysiology of schizophrenia [344].

Serotonin Hypothesis

Serotonin or 5-hydroxytryptamine (5-HT) is a neurotransmitter derived from tryptophan. The serotonin hypothesis is supported by several observations, *viz.*:

- Number of cortical 5-HT2A and 5-HT1A receptors is altered in schizophrenic brains.
- Interactions between the hallucinogenic drug LSD (D-lysergic acid diethylamide) and 5-HT are found in peripheral systems.
- Certain polymorphisms of the 5-HT2A receptor gene are associated with schizophrenia.
- Trophic role of serotonin has been found in neurodevelopment.
- 5-HT2A receptor–mediated activation of the prefrontal cortex found to be impaired in some schizophrenic patients [345, 346].

TREATMENT OF SCHIZOPHRENIA

The cause(s) of schizophrenia is still unknown, and treatments have been focussed on eliminating the symptoms of the disease. Schizophrenia requires lifelong treatment even after symptoms are diminished. The condition of a schizophrenic patient can be controlled with medications and psychosocial therapy. During immense condition, hospitalization may be necessary to ensure safety, adequate sleep, proper nutrition and basic hygiene. Medications are the cornerstone of schizophrenia treatment. Antipsychotic medications are the most commonly prescribed drugs to treat schizophrenia. These are thought to control symptoms by affecting the brain neurotransmitters, dopamine and serotonin [347]. Antipsychotic medications can be typical (First Generation) and atypical (Second Generation). Typical or conventional antipsychotic are the first drug developed in 1950s to treat psychosis. These include haldol (haloperidol) and thorazine (chlorpromazine). Atypical antipsychotic are new medications developed in the 1990s. Clozapine, risperidone, olanzapine, paliperidone, sertindole, ziprasidone, quetiapine, zotepine, asenapine and aripiprazole are atypical antipsychotic drugs

[348]. Besides medication, psychosocial therapy can also help in treating schizophrenia. Psychiatric care can reduce psychotic symptoms and improve patient's condition and reduce illness progression. Five main approaches to psychosocial intervention have been used for the treatment of schizophrenia: cognitive therapy (cognitive behavioral and cognitive remediation therapy), psychoeducation, family intervention, social skills training and assertive community treatment [349].

DATABASES FOR SCHIZOPHRENIA

VSD

VSD is a database for schizophrenia candidate genes that focuses on the variations. It can be accessed via www.chgb.org.cn/vsd.htm. Genetic evidence suggested schizophrenia as the polygenic order and various studies have suggested a number of schizophrenia susceptibility loci. VSD was developed to provide variation data for genes with small effect in the development of schizophrenia. Most of the genes encode neurotransmitter receptors, neurotransmitter transporters and the enzymes involved in their metabolism. These are extracted from published literature and databases such as dbSNP, HGVbase and OMIM with single nucleotide polymorphism (SNP). The latest version of VSD contains 23,648 variations assigned to a total of 186 genes. Five hundred and eighty eight domains and sites annotated in the SWISS-PROT and InterPro databases are found to contain nsSNPs. In addition to variation data, gene descriptions, enzyme information and other biological information for each gene locus are also included [350].

SZGene

Worldwide researchers have published over 1,000 genetic association studies for schizophrenia with largely inconsistent results, so to facilitate the interpretation; a database has been created with all published genetic association studies for schizophrenia. SZGene can be accessed via http://www.szgene.org/. It is the first comprehensive online resource for systematically synthesized and graded evidence of genetic association studies in schizophrenia. Currently, SZGene contains information from about 1727 studies and has information of about 1008 genes, 8788 Polymorphisms and 287 Meta-analyses. This database can serve as a model for field synopses of genetic associations in other common and genetically complex disorders [351].

SZGR

Schizophrenia Gene Resource (SZGR) provides a comprehensive online database for schizophrenia genetics studies. The SZGR database is available at http://bioinfo.mc.vanderbilt.edu/SZGR/. SZGR deposits genetic data from all available sources including those from association studies, linkage scans, gene expression, literature, gene ontology (GO) annotations, gene networks, cellular and regulatory pathways, microRNAs and their target sites. SZGR also provides an online tool for data browse and search, data integration, custom gene ranking and graphical presentation and tool for candidate gene ranking to help the user prioritize candidate genes by pre-optimized or custom weight scheme [352].

FUTURE PERSPECTIVES

There is much hope from bioinformaticians who are engaged in predicting specific drug targets using various methodologies like interactome analysis, flux analysis, pathway analysis, docking studies, *etc*. Besides, Molecular biologists are engaged in identifying defects/ mutations in various genes responsible for different neurodegenerative diseases. On the other hand, some biologists are hopeful for search of natural plant metabolites as therapeutic agents for treatment of AD, PD as well as Schizophrenia. Work may also be carried out in the direction of diagnosis of these diseases at an early stage and efforts may be done to control the symptoms of the diseases. There is scope of doing more work in unraveling the pathobiology of all these diseases. For effective dealing, there is requirement of close collaboration between basic scientists, clinical scientists and pharmaceutical industries.

CONCLUSION

Neurodegenerative disorders are convoluted problems with no elementary solutions. The AD, PD and Schizophrenia are the most prevalent examples of complexity. Although with the efforts of leading researchers in various disciplines, several significant characteristics of these baffling maladies are untangled. However, still much work has to be done to translate this comprehension into effective treatments for the diseases. It is being considered that bioinformatics tools may play an important role in predicting effective specific drugs for neurodegenerative diseases. The various therapeutic strategies described in this chapter may provide new insights for the treatments of AD.

CONFLICT OF INTEREST

The authors declare no conflict of interest, financial or otherwise.

ACKNOWLEDGEMENTS

The authors gratefully acknowledge the facilities of the Department of

Biotechnology, Government of India, New Delhi under its Bioinformatics sub centre used in the present work. Sarika Garg also acknowledges the facilities of CRCHUM used in the present work.

REFRENCES

[1] Kovacs G. Current concepts of neurodegenerative diseases. EMJ Neurol 2014; 1: 78-86.

[2] Waldemar G, Dubois B, Emre M, *et al.* Recommendations for the diagnosis and management of Alzheimer's disease and other disorders associated with dementia: EFNS guideline. Eur J Neurol 2007; 14(1): e1-e26.
[http://dx.doi.org/10.1111/j.1468-1331.2006.01605.x] [PMID: 17222085]

[3] Tabert MH, Liu X, Doty RL, *et al.* A 10-item smell identification scale related to risk for Alzheimer's disease. Ann Neurol 2005; 58(1): 155-60.
[http://dx.doi.org/10.1002/ana.20533] [PMID: 15984022]

[4] Giacobini E. Cholinesterase inhibitors stabilize Alzheimer's disease. Ann N Y Acad Sci 2000; 920: 321-7.
[http://dx.doi.org/10.1111/j.1749-6632.2000.tb06942.x] [PMID: 11193171]

[5] Chaudhuri KR, Healy DG, Schapira AH. Non-motor symptoms of Parkinson's disease: diagnosis and management. Lancet Neurol 2006; 5(3): 235-45.
[http://dx.doi.org/10.1016/S1474-4422(06)70373-8] [PMID: 16488379]

[6] Beitz JM. Parkinson's disease: a review. Front Biosci (Schol Ed) 2014; 6: 65-74.
[http://dx.doi.org/10.2741/S415] [PMID: 24389262]

[7] Aminoff MJ. Treatment of Parkinson's disease. West J Med 1994; 161(3): 303-8.
[PMID: 7975571]

[8] Benabid AL, Chabardes S, Mitrofanis J, Pollak P. Deep brain stimulation of the subthalamic nucleus for the treatment of Parkinson's disease. Lancet Neurol 2009; 8(1): 67-81.
[http://dx.doi.org/10.1016/S1474-4422(08)70291-6] [PMID: 19081516]

[9] Häfner H, Maurer K, Löffler W, Riecher-Rössler A. The influence of age and sex on the onset and early course of schizophrenia. Br J Psychiatry 1993; 162(1): 80-6.
[http://dx.doi.org/10.1192/bjp.162.1.80] [PMID: 8425144]

[10] Messias EL, Chen CY, Eaton WW. Epidemiology of schizophrenia: review of findings and myths. Psychiatr Clin North Am 2007; 30(3): 323-38.
[http://dx.doi.org/10.1016/j.psc.2007.04.007] [PMID: 17720026]

[11] Rummel-Kluge C, Komossa K, Schwarz S, *et al.* Head-to-head comparisons of metabolic side effects of second generation antipsychotics in the treatment of schizophrenia: a systematic review and meta-analysis. Schizophr Res 2010; 123(2-3): 225-33.
[http://dx.doi.org/10.1016/j.schres.2010.07.012] [PMID: 20692814]

[12] Cannon TD, Cornblatt B, McGorry P. The empirical status of the ultra high-risk (prodromal) research paradigm. Schizophr Bull 2007; 33(3): 661-4.
[http://dx.doi.org/10.1093/schbul/sbm031] [PMID: 17470445]

[13] Gupta S, Kulhara P. What is schizophrenia: A neurodevelopmental or neurodegenerative disorder or a combination of both? A critical analysis. Indian J Psychiatry 2010; 52(1): 21-7.
[http://dx.doi.org/10.4103/0019-5545.58891] [PMID: 20174514]

[14] Alzheimer A, Stelzmann RA, Schnitzlein HN, Murtagh FR. Uber eine eigenartige Erkankung der Hirnrinde. Allg Zschr f Psychiatr Psychisch-Gerichtl Mediz 1907; 64: 146-8.

[15] Simchowicz T. Histologische studien uber der senile demenz. Nissl-Alzheimer Histologische histopathologische. Arbeiten 1911; 4(2): 267-444.

[16] Gatz M, Pedersen NL, Berg S, *et al.* Heritability for Alzheimer's disease: the study of dementia in Swedish twins. J Gerontol A Biol Sci Med Sci 1997; 52(2): M117-25. [http://dx.doi.org/10.1093/gerona/52A.2.M117] [PMID: 9060980]

[17] Tanzi RE. A genetic dichotomy model for the inheritance of Alzheimer's disease and common age-related disorders. J Clin Invest 1999; 104(9): 1175-9. [http://dx.doi.org/10.1172/JCI8593] [PMID: 10545516]

[18] Rocchi A, Pellegrini S, Siciliano G, Murri L. Causative and susceptibility genes for Alzheimer's disease: a review. Brain Res Bull 2003; 61(1): 1-24. [http://dx.doi.org/10.1016/S0361-9230(03)00067-4] [PMID: 12788204]

[19] Bertram L, Tanzi RE. The genetic epidemiology of neurodegenerative disease. J Clin Invest 2005; 115(6): 1449-57. [http://dx.doi.org/10.1172/JCI24761] [PMID: 15931380]

[20] McGowan E, Eriksen J, Hutton M. A decade of modeling Alzheimer's disease in transgenic mice. Trends Genet 2006; 22(5): 281-9. [http://dx.doi.org/10.1016/j.tig.2006.03.007] [PMID: 16567017]

[21] Delacourte A, Sergeant N, Champain D, *et al.* Nonoverlapping but synergetic tau and APP pathologies in sporadic Alzheimer's disease. Neurology 2002; 59(3): 398-407. [http://dx.doi.org/10.1212/WNL.59.3.398] [PMID: 12177374]

[22] Sherrington R, Rogaev EI, Liang Y, *et al.* Cloning of a gene bearing missense mutations in early-onset familial Alzheimer's disease. Nature 1995; 375(6534): 754-60. [http://dx.doi.org/10.1038/375754a0] [PMID: 7596406]

[23] Rogaev EI, Sherrington R, Rogaeva EA, *et al.* Familial Alzheimer's disease in kindreds with missense mutations in a gene on chromosome 1 related to the Alzheimer's disease type 3 gene. Nature 1995; 376(6543): 775-8. [http://dx.doi.org/10.1038/376775a0] [PMID: 7651536]

[24] Hutton M, Lendon CL, Rizzu P, *et al.* Association of missense and 5′-splice-site mutations in tau with the inherited dementia FTDP-17. Nature 1998; 393(6686): 702-5. [http://dx.doi.org/10.1038/31508] [PMID: 9641683]

[25] Poorkaj P, Bird TD, Wijsman E, *et al.* Tau is a candidate gene for chromosome 17 frontotemporal dementia. Ann Neurol 1998; 43(6): 815-25. [http://dx.doi.org/10.1002/ana.410430617] [PMID: 9629852]

[26] Spillantini MG, Murrell JR, Goedert M, Farlow MR, Klug A, Ghetti B. Mutation in the tau gene in familial multiple system tauopathy with presenile dementia. Proc Natl Acad Sci USA 1998; 95(13): 7737-41. b [http://dx.doi.org/10.1073/pnas.95.13.7737] [PMID: 9636220]

[27] Braak H, Braak E. Diagnostic criteria for neuropathologic assessment of Alzheimer's disease. Neurobiol Aging 1997; 18(4) (Suppl.): S85-8. [http://dx.doi.org/10.1016/S0197-4580(97)00062-6] [PMID: 9330992]

[28] Rosenwald A, Reusche E, Ogomori K, Teichert HM. Comparison of silver stainings and immunohistology for the detection of neurofibrillary tangles and extracellular cerebral amyloid in paraffin sections. Acta Neuropathol 1993; 86(2): 182-6. [http://dx.doi.org/10.1007/BF00334887] [PMID: 7692696]

[29] Tiraboschi P, Hansen LA, Thal LJ, Corey-Bloom J. The importance of neuritic plaques and tangles to the development and evolution of AD. Neurology 2004; 62(11): 1984-9. [http://dx.doi.org/10.1212/01.WNL.0000129697.01779.0A] [PMID: 15184601]

[30] Ballatore C, Lee VM, Trojanowski JQ. Tau-mediated neurodegeneration in Alzheimer's disease and related disorders. Nat Rev Neurosci 2007; 8(9): 663-72. [http://dx.doi.org/10.1038/nrn2194] [PMID: 17684513]

[31] Haass C, Selkoe DJ. Soluble protein oligomers in neurodegeneration: lessons from the Alzheimer's amyloid beta-peptide. Nat Rev Mol Cell Biol 2007; 8(2): 101-12. [http://dx.doi.org/10.1038/nrm2101] [PMID: 17245412]

[32] Grundke-Iqbal I, Iqbal K, Quinlan M, Tung YC, Zaidi MS, Wisniewski HM. Microtubule-associated protein tau. A component of Alzheimer paired helical filaments. J Biol Chem 1986; 261(13): 6084-9. a [PMID: 3084478]

[33] Goedert M, Jakes R, Spillantini MG, Hasegawa M, Smith MJ, Crowther RA. Assembly of microtubule-associated protein tau into Alzheimer-like filaments induced by sulphated glycosaminoglycans. Nature 1996; 383(6600): 550-3. a [http://dx.doi.org/10.1038/383550a0] [PMID: 8849730]

[34] Lee G. Non-motor microtubule-associated proteins. Curr Opin Cell Biol 1993; 5(1): 88-94. [http://dx.doi.org/10.1016/S0955-0674(05)80013-4] [PMID: 8448035]

[35] Mandelkow E. Alzheimer's disease. The tangled tale of tau. Nature 1999; 402(6762): 588-9. [http://dx.doi.org/10.1038/45095] [PMID: 10604460]

[36] Mandelkow EM, Mandelkow E. Tau in Alzheimer's disease. Trends Cell Biol 1998; 8(11): 425-7. [http://dx.doi.org/10.1016/S0962-8924(98)01368-3] [PMID: 9854307]

[37] Kosik KS. Alzheimer's disease: a cell biological perspective. Science 1992; 256(5058): 780-3. [http://dx.doi.org/10.1126/science.1589757] [PMID: 1589757]

[38] Glenner GG, Wong CW. Alzheimer's disease: initial report of the purification and characterization of a novel cerebrovascular amyloid protein. Biochem Biophys Res Commun 1984; 120(3): 885-90. [http://dx.doi.org/10.1016/S0006-291X(84)80190-4] [PMID: 6375662]

[39] Masters CL, Multhaup G, Simms G, Pottgiesser J, Martins RN, Beyreuther K. Neuronal origin of a cerebral amyloid: neurofibrillary tangles of Alzheimer's disease contain the same protein as the amyloid of plaque cores and blood vessels. EMBO J 1985; 4(11): 2757-63. [PMID: 4065091]

[40] Hardy J, Selkoe DJ. The amyloid hypothesis of Alzheimer's disease: progress and problems on the road to therapeutics. Science 2002; 297(5580): 353-6. [http://dx.doi.org/10.1126/science.1072994] [PMID: 12130773]

[41] Medeiros R, Baglietto-Vargas D, LaFerla FM. The role of tau in Alzheimer's disease and related disorders. CNS Neurosci Ther 2011; 17(5): 514-24. [http://dx.doi.org/10.1111/j.1755-5949.2010.00177.x] [PMID: 20553310]

[42] Kidd M. Paired helical filaments in electron microscopy of Alzheimer's disease. Nature 1963; 197: 192-3. [http://dx.doi.org/10.1038/197192b0] [PMID: 14032480]

[43] Terry RD. The fine structure of neurofibrillary tangles in Alzheimer's disease. J Neuropathol Exp Neurol 1963; 22: 629-42. [http://dx.doi.org/10.1097/00005072-196310000-00005] [PMID: 14069842]

[44] Weingarten MD, Lockwood AH, Hwo SY, Kirschner MW. A protein factor essential for microtubule assembly. Proc Natl Acad Sci USA 1975; 72(5): 1858-62. [http://dx.doi.org/10.1073/pnas.72.5.1858] [PMID: 1057175]

[45] Delacourte A, Défossez A. [Biochemical characterization of an immune serum which specifically marks neurons in neurofibrillary degeneration in Alzheimer's disease]. C R Acad Sci III 1986; 303(11): 439-44. [PMID: 3096503]

[46] Kosik KS, Joachim CL, Selkoe DJ. Microtubule-associated protein tau (tau) is a major antigenic component of paired helical filaments in Alzheimer disease. Proc Natl Acad Sci USA 1986; 83(11): 4044-8.

[http://dx.doi.org/10.1073/pnas.83.11.4044] [PMID: 2424016]

[47] Grundke-Iqbal I, Iqbal K, Tung YC, Quinlan M, Wisniewski HM, Binder LI. Abnormal phosphorylation of the microtubule-associated protein tau (tau) in Alzheimer cytoskeletal pathology. Proc Natl Acad Sci USA 1986; 83(13): 4913-7. [http://dx.doi.org/10.1073/pnas.83.13.4913] [PMID: 3088567]

[48] Iqbal K, Grundke-Iqbal I, Zaidi T, *et al.* Defective brain microtubule assembly in Alzheimer's disease. Lancet 1986; 2(8504): 421-6. [http://dx.doi.org/10.1016/S0140-6736(86)92134-3] [PMID: 2874414]

[49] Goedert M, Wischik CM, Crowther RA, Walker JE, Klug A. Cloning and sequencing of the cDNA encoding a core protein of the paired helical filament of Alzheimer disease: identification as the microtubule-associated protein tau. Proc Natl Acad Sci USA 1988; 85(11): 4051-5. [http://dx.doi.org/10.1073/pnas.85.11.4051] [PMID: 3131773]

[50] Wischik CM, Novak M, Thøgersen HC, *et al.* Isolation of a fragment of tau derived from the core of the paired helical filament of Alzheimer disease. Proc Natl Acad Sci USA 1988; 85(12): 4506-10. b [http://dx.doi.org/10.1073/pnas.85.12.4506] [PMID: 3132715]

[51] Harada A, Oguchi K, Okabe S, *et al.* Altered microtubule organization in small-calibre axons of mice lacking tau protein. Nature 1994; 369(6480): 488-91. [http://dx.doi.org/10.1038/369488a0] [PMID: 8202139]

[52] Alonso AC, Zaidi T, Grundke-Iqbal I, Iqbal K. Role of abnormally phosphorylated tau in the breakdown of microtubules in Alzheimer disease. Proc Natl Acad Sci USA 1994; 91(12): 5562-6. [http://dx.doi.org/10.1073/pnas.91.12.5562] [PMID: 8202528]

[53] Busciglio J, Lorenzo A, Yeh J, Yankner BA. Beta-amyloid fibrils induce tau phosphorylation and loss of microtubule binding. Neuron 1995; 14(4): 879-88. [http://dx.doi.org/10.1016/0896-6273(95)90232-5] [PMID: 7718249]

[54] Mori H, Hosoda K, Matsubara E, *et al.* Tau in cerebrospinal fluids: establishment of the sandwich ELISA with antibody specific to the repeat sequence in tau. Neurosci Lett 1995; 186(2-3): 181-3. [http://dx.doi.org/10.1016/0304-3940(95)11291-4] [PMID: 7777192]

[55] Jensen M, Basun H, Lannfelt L. Increased cerebrospinal fluid tau in patients with Alzheimer's disease. Neurosci Lett 1995; 186(2-3): 189-91. [http://dx.doi.org/10.1016/0304-3940(95)11297-A] [PMID: 7777193]

[56] Smith MA, Siedlak SL, Richey PL, *et al.* Tau protein directly interacts with the amyloid beta-protein precursor: implications for Alzheimer's disease. Nat Med 1995; 1(4): 365-9. [http://dx.doi.org/10.1038/nm0495-365] [PMID: 7585068]

[57] Götz J, Probst A, Spillantini MG, *et al.* Somatodendritic localization and hyperphosphorylation of tau protein in transgenic mice expressing the longest human brain tau isoform. EMBO J 1995; 14(7): 1304-13. [PMID: 7729409]

[58] Alonso AD, Grundke-Iqbal I, Barra HS, Iqbal K. Abnormal phosphorylation of tau and the mechanism of Alzheimer neurofibrillary degeneration: sequestration of microtubule-associated proteins 1 and 2 and the disassembly of microtubules by the abnormal tau. Proc Natl Acad Sci USA 1997; 94(1): 298-303. [http://dx.doi.org/10.1073/pnas.94.1.298] [PMID: 8990203]

[59] Götz J, Chen F, van Dorpe J, Nitsch RM. Formation of neurofibrillary tangles in P301l tau transgenic mice induced by Abeta 42 fibrils. Science 2001; 293(5534): 1491-5. [http://dx.doi.org/10.1126/science.1062097] [PMID: 11520988]

[60] Rapoport M, Dawson HN, Binder LI, Vitek MP, Ferreira A. Tau is essential to beta -amyloid-induced neurotoxicity. Proc Natl Acad Sci USA 2002; 99(9): 6364-9. [http://dx.doi.org/10.1073/pnas.092136199] [PMID: 11959919]

[61] Oddo S, Caccamo A, Kitazawa M, Tseng BP, LaFerla FM. Amyloid deposition precedes tangle formation in a triple transgenic model of Alzheimer's disease. Neurobiol Aging 2003; 24(8): 1063-70. [http://dx.doi.org/10.1016/j.neurobiolaging.2003.08.012] [PMID: 14643377]

[62] Bellucci A, Westwood AJ, Ingram E, Casamenti F, Goedert M, Spillantini MG. Induction of inflammatory mediators and microglial activation in mice transgenic for mutant human P301S tau protein. Am J Pathol 2004; 165(5): 1643-52. [http://dx.doi.org/10.1016/S0002-9440(10)63421-9] [PMID: 15509534]

[63] Santacruz K, Lewis J, Spires T, *et al.* Tau suppression in a neurodegenerative mouse model improves memory function. Science 2005; 309(5733): 476-81. [http://dx.doi.org/10.1126/science.1113694] [PMID: 16020737]

[64] Zilka N, Filipcik P, Koson P, *et al.* Truncated tau from sporadic Alzheimer's disease suffices to drive neurofibrillary degeneration in vivo. FEBS Lett 2006; 580(15): 3582-8. [http://dx.doi.org/10.1016/j.febslet.2006.05.029] [PMID: 16753151]

[65] Roberson ED, Scearce-Levie K, Palop JJ, *et al.* Reducing endogenous tau ameliorates amyloid beta-induced deficits in an Alzheimer's disease mouse model. Science 2007; 316(5825): 750-4. [http://dx.doi.org/10.1126/science.1141736] [PMID: 17478722]

[66] Goedert M, Baur CP, Ahringer J, *et al.* PTL-1, a microtubule-associated protein with tau-like repeats from the nematode Caenorhabditis elegans. J Cell Sci 1996; 109(Pt 11): 2661-72. b [PMID: 8937984]

[67] McDermott JB, Aamodt S, Aamodt E. ptl-1, a Caenorhabditis elegans gene whose products are homologous to the tau microtubule-associated proteins. Biochemistry 1996; 35(29): 9415-23. [http://dx.doi.org/10.1021/bi952646n] [PMID: 8755720]

[68] Cambiazo V, González M, Maccioni RB. DMAP-85: a tau-like protein from Drosophila melanogaster larvae. J Neurochem 1995; 64(3): 1288-97. [http://dx.doi.org/10.1046/j.1471-4159.1995.64031288.x] [PMID: 7861162]

[69] Irminger-Finger I, Laymon RA, Goldstein LS. Analysis of the primary sequence and microtubule-binding region of the Drosophila 205K MAP. J Cell Biol 1990; 111(6 Pt 1): 2563-72. [http://dx.doi.org/10.1083/jcb.111.6.2563] [PMID: 1703540]

[70] Liu Y, Xia J, Ma D, Faber DS, Fischer I. Tau-like proteins in the nervous system of goldfish. Neurochem Res 1997; 22(12): 1511-6. [http://dx.doi.org/10.1023/A:1021914830872] [PMID: 9357018]

[71] Yin HS, Chou HC, Chiu MM. Changes in the microtubule proteins in the developing and transected spinal cords of the bullfrog tadpole: induction of microtubule-associated protein 2c and enhanced levels of Tau and tubulin in regenerating central axons. Neuroscience 1995; 67(3): 763-75. [http://dx.doi.org/10.1016/0306-4522(95)00042-H] [PMID: 7675202]

[72] Kosik KS, Finch EA. MAP2 and tau segregate into dendritic and axonal domains after the elaboration of morphologically distinct neurites: an immunocytochemical study of cultured rat cerebrum. J Neurosci 1987; 7(10): 3142-53. [PMID: 2444675]

[73] Lee G, Cowan N, Kirschner M. The primary structure and heterogeneity of tau protein from mouse brain. Science 1988; 239(4837): 285-8. [http://dx.doi.org/10.1126/science.3122323] [PMID: 3122323]

[74] Himmler A. Structure of the bovine tau gene: alternatively spliced transcripts generate a protein family. Mol Cell Biol 1989; 9(4): 1389-96. a [http://dx.doi.org/10.1128/MCB.9.4.1389] [PMID: 2498650]

[75] Himmler A, Drechsel D, Kirschner MW, Martin DW Jr. Tau consists of a set of proteins with repeated C-terminal microtubule-binding domains and variable N-terminal domains. Mol Cell Biol 1989; 9(4): 1381-8. b

[http://dx.doi.org/10.1128/MCB.9.4.1381] [PMID: 2498649]

[76] Nelson PT, Stefansson K, Gulcher J, Saper CB. Molecular evolution of tau protein: implications for Alzheimer's disease. J Neurochem 1996; 67(4): 1622-32. [http://dx.doi.org/10.1046/j.1471-4159.1996.67041622.x] [PMID: 8858947]

[77] Goedert M, Spillantini MG, Jakes R, Rutherford D, Crowther RA. Multiple isoforms of human microtubule-associated protein Tau: sequences and localization in neurofibrillary tangles of Alzheimer's disease. Neuron 1989; 3(4): 519-26. [http://dx.doi.org/10.1016/0896-6273(89)90210-9]

[78] Goedert M, Spillantini MG, Potier MC, Ulrich J, Crowther RA. Cloning and sequencing of the cDNA encoding an isoform of microtubule-associated protein tau containing four tandem repeats: differential expression of tau protein mRNAs in human brain. EMBO J 1989; 8(2): 393-9. b [PMID: 2498079]

[79] Binder LI, Frankfurter A, Rebhun LI. The distribution of tau in the mammalian central nervous system. J Cell Biol 1985; 101(4): 1371-8. [http://dx.doi.org/10.1083/jcb.101.4.1371] [PMID: 3930508]

[80] Couchie D, Mavilia C, Georgieff IS, Liem RK, Shelanski ML, Nunez J. Primary structure of high molecular weight tau present in the peripheral nervous system. Proc Natl Acad Sci USA 1992; 89(10): 4378-81. [http://dx.doi.org/10.1073/pnas.89.10.4378] [PMID: 1374898]

[81] LoPresti P, Szuchet S, Papasozomenos SC, Zinkowski RP, Binder LI. Functional implications for the microtubule-associated protein tau: localization in oligodendrocytes. Proc Natl Acad Sci USA 1995; 92(22): 10369-73. [http://dx.doi.org/10.1073/pnas.92.22.10369] [PMID: 7479786]

[82] Shin RW, Iwaki T, Kitamoto T, Tateishi J. Hydrated autoclave pretreatment enhances tau immunoreactivity in formalin-fixed normal and Alzheimer's disease brain tissues. Lab Invest 1991; 64(5): 693-702. [PMID: 1903170]

[83] Gu Y, Oyama F, Ihara Y. Tau is widely expressed in rat tissues. J Neurochem 1996; 67(3): 1235-44. [http://dx.doi.org/10.1046/j.1471-4159.1996.67031235.x] [PMID: 8752131]

[84] Ingelson M, Vanmechelen E, Lannfelt L. Microtubule-associated protein tau in human fibroblasts with the Swedish Alzheimer mutation. Neurosci Lett 1996; 220(1): 9-12. [http://dx.doi.org/10.1016/S0304-3940(96)13218-3] [PMID: 8977136]

[85] Vanier MT, Neuville P, Michalik L, Launay JF. Expression of specific tau exons in normal and tumoral pancreatic acinar cells. J Cell Sci 1998; 111(Pt 10): 1419-32. [PMID: 9570759]

[86] Cleveland DW, Hwo SY, Kirschner MW. Purification of tau, a microtubule-associated protein that induces assembly of microtubules from purified tubulin. J Mol Biol 1977; 116(2): 207-25. [http://dx.doi.org/10.1016/0022-2836(77)90213-3] [PMID: 599557]

[87] Drubin DG, Feinstein SC, Shooter EM, Kirschner MW. Nerve growth factor-induced neurite outgrowth in PC12 cells involves the coordinate induction of microtubule assembly and assembly-promoting factors. J Cell Biol 1985; 101(5 Pt 1): 1799-807. [http://dx.doi.org/10.1083/jcb.101.5.1799] [PMID: 2997236]

[88] Drubin DG, Kirschner MW. Tau protein function in living cells. J Cell Biol 1986; 103(6 Pt 2): 2739-46. [http://dx.doi.org/10.1083/jcb.103.6.2739] [PMID: 3098742]

[89] Drubin D, Kobayashi S, Kellogg D, Kirschner M. Regulation of microtubule protein levels during cellular morphogenesis in nerve growth factor-treated PC12 cells. J Cell Biol 1988; 106(5): 1583-91. [http://dx.doi.org/10.1083/jcb.106.5.1583] [PMID: 3131347]

[90] Ferreira A, Busciglio J, Cáceres A. Microtubule formation and neurite growth in cerebellar macroneurons which develop in vitro: evidence for the involvement of the microtubule-associated proteins, MAP-1a, HMW-MAP2 and Tau. Brain Res Dev Brain Res 1989; 49(2): 215-28. [http://dx.doi.org/10.1016/0165-3806(89)90023-0] [PMID: 2509111]

[91] Kanai Y, Takemura R, Oshima T, *et al.* Expression of multiple tau isoforms and microtubule bundle formation in fibroblasts transfected with a single tau cDNA. J Cell Biol 1989; 109(3): 1173-84. [http://dx.doi.org/10.1083/jcb.109.3.1173] [PMID: 2504728]

[92] Drechsel DN, Hyman AA, Cobb MH, Kirschner MW. Modulation of the dynamic instability of tubulin assembly by the microtubule-associated protein tau. Mol Biol Cell 1992; 3(10): 1141-54. [http://dx.doi.org/10.1091/mbc.3.10.1141] [PMID: 1421571]

[93] Caceres A, Kosik KS. Inhibition of neurite polarity by tau antisense oligonucleotides in primary cerebellar neurons. Nature 1990; 343(6257): 461-3. [http://dx.doi.org/10.1038/343461a0] [PMID: 2105469]

[94] Caceres A, Potrebic S, Kosik KS. The effect of tau antisense oligonucleotides on neurite formation of cultured cerebellar macroneurons. J Neurosci 1991; 11(6): 1515-23. [PMID: 1904479]

[95] Ikegami S, Harada A, Hirokawa N. Muscle weakness, hyperactivity, and impairment in fear conditioning in tau-deficient mice. Neurosci Lett 2000; 279(3): 129-32. [http://dx.doi.org/10.1016/S0304-3940(99)00964-7] [PMID: 10688046]

[96] Andreadis A, Brown WM, Kosik KS. Structure and novel exons of the human tau gene. Biochemistry 1992; 31(43): 10626-33. [http://dx.doi.org/10.1021/bi00158a027] [PMID: 1420178]

[97] Goedert M, Jakes R. Expression of separate isoforms of human tau protein: correlation with the tau pattern in brain and effects on tubulin polymerization. EMBO J 1990; 9(13): 4225-30. [PMID: 2124967]

[98] Butner KA, Kirschner MW. Tau protein binds to microtubules through a flexible array of distributed weak sites. J Cell Biol 1991; 115(3): 717-30. [http://dx.doi.org/10.1083/jcb.115.3.717] [PMID: 1918161]

[99] Goode BL, Feinstein SC. Identification of a novel microtubule binding and assembly domain in the developmentally regulated inter-repeat region of tau. J Cell Biol 1994; 124(5): 769-82. [http://dx.doi.org/10.1083/jcb.124.5.769] [PMID: 8120098]

[100] Hong M, Zhukareva V, Vogelsberg-Ragaglia V, *et al.* Mutation-specific functional impairments in distinct tau isoforms of hereditary FTDP-17. Science 1998; 282(5395): 1914-7. [http://dx.doi.org/10.1126/science.282.5395.1914] [PMID: 9836646]

[101] Friedhoff P, von Bergen M, Mandelkow EM, Davies P, Mandelkow E. A nucleated assembly mechanism of Alzheimer paired helical filaments. Proc Natl Acad Sci USA 1998; 95(26): 15712-7. [http://dx.doi.org/10.1073/pnas.95.26.15712] [PMID: 9861035]

[102] Barghorn S, Zheng-Fischhöfer Q, Ackmann M, *et al.* Structure, microtubule interactions, and paired helical filament aggregation by tau mutants of frontotemporal dementias. Biochemistry 2000; 39(38): 11714-21. [http://dx.doi.org/10.1021/bi000850r] [PMID: 10995239]

[103] von Bergen M, Friedhoff P, Biernat J, Heberle J, Mandelkow EM, Mandelkow E. Assembly of tau protein into Alzheimer paired helical filaments depends on a local sequence motif ((306)VQIVYK(311)) forming beta structure. Proc Natl Acad Sci USA 2000; 97(10): 5129-34. [http://dx.doi.org/10.1073/pnas.97.10.5129] [PMID: 10805776]

[104] Khlistunova I, Biernat J, Wang Y, *et al.* Inducible expression of Tau repeat domain in cell models of tauopathy: aggregation is toxic to cells but can be reversed by inhibitor drugs. J Biol Chem 2006; 281(2): 1205-14.

[http://dx.doi.org/10.1074/jbc.M507753200] [PMID: 16246844]

[105] Lindwall G, Cole RD. Phosphorylation affects the ability of tau protein to promote microtubule assembly. J Biol Chem 1984; 259(8): 5301-5.
[PMID: 6425287]

[106] Ishiguro K, Shiratsuchi A, Sato S, *et al.* Glycogen synthase kinase 3 beta is identical to tau protein kinase I generating several epitopes of paired helical filaments. FEBS Lett 1993; 325(3): 167-72.
[http://dx.doi.org/10.1016/0014-5793(93)81066-9] [PMID: 7686508]

[107] Baumann K, Mandelkow EM, Biernat J, Piwnica-Worms H, Mandelkow E. Abnormal Alzheimer-like phosphorylation of tau-protein by cyclin-dependent kinases cdk2 and cdk5. FEBS Lett 1993; 336(3): 417-24.
[http://dx.doi.org/10.1016/0014-5793(93)80849-P] [PMID: 8282104]

[108] Drewes G, Lichtenberg-Kraag B, Döring F, *et al.* Mitogen activated protein (MAP) kinase transforms tau protein into an Alzheimer-like state. EMBO J 1992; 11(6): 2131-8.
[PMID: 1376245]

[109] Lu Q, Soria JP, Wood JG. p44mpk MAP kinase induces Alzheimer type alterations in tau function and in primary hippocampal neurons. J Neurosci Res 1993; 35(4): 439-44.
[http://dx.doi.org/10.1002/jnr.490350411] [PMID: 7689658]

[110] Drewes G, Ebneth A, Preuss U, Mandelkow EM, Mandelkow E. MARK, a novel family of protein kinases that phosphorylate microtubule-associated proteins and trigger microtubule disruption. Cell 1997; 89(2): 297-308.
[http://dx.doi.org/10.1016/S0092-8674(00)80208-1] [PMID: 9108484]

[111] Kishi M, Pan YA, Crump JG, Sanes JR. Mammalian SAD kinases are required for neuronal polarization. Science 2005; 307(5711): 929-32.
[http://dx.doi.org/10.1126/science.1107403] [PMID: 15705853]

[112] Lee G. Tau and src family tyrosine kinases. Biochim Biophys Acta 2005; 1739(2-3): 323-30.
[http://dx.doi.org/10.1016/j.bbadis.2004.09.002] [PMID: 15615649]

[113] Williamson R, Scales T, Clark BR, *et al.* Rapid tyrosine phosphorylation of neuronal proteins including tau and focal adhesion kinase in response to amyloid-beta peptide exposure: involvement of Src family protein kinases. J Neurosci 2002; 22(1): 10-20.
[PMID: 11756483]

[114] Lebouvier T, Scales TM, Hanger DP, *et al.* The microtubule-associated protein tau is phosphorylated by Syk. Biochim Biophys Acta 2008; 1783(2): 188-92.
[http://dx.doi.org/10.1016/j.bbamcr.2007.11.005] [PMID: 18070606]

[115] Lee G, Newman ST, Gard DL, Band H, Panchamoorthy G. Tau interacts with src-family non-receptor tyrosine kinases. J Cell Sci 1998; 111(Pt 21): 3167-77.
[PMID: 9763511]

[116] Lee G, Thangavel R, Sharma VM, *et al.* Phosphorylation of tau by fyn: implications for Alzheimer's disease. J Neurosci 2004; 24(9): 2304-12.
[http://dx.doi.org/10.1523/JNEUROSCI.4162-03.2004] [PMID: 14999081]

[117] Derkinderen P, Scales TM, Hanger DP, *et al.* Tyrosine 394 is phosphorylated in Alzheimer's paired helical filament tau and in fetal tau with c-Abl as the candidate tyrosine kinase. J Neurosci 2005; 25(28): 6584-93.
[http://dx.doi.org/10.1523/JNEUROSCI.1487-05.2005] [PMID: 16014719]

[118] Biernat J, Gustke N, Drewes G, Mandelkow EM, Mandelkow E. Phosphorylation of Ser262 strongly reduces binding of tau to microtubules: distinction between PHF-like immunoreactivity and microtubule binding. Neuron 1993; 11(1): 153-63.
[http://dx.doi.org/10.1016/0896-6273(93)90279-Z] [PMID: 8393323]

[119] Morishima-Kawashima M, Hasegawa M, Takio K, *et al.* Proline-directed and non-proline-directed

phosphorylation of PHF-tau. J Biol Chem 1995; 270(2): 823-9.
[http://dx.doi.org/10.1074/jbc.270.2.823] [PMID: 7822317]

[120] Illenberger S, Zheng-Fischhöfer Q, Preuss U, *et al.* The endogenous and cell cycle-dependent phosphorylation of tau protein in living cells: implications for Alzheimer's disease. Mol Biol Cell 1998; 9(6): 1495-512.
[http://dx.doi.org/10.1091/mbc.9.6.1495] [PMID: 9614189]

[121] Brandt R, Lee G, Teplow DB, Shalloway D, Abdel-Ghany M. Differential effect of phosphorylation and substrate modulation on tau's ability to promote microtubule growth and nucleation. J Biol Chem 1994; 269(16): 11776-82.
[PMID: 8163474]

[122] Sengupta A, Kabat J, Novak M, Wu Q, Grundke-Iqbal I, Iqbal K. Phosphorylation of tau at both Thr 231 and Ser 262 is required for maximal inhibition of its binding to microtubules. Arch Biochem Biophys 1998; 357(2): 299-309.
[http://dx.doi.org/10.1006/abbi.1998.0813] [PMID: 9735171]

[123] Morishima-Kawashima M, Hasegawa M, Takio K, *et al.* Hyperphosphorylation of tau in PHF. Neurobiol Aging 1995; 16(3): 365-71. b
[http://dx.doi.org/10.1016/0197-4580(95)00027-C] [PMID: 7566346]

[124] Kadowaki T, Fujita-Yamaguchi Y, Nishida E, *et al.* Phosphorylation of tubulin and microtubule-associated proteins by the purified insulin receptor kinase. J Biol Chem 1985; 260(7): 4016-20.
[PMID: 3920212]

[125] Sontag E, Nunbhakdi-Craig V, Lee G, Bloom GS, Mumby MC. Regulation of the phosphorylation state and microtubule-binding activity of Tau by protein phosphatase 2A. Neuron 1996; 17(6): 1201-7.
[http://dx.doi.org/10.1016/S0896-6273(00)80250-0] [PMID: 8982166]

[126] Sun L, Liu SY, Zhou XW, *et al.* Inhibition of protein phosphatase 2A- and protein phosphatase 1-induced tau hyperphosphorylation and impairment of spatial memory retention in rats. Neuroscience 2003; 118(4): 1175-82.
[http://dx.doi.org/10.1016/S0306-4522(02)00697-8] [PMID: 12732260]

[127] Ikeda K, Akiyama H, Arai T, *et al.* Alz-50/Gallyas-positive lysosome-like intraneuronal granules in Alzheimer's disease and control brains. Neurosci Lett 1998; 258(2): 113-6.
[http://dx.doi.org/10.1016/S0304-3940(98)00867-2] [PMID: 9875540]

[128] Wang Y, Garg S, Mandelkow EM, Mandelkow E. Proteolytic processing of tau. Biochem Soc Trans 2010; 38(4): 955-61.
[http://dx.doi.org/10.1042/BST0380955] [PMID: 20658984]

[129] Wischik CM, Novak M, Edwards PC, Klug A, Tichelaar W, Crowther RA. Structural characterization of the core of the paired helical filament of Alzheimer disease. Proc Natl Acad Sci USA 1988; 85(13): 4884-8. a
[http://dx.doi.org/10.1073/pnas.85.13.4884] [PMID: 2455299]

[130] Lewis SA, Wang DH, Cowan NJ. Microtubule-associated protein MAP2 shares a microtubule binding motif with tau protein. Science 1988; 242(4880): 936-9.
[http://dx.doi.org/10.1126/science.3142041] [PMID: 3142041]

[131] Jameson L, Frey T, Zeeberg B, Dalldorf F, Caplow M. Inhibition of microtubule assembly by phosphorylation of microtubule-associated proteins. Biochemistry 1980; 19(11): 2472-9.
[http://dx.doi.org/10.1021/bi00552a027] [PMID: 7387985]

[132] Steiner B, Mandelkow EM, Biernat J, *et al.* Phosphorylation of microtubule-associated protein tau: identification of the site for Ca2(+)-calmodulin dependent kinase and relationship with tau phosphorylation in Alzheimer tangles. EMBO J 1990; 9(11): 3539-44.
[PMID: 2120043]

[133] McKinney M, Snider RM, Richelson E. Thrombin binding to human brain and spinal cord. Mayo Clin

Proc 1983; 58(12): 829-31.
[PMID: 6645628]

[134] Deschepper CF, Bigornia V, Berens ME, Lapointe MC. Production of thrombin and antithrombin III by brain and astroglial cell cultures. Brain Res Mol Brain Res 1991; 11(3-4): 355-8.
[http://dx.doi.org/10.1016/0169-328X(91)90045-Y] [PMID: 1661827]

[135] Dihanich M, Kaser M, Reinhard E, Cunningham D, Monard D. Prothrombin mRNA is expressed by cells of the nervous system. Neuron 1991; 6(4): 575-81.
[http://dx.doi.org/10.1016/0896-6273(91)90060-D] [PMID: 2015093]

[136] Wagner SL, Geddes JW, Cotman CW, *et al.* Protease nexin-1, an antithrombin with neurite outgrowth activity, is reduced in Alzheimer disease. Proc Natl Acad Sci USA 1989; 86(21): 8284-8.
[http://dx.doi.org/10.1073/pnas.86.21.8284] [PMID: 2813392]

[137] Igarashi K, Murai H, Asaka J. Proteolytic processing of amyloid β protein precursor (APP) by thrombin. Biochem Biophys Res Commun 1992; 185(3): 1000-4.
[http://dx.doi.org/10.1016/0006-291X(92)91726-7] [PMID: 1627124]

[138] Arai T, Guo JP, McGeer PL. Proteolysis of non-phosphorylated and phosphorylated tau by thrombin. J Biol Chem 2005; 280(7): 5145-53.
[http://dx.doi.org/10.1074/jbc.M409234200] [PMID: 15542598]

[139] Olesen OF. Proteolytic degradation of microtubule associated protein tau by thrombin. Biochem Biophys Res Commun 1994; 201(2): 716-21.
[http://dx.doi.org/10.1006/bbrc.1994.1759] [PMID: 8003007]

[140] Gervais FG, Xu D, Robertson GS, *et al.* Involvement of caspases in proteolytic cleavage of Alzheimer's amyloid-beta precursor protein and amyloidogenic A beta peptide formation. Cell 1999; 97(3): 395-406.
[http://dx.doi.org/10.1016/S0092-8674(00)80748-5] [PMID: 10319819]

[141] Nakagawa T, Zhu H, Morishima N, *et al.* Caspase-12 mediates endoplasmic-reticulum-specific apoptosis and cytotoxicity by amyloid-beta. Nature 2000; 403(6765): 98-103.
[http://dx.doi.org/10.1038/47513] [PMID: 10638761]

[142] Troy CM, Rabacchi SA, Friedman WJ, Frappier TF, Brown K, Shelanski ML. Caspase-2 mediates neuronal cell death induced by β-amyloid. J Neurosci 2000; 20(4): 1386-92.
[PMID: 10662829]

[143] Gamblin TC, Chen F, Zambrano A, *et al.* Caspase cleavage of tau: linking amyloid and neurofibrillary tangles in Alzheimer's disease. Proc Natl Acad Sci USA 2003; 100(17): 10032-7.
[http://dx.doi.org/10.1073/pnas.1630428100] [PMID: 12888622]

[144] Fasulo L, Ugolini G, Visintin M, *et al.* The neuronal microtubule-associated protein tau is a substrate for caspase-3 and an effector of apoptosis. J Neurochem 2000; 75(2): 624-33.
[http://dx.doi.org/10.1046/j.1471-4159.2000.0750624.x] [PMID: 10899937]

[145] Chung CW, Song YH, Kim IK, *et al.* Proapoptotic effects of tau cleavage product generated by caspase-3. Neurobiol Dis 2001; 8(1): 162-72.
[http://dx.doi.org/10.1006/nbdi.2000.0335] [PMID: 11162250]

[146] Rissman RA, Poon WW, Blurton-Jones M, *et al.* Caspase-cleavage of tau is an early event in Alzheimer disease tangle pathology. J Clin Invest 2004; 114(1): 121-30.
[http://dx.doi.org/10.1172/JCI200420640] [PMID: 15232619]

[147] Rohn TT, Rissman RA, Davis MC, Kim YE, Cotman CW, Head E. Caspase-9 activation and caspase cleavage of tau in the Alzheimer's disease brain. Neurobiol Dis 2002; 11(2): 341-54.
[http://dx.doi.org/10.1006/nbdi.2002.0549] [PMID: 12505426]

[148] Lu DC, Rabizadeh S, Chandra S, *et al.* A second cytotoxic proteolytic peptide derived from amyloid beta-protein precursor. Nat Med 2000; 6(4): 397-404.
[http://dx.doi.org/10.1038/74656] [PMID: 10742146]

[149] Canu N, Dus L, Barbato C, *et al.* Tau cleavage and dephosphorylation in cerebellar granule neurons undergoing apoptosis. J Neurosci 1998; 18(18): 7061-74. [PMID: 9736630]

[150] Abraha A, Ghoshal N, Gamblin TC, *et al.* C-terminal inhibition of tau assembly in vitro and in Alzheimer's disease. J Cell Sci 2000; 113(Pt 21): 3737-45. [PMID: 11034902]

[151] LeBlanc A, Liu H, Goodyer C, Bergeron C, Hammond J. Caspase-6 role in apoptosis of human neurons, amyloidogenesis, and Alzheimer's disease. J Biol Chem 1999; 274(33): 23426-36. [http://dx.doi.org/10.1074/jbc.274.33.23426] [PMID: 10438520]

[152] Zhang Y, Goodyer C, LeBlanc A. Selective and protracted apoptosis in human primary neurons microinjected with active caspase-3, -6, -7, and -8. J Neurosci 2000; 20(22): 8384-9. [PMID: 11069945]

[153] Jiang CH, Tsien JZ, Schultz PG, Hu Y. The effects of aging on gene expression in the hypothalamus and cortex of mice. Proc Natl Acad Sci USA 2001; 98(4): 1930-4. [http://dx.doi.org/10.1073/pnas.98.4.1930] [PMID: 11172053]

[154] Guo H, Albrecht S, Bourdeau M, Petzke T, Bergeron C, LeBlanc AC. Active caspase-6 and caspase-6-cleaved tau in neuropil threads, neuritic plaques, and neurofibrillary tangles of Alzheimer's disease. Am J Pathol 2004; 165(2): 523-31. [http://dx.doi.org/10.1016/S0002-9440(10)63317-2] [PMID: 15277226]

[155] Albrecht S, Bourdeau M, Bennett D, Mufson EJ, Bhattacharjee M, LeBlanc AC. Activation of caspase-6 in aging and mild cognitive impairment. Am J Pathol 2007; 170(4): 1200-9. [http://dx.doi.org/10.2353/ajpath.2007.060974] [PMID: 17392160]

[156] Horowitz PM, Patterson KR, Guillozet-Bongaarts AL, *et al.* Early N-terminal changes and caspase-6 cleavage of tau in Alzheimer's disease. J Neurosci 2004; 24(36): 7895-902. [http://dx.doi.org/10.1523/JNEUROSCI.1988-04.2004] [PMID: 15356202]

[157] Perlmutter LS, Gall C, Baudry M, Lynch G. Distribution of calcium-activated protease calpain in the rat brain. J Comp Neurol 1990; 296(2): 269-76. [http://dx.doi.org/10.1002/cne.902960207] [PMID: 2358536]

[158] Siman R, Gall C, Perlmutter LS, Christian C, Baudry M, Lynch G. Distribution of calpain I, an enzyme associated with degenerative activity, in rat brain. Brain Res 1985; 347(2): 399-403. [http://dx.doi.org/10.1016/0006-8993(85)90208-2] [PMID: 2998556]

[159] Johnson GV, Jope RS, Binder LI. Proteolysis of tau by calpain. Biochem Biophys Res Commun 1989; 163(3): 1505-11. [http://dx.doi.org/10.1016/0006-291X(89)91150-9] [PMID: 2551295]

[160] Litersky JM, Scott CW, Johnson GV. Phosphorylation, calpain proteolysis and tubulin binding of recombinant human tau isoforms. Brain Res 1993; 604(1-2): 32-40. [http://dx.doi.org/10.1016/0006-8993(93)90349-R] [PMID: 8384512]

[161] Garg S, Timm T, Mandelkow EM, Mandelkow E, Wang Y. Cleavage of Tau by calpain in Alzheimer's disease: the quest for the toxic 17 kD fragment. Neurobiol Aging 2011; 32(1): 1-14. [http://dx.doi.org/10.1016/j.neurobiolaging.2010.09.008] [PMID: 20961659]

[162] Mandelkow EM, Mandelkow E. Biochemistry and cell biology of tau protein in neurofibrillary degeneration. Cold Spring Harb Perspect Med 2012; 2(7): a006247. [http://dx.doi.org/10.1101/cshperspect.a006247] [PMID: 22762014]

[163] Park SY, Ferreira A. The generation of a 17 kDa neurotoxic fragment: an alternative mechanism by which tau mediates beta-amyloid-induced neurodegeneration. J Neurosci 2005; 25(22): 5365-75. [http://dx.doi.org/10.1523/JNEUROSCI.1125-05.2005] [PMID: 15930385]

[164] Marks N, Lajtha A. Separation of acid and neutral proteinases of brain. Biochem J 1965; 97(1): 74-83.

[http://dx.doi.org/10.1042/bj0970074] [PMID: 16749127]

[165] Whitaker JN, Terry LC, Whetsell WO Jr. Immunocytochemical localization of cathepsin D in rat neural tissue. Brain Res 1981; 216(1): 109-24.
[http://dx.doi.org/10.1016/0006-8993(81)91281-6] [PMID: 7020877]

[166] Bernstein HG, Wiederanders B, Rinne A, Dorn A. Distribution of cathepsin D immunoreactivity in the central nervous system of rat and selected brain regions of man. Acta Histochem 1985; 77(2): 139-42.
[http://dx.doi.org/10.1016/S0065-1281(85)80073-8] [PMID: 3938170]

[167] Cataldo AM, Nixon RA. Enzymatically active lysosomal proteases are associated with amyloid deposits in Alzheimer brain. Proc Natl Acad Sci USA 1990; 87(10): 3861-5.
[http://dx.doi.org/10.1073/pnas.87.10.3861] [PMID: 1692625]

[168] Mercken M, Grynspan F, Nixon RA. Differential sensitivity to proteolysis by brain calpain of adult human tau, fetal human tau and PHF-tau. FEBS Lett 1995; 368(1): 10-4.
[http://dx.doi.org/10.1016/0014-5793(95)00590-6] [PMID: 7615058]

[169] Bednarski E, Lynch G. Cytosolic proteolysis of tau by cathepsin D in hippocampus following suppression of cathepsins B and L. J Neurochem 1996; 67(5): 1846-55.
[http://dx.doi.org/10.1046/j.1471-4159.1996.67051846.x] [PMID: 8863489]

[170] Kenessey A, Nacharaju P, Ko LW, Yen SH. Degradation of tau by lysosomal enzyme cathepsin D: implication for Alzheimer neurofibrillary degeneration. J Neurochem 1997; 69(5): 2026-38.
[http://dx.doi.org/10.1046/j.1471-4159.1997.69052026.x] [PMID: 9349548]

[171] Selkoe DJ. Normal and abnormal biology of the beta-amyloid precursor protein. Annu Rev Neurosci 1994; 17: 489-517.
[http://dx.doi.org/10.1146/annurev.ne.17.030194.002421] [PMID: 8210185]

[172] Esler WP, Wolfe MS. A portrait of Alzheimer secretases--new features and familiar faces. Science 2001; 293(5534): 1449-54.
[http://dx.doi.org/10.1126/science.1064638] [PMID: 11520976]

[173] Haass C. Take five--BACE and the gamma-secretase quartet conduct Alzheimer's amyloid beta-peptide generation. EMBO J 2004; 23(3): 483-8.
[http://dx.doi.org/10.1038/sj.emboj.7600061] [PMID: 14749724]

[174] Kim TW, Tanzi RE. Presenilins and Alzheimer's disease. Curr Opin Neurobiol 1997; 7(5): 683-8.
[http://dx.doi.org/10.1016/S0959-4388(97)80089-X] [PMID: 9384549]

[175] De Strooper B, Saftig P, Craessaerts K, *et al.* Deficiency of presenilin-1 inhibits the normal cleavage of amyloid precursor protein. Nature 1998; 391(6665): 387-90.
[http://dx.doi.org/10.1038/34910] [PMID: 9450754]

[176] Herreman A, Serneels L, Annaert W, Collen D, Schoonjans L, De Strooper B. Total inactivation of gamma-secretase activity in presenilin-deficient embryonic stem cells. Nat Cell Biol 2000; 2(7): 461-2.
[http://dx.doi.org/10.1038/35017105] [PMID: 10878813]

[177] Goodman Y, Mattson MP. Secreted forms of beta-amyloid precursor protein protect hippocampal neurons against amyloid beta-peptide-induced oxidative injury. Exp Neurol 1994; 128(1): 1-12.
[http://dx.doi.org/10.1006/exnr.1994.1107] [PMID: 8070512]

[178] O'Mahony S, Harkany T, Rensink AA, *et al.* Beta-amyloid-induced cholinergic denervation correlates with enhanced nitric oxide synthase activity in rat cerebral cortex: reversal by NMDA receptor blockade. Brain Res Bull 1998; 45(4): 405-11.
[http://dx.doi.org/10.1016/S0361-9230(97)00405-X] [PMID: 9527015]

[179] Lustbader JW, Cirilli M, Lin C, *et al.* ABAD directly links Abeta to mitochondrial toxicity in Alzheimer's disease. Science 2004; 304(5669): 448-52.
[http://dx.doi.org/10.1126/science.1091230] [PMID: 15087549]

[180] Caricasole A, Copani A, Caruso A, *et al.* The Wnt pathway, cell-cycle activation and beta-amyloid: novel therapeutic strategies in Alzheimer's disease? Trends Pharmacol Sci 2003; 24(5): 233-8. [http://dx.doi.org/10.1016/S0165-6147(03)00100-7] [PMID: 12767722]

[181] Bamberger ME, Landreth GE. Microglial interaction with beta-amyloid: implications for the pathogenesis of Alzheimer's disease. Microsc Res Tech 2001; 54(2): 59-70. [http://dx.doi.org/10.1002/jemt.1121] [PMID: 11455613]

[182] Harris ME, Wang Y, Pedigo NW Jr, Hensley K, Butterfield DA, Carney JM. Amyloid beta peptide (25-35) inhibits Na+-dependent glutamate uptake in rat hippocampal astrocyte cultures. J Neurochem 1996; 67(1): 277-86. [http://dx.doi.org/10.1046/j.1471-4159.1996.67010277.x] [PMID: 8667003]

[183] Folch J, Petrov D, Ettcheto M, *et al.* Current research therapeutic strategies for alzheimer's disease treatment. Neural Plast 2016; 2016: 8501693. [http://dx.doi.org/10.1155/2016/8501693] [PMID: 26881137]

[184] Godyń J, Jończyk J, Panek D, Malawska B. Therapeutic strategies for Alzheimer's disease in clinical trials. Pharmacol Rep 2016; 68(1): 127-38. [http://dx.doi.org/10.1016/j.pharep.2015.07.006] [PMID: 26721364]

[185] Lovestone S, Boada M, Dubois B, *et al.* A phase II trial of tideglusib in Alzheimer's disease. J Alzheimers Dis 2015; 45(1): 75-88. [PMID: 25537011]

[186] Camins A, Verdaguer E, Folch J, Canudas AM, Pallàs M. The role of CDK5/P25 formation/inhibition in neurodegeneration. Drug News Perspect 2006; 19(8): 453-60. [http://dx.doi.org/10.1358/dnp.2006.19.8.1043961] [PMID: 17160145]

[187] de la Torre AV, Junyent F, Folch J, *et al.* GSK3β inhibition is involved in the neuroprotective effects of cyclin-dependent kinase inhibitors in neurons. Pharmacol Res 2012; 65(1): 66-73. [http://dx.doi.org/10.1016/j.phrs.2011.08.006] [PMID: 21875668]

[188] Gourmaud S, Paquet C, Dumurgier J, *et al.* Increased levels of cerebrospinal fluid JNK3 associated with amyloid pathology: links to cognitive decline. J Psychiatry Neurosci 2015; 40(3): 151-61. [http://dx.doi.org/10.1503/jpn.140062] [PMID: 25455349]

[189] Resnick L, Fennell M. Targeting JNK3 for the treatment of neurodegenerative disorders. Drug Discov Today 2004; 9(21): 932-9. [http://dx.doi.org/10.1016/S1359-6446(04)03251-9] [PMID: 15501728]

[190] Zhou Q, Wang M, Du Y, *et al.* Inhibition of c-Jun N-terminal kinase activation reverses Alzheimer disease phenotypes in APPswe/PS1dE9 mice. Ann Neurol 2015; 77(4): 637-54. [http://dx.doi.org/10.1002/ana.24361] [PMID: 25611954]

[191] Hochgräfe K, Sydow A, Matenia D, *et al.* Preventive methylene blue treatment preserves cognition in mice expressing full-length pro-aggregant human Tau. Acta Neuropathol Commun 2015; 3: 25. [http://dx.doi.org/10.1186/s40478-015-0204-4] [PMID: 25958115]

[192] Wischik CM, Staff RT, Wischik DJ, *et al.* Tau aggregation inhibitor therapy: an exploratory phase 2 study in mild or moderate Alzheimer's disease. J Alzheimers Dis 2015; 44(2): 705-20. [PMID: 25550228]

[193] Shemesh OA, Spira ME. Rescue of neurons from undergoing hallmark tau-induced Alzheimer's disease cell pathologies by the antimitotic drug paclitaxel. Neurobiol Dis 2011; 43(1): 163-75. [http://dx.doi.org/10.1016/j.nbd.2011.03.008] [PMID: 21406229]

[194] Wisniewski T, Goñi F. Immunotherapeutic approaches for Alzheimer's disease. Neuron 2015; 85(6): 1162-76. [http://dx.doi.org/10.1016/j.neuron.2014.12.064] [PMID: 25789753]

[195] Haass C, Kaether C, Thinakaran G, Sisodia S. Trafficking and proteolytic processing of APP. Cold

Spring Harb Perspect Med 2012; 2(5): a006270.
[http://dx.doi.org/10.1101/cshperspect.a006270] [PMID: 22553493]

[196] Chiang K, Koo EH. Emerging therapeutics for Alzheimer's disease. Annu Rev Pharmacol Toxicol 2014; 54: 381-405.
[http://dx.doi.org/10.1146/annurev-pharmtox-011613-135932] [PMID: 24392696]

[197] Imbimbo BP, Giardina GA. γ-secretase inhibitors and modulators for the treatment of Alzheimer's disease: disappointments and hopes. Curr Top Med Chem 2011; 11(12): 1555-70.
[http://dx.doi.org/10.2174/156802611795860942] [PMID: 21510832]

[198] Menting KW, Claassen JA. β-secretase inhibitor; a promising novel therapeutic drug in Alzheimer's disease. Front Aging Neurosci 2014; 6: 165.
[http://dx.doi.org/10.3389/fnagi.2014.00165] [PMID: 25100992]

[199] May PC, Willis BA, Lowe SL, *et al.* The potent BACE1 inhibitor LY2886721 elicits robust central Aβ pharmacodynamic responses in mice, dogs, and humans. J Neurosci 2015; 35(3): 1199-210.
[http://dx.doi.org/10.1523/JNEUROSCI.4129-14.2015] [PMID: 25609634]

[200] Vassar R, Kandalepas PC. The β-secretase enzyme BACE1 as a therapeutic target for Alzheimer's disease. Alzheimers Res Ther 2011; 3(3): 20.
[http://dx.doi.org/10.1186/alzrt82] [PMID: 21639952]

[201] Coric V, van Dyck CH, Salloway S, *et al.* Safety and tolerability of the γ-secretase inhibitor avagacestat in a phase 2 study of mild to moderate Alzheimer disease. Arch Neurol 2012; 69(11): 1430-40.
[http://dx.doi.org/10.1001/archneurol.2012.2194] [PMID: 22892585]

[202] Dockens R, Wang JS, Castaneda L, *et al.* A placebo-controlled, multiple ascending dose study to evaluate the safety, pharmacokinetics and pharmacodynamics of avagacestat (BMS-708163) in healthy young and elderly subjects. Clin Pharmacokinet 2012; 51(10): 681-93.
[http://dx.doi.org/10.1007/s40262-012-0005-x] [PMID: 23018531]

[203] Miguel-Álvarez M, Santos-Lozano A, Sanchis-Gomar F, *et al.* Non-steroidal anti-inflammatory drugs as a treatment for Alzheimer's disease: a systematic review and meta-analysis of treatment effect. Drugs Aging 2015; 32(2): 139-47.
[http://dx.doi.org/10.1007/s40266-015-0239-z] [PMID: 25644018]

[204] Pasqualetti P, Bonomini C, Dal Forno G, *et al.* A randomized controlled study on effects of ibuprofen on cognitive progression of Alzheimer's disease. Aging Clin Exp Res 2009; 21(2): 102-10.
[http://dx.doi.org/10.1007/BF03325217] [PMID: 19448381]

[205] Ross J, Sharma S, Winston J, *et al.* CHF5074 reduces biomarkers of neuroinflammation in patients with mild cognitive impairment: a 12-week, double-blind, placebo-controlled study. Curr Alzheimer Res 2013; 10(7): 742-53.
[http://dx.doi.org/10.2174/13892037113149990144] [PMID: 23968157]

[206] Bandyopadhyay S, Goldstein LE, Lahiri DK, Rogers JT. Role of the APP non-amyloidogenic signaling pathway and targeting alpha-secretase as an alternative drug target for treatment of Alzheimer's disease. Curr Med Chem 2007; 14(27): 2848-64.
[http://dx.doi.org/10.2174/092986707782360060] [PMID: 18045131]

[207] Yang HQ, Sun ZK, Ba MW, Xu J, Xing Y. Involvement of proteintrafficking in deprenyl-induced alpha-secretase activity regulation in PC12cells. Eur J Pharmacol 2009; 610(1–3): 37-41.

[208] Vellas B, Sol O, Snyder PJ, *et al.* EHT0202 in Alzheimer's disease: a 3-month, randomized, placebo-controlled, double-blind study. Curr Alzheimer Res 2011; 8(2): 203-12.
[http://dx.doi.org/10.2174/156720511795256053] [PMID: 21222604]

[209] Khan TK, Nelson TJ, Verma VA, Wender PA, Alkon DL. A cellular model of Alzheimer's disease therapeutic efficacy: PKC activation reverses Abeta-induced biomarker abnormality on cultured fibroblasts. Neurobiol Dis 2009; 34(2): 332-9.

[http://dx.doi.org/10.1016/j.nbd.2009.02.003] [PMID: 19233276]

[210] Bilikiewicz A, Gaus W. Colostrinin (a naturally occurring, proline-rich, polypeptide mixture) in the treatment of Alzheimer's disease. J Alzheimers Dis 2004; 6(1): 17-26. [http://dx.doi.org/10.3233/JAD-2004-6103] [PMID: 15004324]

[211] Matlack KE, Tardiff DF, Narayan P, *et al.* Clioquinol promotes the degradation of metal-dependent amyloid-β (Aβ) oligomers to restore endocytosis and ameliorate Aβ toxicity. Proc Natl Acad Sci USA 2014; 111(11): 4013-8. [http://dx.doi.org/10.1073/pnas.1402228111] [PMID: 24591589]

[212] Gilman S, Koller M, Black RS, *et al.* Clinical effects of Abeta immunization (AN1792) in patients with AD in an interrupted trial. Neurology 2005; 64(9): 1553-62. [http://dx.doi.org/10.1212/01.WNL.0000159740.16984.3C] [PMID: 15883316]

[213] Tayeb HO, Murray ED, Price BH, Tarazi FI. Bapineuzumab and solanezumab for Alzheimer's disease: is the 'amyloid cascade hypothesis' still alive? Expert Opin Biol Ther 2013; 13(7): 1075-84. [http://dx.doi.org/10.1517/14712598.2013.789856] [PMID: 23574434]

[214] Colović MB, Krstić DZ, Lazarević-Pašti TD, Bondžić AM, Vasić VM. Acetylcholinesterase inhibitors: pharmacology and toxicology. Curr Neuropharmacol 2013; 11(3): 315-35. [http://dx.doi.org/10.2174/1570159X11311030006] [PMID: 24179466]

[215] Mehta M, Adem A, Sabbagh M. New acetylcholinesterase inhibitors for Alzheimer's disease. Int J Alzheimers Dis 2011; 2012. [PMID: 22216416]

[216] Galimberti D, Scarpini E. Old and new acetylcholinesterase inhibitors for Alzheimer's disease. Expert Opin Investig Drugs 2016; 25(10): 1181-7. [http://dx.doi.org/10.1080/13543784.2016.1216972] [PMID: 27459153]

[217] Liu H, Wang L, Lv M, *et al.* AlzPlatform: an Alzheimer's disease domain-specific chemogenomics knowledgebase for polypharmacology and target identification research. J Chem Inf Model 2014; 54(4): 1050-60. [http://dx.doi.org/10.1021/ci500004h] [PMID: 24597646]

[218] Nikolic K, Mavridis L, Djikic T, *et al.* Drug design for CNS diseases: polypharmacological profiling of compounds using cheminformatic, 3D-QSAR and virtual screening methodologies. Front Neurosci 2016; 10: 265. [http://dx.doi.org/10.3389/fnins.2016.00265] [PMID: 27375423]

[219] Hill JM, Clement C, Pogue AI, Bhattacharjee S, Zhao Y, Lukiw WJ. Pathogenic microbes, the microbiome, and Alzheimer's disease (AD). Front Aging Neurosci 2014; 6: 127. [PMID: 24982633]

[220] Bhattacharjee S, Lukiw WJ. Alzheimer's disease and the microbiome. Front Cell Neurosci 2013; 7: 153. [http://dx.doi.org/10.3389/fncel.2013.00153] [PMID: 24062644]

[221] Honjo K, van Reekum R, Verhoeff NP. Alzheimer's disease and infection: do infectious agents contribute to progression of Alzheimer's disease? Alzheimers Dement 2009; 5(4): 348-60. [http://dx.doi.org/10.1016/j.jalz.2008.12.001] [PMID: 19560105]

[222] Itzhaki R. Herpes simplex virus type 1, apolipoprotein E and Alzheimer's disease. Herpes: the journal of the IHMF 2004; 11: 77A-82A.

[223] Contini C, Seraceni S, Cultrera R, Castellazzi M, Granieri E, Fainardi E. Chlamydophila pneumoniae infection and its role in neurological disorders. Interdiscip Perspect Infect Dis 2010; 2010: 273573. [http://dx.doi.org/10.1155/2010/273573] [PMID: 20182626]

[224] Bu XL, Yao XQ, Jiao SS, *et al.* A study on the association between infectious burden and Alzheimer's disease. Eur J Neurol 2015; 22(12): 1519-25. [http://dx.doi.org/10.1111/ene.12477] [PMID: 24910016]

[225] Bertram L, McQueen MB, Mullin K, Blacker D, Tanzi RE. Systematic meta-analyses of Alzheimer disease genetic association studies: the AlzGene database. Nat Genet 2007; 39(1): 17-23. [http://dx.doi.org/10.1038/ng1934] [PMID: 17192785]

[226] Olsson B, Lautner R, Andreasson U, Öhrfelt A, Portelius E, Bjerke M, *et al.* Alzbiomarker database on established and novel CSF and plasma biomarkers for Alzheimer's disease. Alzheimer's & Dementia. Journal of the Alzheimer's Association 2015; 11(7): 302. [http://dx.doi.org/10.1016/j.jalz.2015.07.422]

[227] Weuve J, McQueen MB, Harrington M, O'Brien J, Li S, Power M, *et al.* The AlzRisk database: Web-based catalogue and meta-analysis of findings from epidemiologic studies of non-genetic risk factors for Alzheimer's disease. Alzheimers Dement 2010; 6(4): S125. [http://dx.doi.org/10.1016/j.jalz.2010.05.392]

[228] Gangadharan P, Partch AB, Valladares O, Greenfest-Allen E, Childress DM, Cweibel R, *et al.* NIA GENETICS OF ALZHEIMER'S DISEASE DATA STORAGE SITE (NIAGADS): 2016 UPDATE. Alzheimer's & Dementia. Journal of the Alzheimer's Association 2016; 12(7): 855-P856. [http://dx.doi.org/10.1016/j.jalz.2016.06.1752]

[229] James P. An Essay on the Shaking Palsy. J Nerv Ment Dis 1924; 60(4): 441. [http://dx.doi.org/10.1097/00005053-192410000-00124]

[230] Pollock M, Hornabrook RW. The prevalence, natural history and dementia of Parkinson's disease. Brain 1966; 89(3): 429-48. [http://dx.doi.org/10.1093/brain/89.3.429] [PMID: 5921126]

[231] Ehringer H, Hornykiewicz O. Verteilung von noradrenalin and dopamin im gehirn des menschen und ihr verhalten bei erkrankungen des extrapyramidalen systems. Klin Wochenschr 1960; 38: 1126-239. [http://dx.doi.org/10.1007/BF01485901]

[232] Jankovic J. Parkinson's disease: clinical features and diagnosis. J Neurol Neurosurg Psychiatry 2008; 79(4): 368-76. [http://dx.doi.org/10.1136/jnnp.2007.131045] [PMID: 18344392]

[233] Helmich RC, Hallett M, Deuschl G, Toni I, Bloem BR. Cerebral causes and consequences of parkinsonian resting tremor: a tale of two circuits? Brain 2012; 135(Pt 11): 3206-26. [http://dx.doi.org/10.1093/brain/aws023] [PMID: 22382359]

[234] Hoehn MM, Yahr MD. Parkinsonism: onset, progression, and mortality. 1967. Neurology 2001; 57(10) (Suppl. 3): S11-26. [PMID: 11775596]

[235] Berardelli A, Rothwell JC, Thompson PD, Hallett M. Pathophysiology of bradykinesia in Parkinson's disease. Brain 2001; 124(Pt 11): 2131-46. [http://dx.doi.org/10.1093/brain/124.11.2131] [PMID: 11673316]

[236] Kim SD, Allen NE, Canning CG, Fung VS. Postural instability in patients with Parkinson's disease. Epidemiology, pathophysiology and management. CNS Drugs 2013; 27(2): 97-112. [http://dx.doi.org/10.1007/s40263-012-0012-3] [PMID: 23076544]

[237] Gollob MH, Green MS, Tang AS, *et al.* Identification of a gene responsible for familial Wolff-Parkinson-White syndrome. N Engl J Med 2001; 344(24): 1823-31. [http://dx.doi.org/10.1056/NEJM200106143442403] [PMID: 11407343]

[238] Nuytemans K, Theuns J, Cruts M, Van Broeckhoven C. Genetic etiology of Parkinson disease associated with mutations in the SNCA, PARK2, PINK1, PARK7, and LRRK2 genes: a mutation update. Hum Mutat 2010; 31(7): 763-80. [http://dx.doi.org/10.1002/humu.21277] [PMID: 20506312]

[239] Klein C, Chuang R, Marras C, Lang AE. The curious case of phenocopies in families with genetic Parkinson's disease. Mov Disord 2011; 26(10): 1793-802. [http://dx.doi.org/10.1002/mds.23853] [PMID: 21735483]

[240] Li J-Q, Tan L, Yu J-T. The role of the LRRK2 gene in Parkinsonism. Mol Neurodegener 2014; 9: 47. [http://dx.doi.org/10.1186/1750-1326-9-47] [PMID: 25391693]

[241] MacLeod D, Dowman J, Hammond R, Leete T, Inoue K, Abeliovich A. The familial Parkinsonism gene LRRK2 regulates neurite process morphology. Neuron 2006; 52(4): 587-93. [http://dx.doi.org/10.1016/j.neuron.2006.10.008] [PMID: 17114044]

[242] Miklya I, Göltl P, Hafenscher F, Pencz N. The role of parkin in Parkinson's disease. Neuropsychopharmacologia Hungarica: a Magyar Pszichofarmakologiai Egyesulet lapja 2014; 16(2): 67-76.

[243] Dawson TM, Dawson VL. The role of parkin in familial and sporadic Parkinson's disease. Mov Disord 2010; 25(S1) (Suppl. 1): S32-9. [http://dx.doi.org/10.1002/mds.22798] [PMID: 20187240]

[244] Valente EM, Salvi S, Ialongo T, *et al.* PINK1 mutations are associated with sporadic early-onset parkinsonism. Ann Neurol 2004; 56(3): 336-41. [http://dx.doi.org/10.1002/ana.20256] [PMID: 15349860]

[245] Morais VA, Verstreken P, Roethig A, *et al.* Parkinson's disease mutations in PINK1 result in decreased Complex I activity and deficient synaptic function. EMBO Mol Med 2009; 1(2): 99-111. [http://dx.doi.org/10.1002/emmm.200900006] [PMID: 20049710]

[246] Kumazawa R, Tomiyama H, Li Y, *et al.* Mutation analysis of the PINK1 gene in 391 patients with Parkinson disease. Arch Neurol 2008; 65(6): 802-8. [http://dx.doi.org/10.1001/archneur.65.6.802] [PMID: 18541801]

[247] Song S, Jang S, Park J, *et al.* Characterization of PINK1 (PTEN-induced putative kinase 1) mutations associated with Parkinson disease in mammalian cells and Drosophila. J Biol Chem 2013; 288(8): 5660-72. [http://dx.doi.org/10.1074/jbc.M112.430801] [PMID: 23303188]

[248] Ariga H, Takahashi-Niki K, Kato I, Maita H, Niki T, Iguchi-Ariga SM. Neuroprotective function of DJ-1 in Parkinson's disease. Oxid Med Cell Longev 2013; 2013: 683920. [http://dx.doi.org/10.1155/2013/683920] [PMID: 23766857]

[249] Lev N, Roncevic D, Ickowicz D, Melamed E, Offen D. Role of DJ-1 in Parkinson's disease. J Mol Neurosci 2006; 29(3): 215-25. [http://dx.doi.org/10.1385/JMN:29:3:215] [PMID: 17085780]

[250] Takahashi-Niki K, Niki T, Taira T, Iguchi-Ariga SM, Ariga H. Reduced anti-oxidative stress activities of DJ-1 mutants found in Parkinson's disease patients. Biochem Biophys Res Commun 2004; 320(2): 389-97. [http://dx.doi.org/10.1016/j.bbrc.2004.05.187] [PMID: 15219840]

[251] Malgieri G, Eliezer D. Structural effects of Parkinson's disease linked DJ-1 mutations. Protein Sci 2008; 17(5): 855-68. [http://dx.doi.org/10.1110/ps.073411608] [PMID: 18436956]

[252] Willis AW, Evanoff BA, Lian M, *et al.* Metal emissions and urban incident Parkinson disease: a community health study of Medicare beneficiaries by using geographic information systems. Am J Epidemiol 2010; 172(12): 1357-63. [http://dx.doi.org/10.1093/aje/kwq303] [PMID: 20959505]

[253] Koller W, Vetere-Overfield B, Gray C, *et al.* Environmental risk factors in Parkinson's disease. Neurology 1990; 40(8): 1218-21. [http://dx.doi.org/10.1212/WNL.40.8.1218] [PMID: 2381528]

[254] Gorell JM, Johnson CC, Rybicki BA, Peterson EL, Richardson RJ. The risk of Parkinson's disease with exposure to pesticides, farming, well water, and rural living. Neurology 1998; 50(5): 1346-50. [http://dx.doi.org/10.1212/WNL.50.5.1346] [PMID: 9595985]

[255] Firestone JA, Lundin JI, Powers KM, *et al.* Occupational factors and risk of Parkinson's disease: A population-based case-control study. Am J Ind Med 2010; 53(3): 217-23. [PMID: 20025075]

[256] Park J, Yoo CI, Sim CS, *et al.* Occupations and Parkinson's disease: a multi-center case-control study in South Korea. Neurotoxicology 2005; 26(1): 99-105. [http://dx.doi.org/10.1016/j.neuro.2004.07.001] [PMID: 15527877]

[257] Hertzman C, Wiens M, Bowering D, Snow B, Calne D. Parkinson's disease: a case-control study of occupational and environmental risk factors. Am J Ind Med 1990; 17(3): 349-55. [http://dx.doi.org/10.1002/ajim.4700170307] [PMID: 2305814]

[258] Chen H, Schernhammer E, Schwarzschild MA, Ascherio A. A prospective study of night shift work, sleep duration, and risk of Parkinson's disease. Am J Epidemiol 2006; 163(8): 726-30. [http://dx.doi.org/10.1093/aje/kwj096] [PMID: 16495472]

[259] Uversky VN, Li J, Fink AL. Metal-triggered structural transformations, aggregation, and fibrillation of human α-synuclein. A possible molecular NK between Parkinson's disease and heavy metal exposure. J Biol Chem 2001; 276(47): 44284-96. [http://dx.doi.org/10.1074/jbc.M105343200] [PMID: 11553618]

[260] Giasson BI, Lee VM. A new link between pesticides and Parkinson's disease. Nat Neurosci 2000; 3(12): 1227-8. [http://dx.doi.org/10.1038/81737] [PMID: 11100135]

[261] Goldstein DS, Sullivan P, Cooney A, Jinsmaa Y, Kopin IJ, Sharabi Y. Rotenone decreases intracellular aldehyde dehydrogenase activity: implications for the pathogenesis of Parkinson's disease. J Neurochem 2015; 133(1): 14-25. [http://dx.doi.org/10.1111/jnc.13042] [PMID: 25645689]

[262] Qi Z, Miller GW, Voit EO. Rotenone and paraquat perturb dopamine metabolism: A computational analysis of pesticide toxicity. Toxicology 2014; 315: 92-101. [http://dx.doi.org/10.1016/j.tox.2013.11.003] [PMID: 24269752]

[263] Fujita KA, Ostaszewski M, Matsuoka Y, *et al.* Integrating pathways of Parkinson's disease in a molecular interaction map. Mol Neurobiol 2014; 49(1): 88-102. [http://dx.doi.org/10.1007/s12035-013-8489-4] [PMID: 23832570]

[264] Winklhofer KF, Haass C. Mitochondrial dysfunction in Parkinson's disease. Biochimica et Biophysica Acta (BBA)-. Molecular Basis of Disease 2010; 1802(1): 29-44. [http://dx.doi.org/10.1016/j.bbadis.2009.08.013]

[265] Breydo L, Wu JW, Uversky VN. A-synuclein misfolding and Parkinson's disease. Biochimica et Biophysica Acta (BBA)-. Molecular Basis of Disease 2012; 1822(2): 261-85. [http://dx.doi.org/10.1016/j.bbadis.2011.10.002]

[266] Stefanis L. α-Synuclein in Parkinson's disease. Cold Spring Harb Perspect Med 2012; 2(2): a009399. [http://dx.doi.org/10.1101/cshperspect.a009399] [PMID: 22355802]

[267] Malkus KA, Tsika E, Ischiropoulos H. Oxidative modifications, mitochondrial dysfunction, and impaired protein degradation in Parkinson's disease: how neurons are lost in the Bermuda triangle. Mol Neurodegener 2009; 4(24): 24. [http://dx.doi.org/10.1186/1750-1326-4-24] [PMID: 19500376]

[268] Tansey MG, Goldberg MS. Neuroinflammation in Parkinson's disease: its role in neuronal death and implications for therapeutic intervention. Neurobiol Dis 2010; 37(3): 510-8. [http://dx.doi.org/10.1016/j.nbd.2009.11.004] [PMID: 19913097]

[269] Frank-Cannon TC, Tran T, Ruhn KA, *et al.* Parkin deficiency increases vulnerability to inflammation-related nigral degeneration. J Neurosci 2008; 28(43): 10825-34. [http://dx.doi.org/10.1523/JNEUROSCI.3001-08.2008] [PMID: 18945890]

[270] Brooks DJ. Parkinson's disease: diagnosis. Parkinsonism Relat Disord 2012; 18 (Suppl. 1): S31-3. [http://dx.doi.org/10.1016/S1353-8020(11)70012-8] [PMID: 22166447]

[271] Stoessl AJ. Neuroimaging in Parkinson's disease: from pathology to diagnosis. Parkinsonism Relat Disord 2012; 18 (Suppl. 1): S55-9. [http://dx.doi.org/10.1016/S1353-8020(11)70019-0] [PMID: 22166455]

[272] Fahn S, Oakes D, Shoulson I, *et al.* Levodopa and the progression of Parkinson's disease. N Engl J Med 2004; 351(24): 2498-508. [http://dx.doi.org/10.1056/NEJMoa033447] [PMID: 15590952]

[273] Carlson JH, Bergstrom DA, Walters JR. Stimulation of both D1 and D2 dopamine receptors appears necessary for full expression of postsynaptic effects of dopamine agonists: a neurophysiological study. Brain Res 1987; 400(2): 205-18. [http://dx.doi.org/10.1016/0006-8993(87)90619-6] [PMID: 2880637]

[274] Youdim MB, Bakhle YS. Monoamine oxidase: isoforms and inhibitors in Parkinson's disease and depressive illness. Br J Pharmacol 2006; 147(S1) (Suppl. 1): S287-96. [http://dx.doi.org/10.1038/sj.bjp.0706464] [PMID: 16402116]

[275] Ruottinen HM, Rinne UK. COMT inhibition in the treatment of Parkinson's disease. J Neurol 1998; 245(11) (Suppl. 3): 25-34. [http://dx.doi.org/10.1007/PL00007743] [PMID: 9808337]

[276] Brocks DR. Anticholinergic drugs used in Parkinson's disease: An overlooked class of drugs from a pharmacokinetic perspective. J Pharm Pharm Sci 1999; 2(2): 39-46. [PMID: 10952768]

[277] Warren N, Burn DJ. The Use of Amantadine in Parkinson's Disease and other Akinetic-Rigid Disorders. Drugs in Neurology 2004; 4-41.(5): 38-41.

[278] Stocchi F. Use of apomorphine in Parkinson's disease. Neurol Sci 2008; 29(5) (Suppl. 5): S383-6. [http://dx.doi.org/10.1007/s10072-008-1053-8] [PMID: 19381769]

[279] Chen S, Le W. Neuroprotective therapy in Parkinson disease. Am J Ther 2006; 13(5): 445-57. [http://dx.doi.org/10.1097/01.mjt.0000174353.28012.a7] [PMID: 16988541]

[280] Sullivan AM, Toulouse A. Neurotrophic factors for the treatment of Parkinson's disease. Cytokine Growth Factor Rev 2011; 22(3): 157-65. [http://dx.doi.org/10.1016/j.cytogfr.2011.05.001] [PMID: 21689963]

[281] Szigeti E. Nursing care of patients with Parkinson's disease. Neurosci Biobehav Rev 1988; 12(3-4): 307-9. [http://dx.doi.org/10.1016/S0149-7634(88)80063-0] [PMID: 3226657]

[282] Seidl SE, Santiago JA, Bilyk H, Potashkin JA. The emerging role of nutrition in Parkinson's disease. Front Aging Neurosci 2014; 6: 36. [http://dx.doi.org/10.3389/fnagi.2014.00036] [PMID: 24639650]

[283] Aminoff MJ. Treatment of Parkinson's disease. West J Med 1994; 161(3): 303-8. [PMID: 7975571]

[284] Lang AE. Surgery for Parkinson disease: A critical evaluation of the state of the art. Arch Neurol 2000; 57(8): 1118-25. [http://dx.doi.org/10.1001/archneur.57.8.1118] [PMID: 10927791]

[285] Yang JO, Kim WY, Jeong SY, *et al.* PDbase: a database of Parkinson's disease-related genes and genetic variation using substantia nigra ESTs. BMC Genomics 2009; 10 (Suppl. 3): S32. [http://dx.doi.org/10.1186/1471-2164-10-S3-S32] [PMID: 19958497]

[286] Cruts M, Theuns J, Van Broeckhoven C. Locus-specific mutation databases for neurodegenerative brain diseases. Hum Mutat 2012; 33(9): 1340-4. [http://dx.doi.org/10.1002/humu.22117] [PMID: 22581678]

[287] Lill CM, Roehr JT, McQueen MB, *et al.* Comprehensive research synopsis and systematic meta-analyses in Parkinson's disease genetics: The PDGene database. PLoS Genet 2012; 8(3): e1002548. [http://dx.doi.org/10.1371/journal.pgen.1002548] [PMID: 22438815]

[288] Taccioli C, Tegnér J, Maselli V, *et al.* ParkDB: a Parkinson's disease gene expression database. The Journal of Biological Databases and Curation 2011; bar007. [http://dx.doi.org/10.1093/database/bar007]

[289] Tang S, Zhang Z, Kavitha G, Tan E-K, Ng SK. MDPD: an integrated genetic information resource for Parkinson's disease. Nucleic Acids Res 2009; 37(Database issue): D858-62. [http://dx.doi.org/10.1093/nar/gkn770] [PMID: 18948286]

[290] Owen R. Schizophrenia–From devilry to disease. Resen Med 2014; 22(1): 126-32.

[291] Kyziridis TC. Notes on the history of schizophrenia. Ger J Psychiatry 2005; 8(3): 8-42.

[292] Kirkpatrick B, Messias E, Harvey PD, Fernandez-Egea E, Bowie CR. Is schizophrenia a syndrome of accelerated aging? Schizophr Bull 2008; 34(6): 1024-32. [http://dx.doi.org/10.1093/schbul/sbm140] [PMID: 18156637]

[293] Shibre T, Kebede D, Alem A, *et al.* Schizophrenia: illness impact on family members in a traditional society--rural Ethiopia. Soc Psychiatry Psychiatr Epidemiol 2003; 38(1): 27-34. [http://dx.doi.org/10.1007/s00127-003-0594-7] [PMID: 12563556]

[294] McNally K. Schizophrenia as split personality/Jekyll and Hyde: the origins of the informal usage in the English language. J Hist Behav Sci 2007; 43(1): 69-79. [http://dx.doi.org/10.1002/jhbs.20209] [PMID: 17205539]

[295] Kochunov P, Hong LE. Neurodevelopmental and neurodegenerative models of schizophrenia: white matter at the center stage. Schizophr Bull 2014; 40(4): 721-8. [http://dx.doi.org/10.1093/schbul/sbu070] [PMID: 24870447]

[296] Rapoport JL, Addington AM, Frangou S, Psych MR. The neurodevelopmental model of schizophrenia: update 2005. Mol Psychiatry 2005; 10(5): 434-49. [http://dx.doi.org/10.1038/sj.mp.4001642] [PMID: 15700048]

[297] Marenco S, Weinberger DR. The neurodevelopmental hypothesis of schizophrenia: following a trail of evidence from cradle to grave. Dev Psychopathol 2000; 12(3): 501-27. [http://dx.doi.org/10.1017/S0954579400003138] [PMID: 11014750]

[298] Niemi LT, Suvisaari JM, Tuulio-Henriksson A, Lönnqvist JK. Childhood developmental abnormalities in schizophrenia: evidence from high-risk studies. Schizophr Res 2003; 60(2-3): 239-58. [http://dx.doi.org/10.1016/S0920-9964(02)00234-7] [PMID: 12591587]

[299] Schiffman J, LaBrie J, Carter J, *et al.* Perception of parent-child relationships in high-risk families, and adult schizophrenia outcome of offspring. J Psychiatr Res 2002; 36(1): 41-7. [http://dx.doi.org/10.1016/S0022-3956(01)00046-2] [PMID: 11755460]

[300] Erlenmeyer-Kimling L. Neurobehavioral deficits in offspring of schizophrenic parents: liability indicators and predictors of illness. Am J Med Genet 2000; 97(1): 65-71. [http://dx.doi.org/10.1002/(SICI)1096-8628(200021)97:1<65::AID-AJMG9>3.0.CO;2-V] [PMID: 10813806]

[301] Rapoport JL, Giedd JN, Blumenthal J, *et al.* Progressive cortical change during adolescence in childhood-onset schizophrenia. A longitudinal magnetic resonance imaging study. Arch Gen Psychiatry 1999; 56(7): 649-54. [http://dx.doi.org/10.1001/archpsyc.56.7.649] [PMID: 10401513]

[302] Thompson PM, Vidal C, Giedd JN, *et al.* Mapping adolescent brain change reveals dynamic wave of accelerated gray matter loss in very early-onset schizophrenia. Proc Natl Acad Sci USA 2001; 98(20): 11650-5. [http://dx.doi.org/10.1073/pnas.201243998] [PMID: 11573002]

[303] Harrison PJ. Postmortem studies in schizophrenia. Dialogues Clin Neurosci 2000; 2(4): 349-57. [PMID: 22033474]

[304] Pino O, Guilera G, Gómez-Benito J, Najas-García A, Rufián S, Rojo E. Neurodevelopment or neurodegeneration: review of theories of schizophrenia. Actas Esp Psiquiatr 2014; 42(4): 185-95. [PMID: 25017496]

[305] McClure RK, Lieberman JA. Neurodevelopmental and neurodegenerative hypotheses of schizophrenia: a review and critique. Curr Opin Psychiatry 2003; 16: S15-28. [http://dx.doi.org/10.1097/00001504-200304002-00004]

[306] Andreasen NC, Flaum M. Schizophrenia: the characteristic symptoms. Schizophr Bull 1991; 17(1): 27-49. [http://dx.doi.org/10.1093/schbul/17.1.27] [PMID: 2047788]

[307] Picchioni MM, Murray RM. Schizophrenia. BMJ 2007; 335(7610): 91-5. [http://dx.doi.org/10.1136/bmj.39227.616447.BE] [PMID: 17626963]

[308] Owen MJ, Williams NM, O'Donovan MC. The molecular genetics of schizophrenia: new findings promise new insights. Mol Psychiatry 2004; 9(1): 14-27. [http://dx.doi.org/10.1038/sj.mp.4001444] [PMID: 14581932]

[309] Dean K, Murray RM. Environmental risk factors for psychosis. Dialogues Clin Neurosci 2005; 7(1): 69-80. [PMID: 16060597]

[310] Cannon M, Tarrant CJ, Huttunen MO, Jones P. Childhood development and later schizophrenia: evidence from genetic high-risk and birth cohort studies. Cambridge University Press 2003; pp. 100-23.

[311] Bradbury TN, Miller GA. Season of birth in schizophrenia: a review of evidence, methodology, and etiology. Psychol Bull 1985; 98(3): 569-94. [http://dx.doi.org/10.1037/0033-2909.98.3.569] [PMID: 4080898]

[312] Brown AS. Prenatal infection and adult schizophrenia: a review and synthesis, int. J Ment Health 2001; 29: 22-37. [http://dx.doi.org/10.1080/00207411.2000.11449501]

[313] Kinney D. Prenatal stress and risk for schizophrenia. Int J Ment Health 2001; 29: 62-72. [http://dx.doi.org/10.1080/00207411.2000.11449503]

[314] Susser E, Hoek HW, Brown A. Neurodevelopmental disorders after prenatal famine: The story of the Dutch Famine Study. Am J Epidemiol 1998; 147(3): 213-6. [http://dx.doi.org/10.1093/oxfordjournals.aje.a009439] [PMID: 9482494]

[315] Hollister JM, Laing P, Mednick SA. Rhesus incompatibility as a risk factor for schizophrenia in male adults. Arch Gen Psychiatry 1996; 53(1): 19-24. [http://dx.doi.org/10.1001/archpsyc.1996.01830010021004] [PMID: 8540773]

[316] Cannon M, Caspi A, Moffitt TE, *et al.* Evidence for early-childhood, pan-developmental impairment specific to schizophreniform disorder: results from a longitudinal birth cohort. Arch Gen Psychiatry 2002; 59(5): 449-56. [http://dx.doi.org/10.1001/archpsyc.59.5.449] [PMID: 11982449]

[317] Agid O, Shapira B, Zislin J, *et al.* Environment and vulnerability to major psychiatric illness: a case control study of early parental loss in major depression, bipolar disorder and schizophrenia. Mol Psychiatry 1999; 4(2): 163-72. [http://dx.doi.org/10.1038/sj.mp.4000473] [PMID: 10208448]

[318] Jones P, Rodgers B, Murray R, Marmot M. Child development risk factors for adult schizophrenia in the British 1946 birth cohort. Lancet 1994; 344(8934): 1398-402. [http://dx.doi.org/10.1016/S0140-6736(94)90569-X] [PMID: 7968076]

[319] Sachdev P. Schizophrenia-like psychosis following traumatic brain injury. J Neuropsychiatry Clin Neurosci 2001; 13(4): 533-4.
[http://dx.doi.org/10.1176/jnp.13.4.533] [PMID: 11748328]

[320] Chen CK, Lin SK, Sham PC, *et al.* Pre-morbid characteristics and co-morbidity of methamphetamine users with and without psychosis. Psychol Med 2003; 33(8): 1407-14.
[http://dx.doi.org/10.1017/S0033291703008353] [PMID: 14672249]

[321] D'Souza DC, Abi-Saad W, Madonick S, *et al.* Cannabinoids and psychosis: evidence from studies with iv THC in schizophrenia patients and controls. Schizophr Res 2000; 41(special issue): 33.
[http://dx.doi.org/10.1016/S0920-9964(00)90371-2]

[322] Freeman H. Schizophrenia and city residence. Br J Psychiatry Suppl 1994; (23): 39-50.
[PMID: 8037900]

[323] Selten JP, Cantor-Graae E. Schizophrenia and migration. In: Gattaz WF, Hafner H, Eds. Search for the Causes of Schizophrenia. Berlin, Germany: Steinkopff Verlag 2004; pp. 3-25.
[http://dx.doi.org/10.1007/978-3-7985-1953-4_1]

[324] Sharpley M, Hutchinson G, McKenzie K, Murray RM. Understanding the excess of psychosis among the African-Caribbean population in England. Review of current hypotheses. Br J Psychiatry Suppl 2001; 40: s60-8.
[http://dx.doi.org/10.1192/bjp.178.40.s60] [PMID: 11315227]

[325] Malla AK, Norman RM. Relationship of major life events and daily stressors to symptomatology in schizophrenia. J Nerv Ment Dis 1992; 180(10): 664-7.
[http://dx.doi.org/10.1097/00005053-199210000-00011] [PMID: 1402848]

[326] Brisch R, Saniotis A, Wolf R, *et al.* The role of dopamine in schizophrenia from a neurobiological and evolutionary perspective: old fashioned, but still in vogue. Front Psychiatry 2014; 19(5): 47.
[http://dx.doi.org/10.3389/fpsyt.2014.00047]

[327] Hökfelt T, Ljungdahl A, Fuxe K, Johansson O. Dopamine nerve terminals in the rat limbic cortex: aspects of the dopamine hypothesis of schizophrenia. Science 1974; 184(4133): 177-9.
[http://dx.doi.org/10.1126/science.184.4133.177] [PMID: 4856104]

[328] da Silva Alves F, Figee M, van Amelsvoort T, Veltman D, de Haan L. The revised dopamine hypothesis of schizophrenia: evidence from pharmacological MRI studies with atypical antipsychotic medication. Psychopharmacol Bull 2008; 41(1): 121-32.
[PMID: 18362875]

[329] Domyo T, Kurumaji A, Toru M. An increase in [3H]SCH23390 binding in the cerebral cortex of postmortem brains of chronic schizophrenics. J Neural Transm (Vienna) 2001; 108(12): 1475-84.
[http://dx.doi.org/10.1007/s007020100021] [PMID: 11810409]

[330] Tallerico T, Novak G, Liu IS, Ulpian C, Seeman P. Schizophrenia: elevated mRNA for dopamine D2(Longer) receptors in frontal cortex. Brain Res Mol Brain Res 2001; 87(2): 160-5.
[http://dx.doi.org/10.1016/S0169-328X(00)00293-X] [PMID: 11245917]

[331] Takahashi H, Higuchi M, Suhara T. The role of extrastriatal dopamine D2 receptors in schizophrenia. Biol Psychiatry 2006; 59(10): 919-28.
[http://dx.doi.org/10.1016/j.biopsych.2006.01.022] [PMID: 16682269]

[332] Jardemark K, Wadenberg ML, Grillner P, Svensson TH. Dopamine D3 and D4 receptor antagonists in the treatment of schizophrenia. Curr Opin Investig Drugs 2002; 3(1): 101-5.
[PMID: 12054059]

[333] Hashimoto K, Okamura N, Shimizu E, Iyo M. Glutamate hypothesis of schizophrenia and approach for possible therapeutic drugs. Curr Med Chem Cent Nerv Syst Agents 2004; 4(2): 147-54.
[http://dx.doi.org/10.2174/1568015043357011]

[334] Kim JS, Kornhuber HH, Schmid-Burgk W, Holzmüller B. Low cerebrospinal fluid glutamate in

schizophrenic patients and a new hypothesis on schizophrenia. Neurosci Lett 1980; 20(3): 379-82. [http://dx.doi.org/10.1016/0304-3940(80)90178-0] [PMID: 6108541]

[335] Moghaddam B, Javitt D. From revolution to evolution: the glutamate hypothesis of schizophrenia and its implication for treatment. Neuropsychopharmacology 2012; 37(1): 4-15. [http://dx.doi.org/10.1038/npp.2011.181] [PMID: 21956446]

[336] Clinton SM, Meador-Woodruff JH. Abnormalities of the NMDA Receptor and Associated Intracellular Molecules in the Thalamus in Schizophrenia and Bipolar Disorder. Neuropsychopharmacology 2004; 29(7): 1353-62. [http://dx.doi.org/10.1038/sj.npp.1300451] [PMID: 15054476]

[337] Tsai G, Passani LA, Slusher BS, *et al.* Abnormal excitatory neurotransmitter metabolism in schizophrenic brains. Arch Gen Psychiatry 1995; 52(10): 829-36. [http://dx.doi.org/10.1001/archpsyc.1995.03950220039008] [PMID: 7575102]

[338] Pilowsky LS, Bressan RA, Stone JM, *et al.* First in vivo evidence of an NMDA receptor deficit in medication-free schizophrenic patients. Mol Psychiatry 2006; 11(2): 118-9. [http://dx.doi.org/10.1038/sj.mp.4001751] [PMID: 16189506]

[339] Varju P, Katarova Z, Madarász E, Szabó G. GABA signalling during development: new data and old questions. Cell Tissue Res 2001; 305(2): 239-46. [http://dx.doi.org/10.1007/s004410100356] [PMID: 11545261]

[340] Koella WP. GABA systems and behavior. Adv Biochem Psychopharmacol 1981; 29: 11-21. [PMID: 6266210]

[341] Hinton T, Johnston GA. Role of GABAA Receptors in Schizophrenia 2008; 5: 180-94.

[342] Scarr E, Cowie TF, Kanellakis S, Sundram S, Pantelis C, Dean B. Decreased cortical muscarinic receptors define a subgroup of subjects with schizophrenia. Mol Psychiatry 2009; 14(11): 1017-23. [http://dx.doi.org/10.1038/mp.2008.28] [PMID: 18317461]

[343] Jones CK, Byun N, Bubser M. Muscarinic and nicotinic acetylcholine receptor agonists and allosteric modulators for the treatment of schizophrenia. Neuropsychopharmacology 2012; 37(1): 16-42. [http://dx.doi.org/10.1038/npp.2011.199] [PMID: 21956443]

[344] Raedler TJ, Bymaster FP, Tandon R, Copolov D, Dean B. Towards a muscarinic hypothesis of schizophrenia. Mol Psychiatry 2007; 12(3): 232-46. [PMID: 17146471]

[345] Akhondzadeh S. The 5-HT hypothesis of schizophrenia. IDrugs: the investigational drugs journal 2001; 4(3): 295-300.

[346] Aghajanian GK, Marek GJ. Serotonin model of schizophrenia: emerging role of glutamate mechanisms. Brain Res Brain Res Rev 2000; 31(2-3): 302-12. [http://dx.doi.org/10.1016/S0165-0173(99)00046-6] [PMID: 10719157]

[347] Geddes J, Freemantle N, Harrison P, Bebbington P. Atypical antipsychotics in the treatment of schizophrenia: systematic overview and meta-regression analysis. BMJ 2000; 321(7273): 1371-6. [http://dx.doi.org/10.1136/bmj.321.7273.1371] [PMID: 11099280]

[348] Luft B, Taylor D. A review of atypical antipsychotic drugs versus conventional medication in schizophrenia. Expert Opin Pharmacother 2006; 7(13): 1739-48. [http://dx.doi.org/10.1517/14656566.7.13.1739] [PMID: 16925501]

[349] Chien WT, Leung SF, Yeung FK, Wong WK. Current approaches to treatments for schizophrenia spectrum disorders, part II: psychosocial interventions and patient-focused perspectives in psychiatric care. Neuropsychiatr Dis Treat 2013; 9: 1463-81. [http://dx.doi.org/10.2147/NDT.S49263] [PMID: 24109184]

[350] Zhou M, Zhuang YL, Xu Q, Li YD, Shen Y. VSD: a database for schizophrenia candidate genes focusing on variations. Hum Mutat 2004; 23(1): 1-7.

[http://dx.doi.org/10.1002/humu.10289] [PMID: 14695526]

[351] Allen NC, Bagade S, McQueen MB, *et al.* Systematic meta-analyses and field synopsis of genetic association studies in schizophrenia: the SzGene database. Nat Genet 2008; 40(7): 827-34. [http://dx.doi.org/10.1038/ng.171] [PMID: 18583979]

[352] Jia P, Sun J, Guo AY, Zhao Z. SZGR: a comprehensive schizophrenia gene resource. Mol Psychiatry 2010; 15(5): 453-62. [http://dx.doi.org/10.1038/mp.2009.93] [PMID: 20424623]

CHAPTER 4

Neuroimmune Regulation of Pain and Inflammation: Targeting Glial Cells and Nociceptor Sensory Neurons Interaction

Victor Fattori[1], Sergio M. Borghi[1], Ana C. Rossaneis[1], Mariana M. Bertozzi[1], Thiago M. Cunha[2] and Waldiceu A. Verri, Jr[1,*]

[1] *Departamento de Ciências Patológicas, Centro de Ciências Biológicas, Universidade Estadual de Londrina, Rodovia Celso Garcia Cid KM480 PR445, Caixa Postal 10.011, CEP 86057-970, Londrina, Paraná, Brazil*

[2] *Department of Pharmacology, Ribeirão Preto Medical School, University of São Paulo, Avenida do Café 3900, CEP 14049-900, Ribeirão Preto, São Paulo, Brazil*

Abstract: Chronic pain, differently from nociceptive pain, results from a maladaptive response of the body. Accumulating evidence shows that the mechanism of persistent pathological pain is mediated by complex interactions between sensory neurons and glial cells, namely astrocytes, microglia, and oligodendrocytes. In this chapter, we focus on the current understanding of the neuroimmune contribution to pathological pain and the mechanisms by which glial cells interact with sensory neurons to modulate pain and inflammation. The glial cells biology and how sensory neurons can modulate inflammatory response are also highlighted topics in this chapter. Given the heterogeneous immune functions of different cells in the spinal cord and the sex differential role of glial cells in chronic pain, we also explore how this could be harnessed to develop new therapeutic approaches for pain relief.

Keywords: Allodynia, Analgesia, Clinical trials, Chronic pain, Cytokines, Depression, Hyperalgesia, Hypersensitivity, Inflammation, JNK, MAPK, Neuropathy, NF-κB, p38, Sex dimorphism.

INTRODUCTION

In the 19th century, with the necessity of sanitation and modernization of urban centers, the health regulation was on the forefront of the agenda of many governments. The advance in health regulatory issues allowed the implementation of policies that contributed to the cure/eradication of several diseases (smallpox

* **Corresponding author Waldiceu A. Verri, Jr:** Departamento de Ciências Patológicas, Centro de Ciências Biológicas, Universidade Estadual de Londrina, Rodovia Celso Garcia Cid KM480 PR445, Caixa Postal 10.011, CEP 86057-970, Londrina, Paraná, Brazil; Tel: + 55 43 3371-4979; Fax: +55 43 3371 4387; E-mail: waverri@uel.br; waldiceujr@yahoo.com.br

Atta-ur-Rahman & M. Iqbal Choudhary (Eds.)

and polio, for instance) favoring the increase of human life expectancy and (paradoxically, but inevitably) the emergence of diseases that once did not exist. The progressive increase in human survival is one of the society's greatest achievements and a considerable challenge faced in this new phase of society is to deal with the fact that many of chronic diseases are followed by chronic pain. Differently from nociceptive pain, chronic pain results from a maladaptive response of the body. Nociceptive pain is a high threshold type of pain, *i.e.* it requires a stimulus of high intensity to induce pain. This type of pain possesses protective character with a learning component that helps to avoid potential tissue damage. In fact, individuals that are unable to feel pain (diagnosed with congenital insensitivity to pain) rarely get to adult life as they cannot differentiate non-noxious from noxious stimuli. Chronic pain, on the other hand, is a public health problem and has a negative impact on the quality life of affected patients. In fact, chronic pain is a consistent factor that leads to suicidal thoughts and behaviors [1] and has a straight relationship with depression [2] given that it occurs alongside with allodynia which impairs normal daily activities, such as walking. Of note, acute pain can also be pathological and thereby different from nociceptive pain. For instance, acute inflammatory pain is a type of acute pain that is detrimental if not managed with NSAIDs – in spite of possessing protective nature (*e.g.* in a case of ankle sprain, pain contributes by limiting the movement of the injured member). Thus, pathological pain is mainly characterized by the shift from a high threshold type of pain to a low threshold pain, *i.e.*, non-noxious stimuli can now induce pain.

The modern understanding of the physiology of pain starts with Treatise of Man's René Descartes, 1664. Descartes describes the pain as a perception that exists in the brain and he made distinction between the neural phenomenon of sensory transduction (nowadays known as nociception) and the perceptual experience of pain. To Descartes, the pain was a consequence of linear peripheral activation to the brain as observed by its iconic diagram of a boy near the bonfire [3]. Much has evolved since then. This evolution is exemplified by the definition of pain by the taxonomy committee of the International Association for the Study of Pain (IASP): "an unpleasant sensory and emotional experience associated with actual or potential tissue damage, or described in terms of such damage." Therefore, each person interprets pain accordingly to the experiences during life with varied emotional shades, which makes inconceivable the dissociation of the emotional character for the understanding of pain. Further, the emotional character influences on how patients with chronic pain feel it. Thus, chronic pain should be treated as the disease itself and not as a symptom, and this should be taken as relevant, especially by clinicians. In fact, previous pain-related experiences during life and expectancy regarding a stimulus change our nervous system and therefore the neuronal activity after an injury [4]. In this sense, the perception of pain involves regulation by excitatory and inhibitory circuits in the spinal cord that can either diminish or increase pain depending on mood, cognitive function, and memories. These elements also provide the neurobiological basis for the efficacy of placebo and suggestion. Other factors contribute importantly to the perception of pain such as the state of humor, the attention [5], and the expectations regarding the intensity of the stimulus [6]. The contemporary understanding of pain physiology includes peripheral and spinal cord sensitization of nociceptor neurons and change in the immune cells phenotypes. Mounting evidence shows that the mechanism of persistent pathological pain is mediated by complex interactions between sensory neurons and immune cells, namely astrocytes, microglia, and oligodendrocytes (Fig. **1**) [7, 8]. As such, in this chapter, we focus on the current understanding of the neuroimmune contribution to pathological pain and the mechanisms by which glial cells interact with sensory neurons to modulate pain and inflammation.

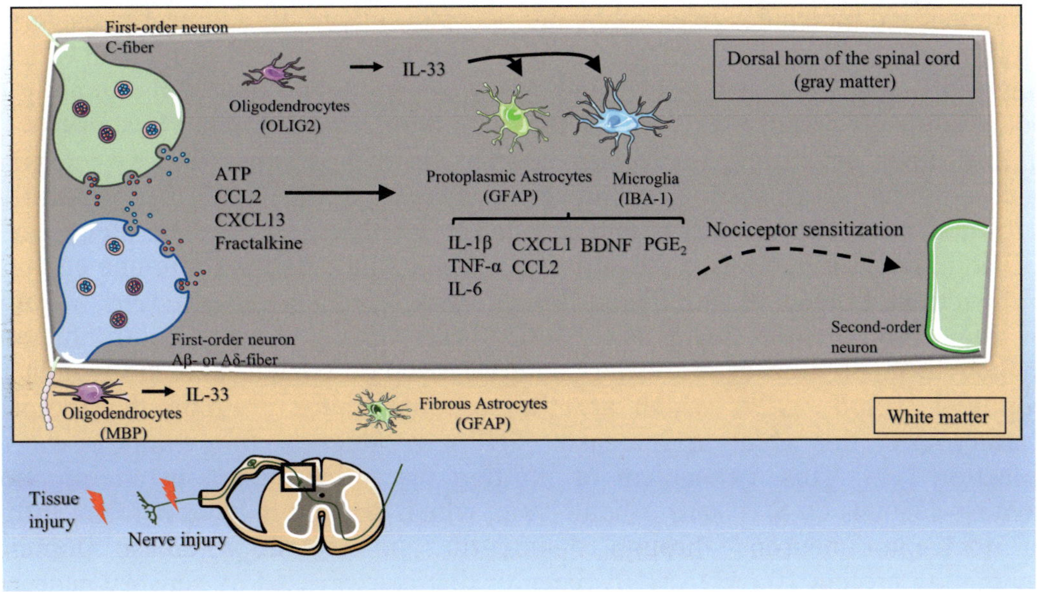

Fig. (1). Glial cells distribution in the spinal cord and overview of the interaction between glial cells and nociceptor neurons.
Upon tissue or nerve injury, astrocyte, microglia, and oligodendrocyte, modulate primary afferent nociceptors activity through the release of cytokines (*e.g.* IL-33, IL-1β, TNF-α, and IL-6), chemokines (*e.g.* CXCL1 and CCL2), growth factors (*e.g.* BDNF), and lipid mediators (*e.g.* PGE_2). Altogether, these molecules can trigger the activation or sensitization of post-synaptic neurons by binding specific receptors expressed by these nociceptors [7, 8].

MODULATION OF PERIPHERAL INFLAMMATION BY NOCICEPTOR NEURONS

In the past few years, the role of nociceptor neurons in the regulation of peripheral inflammation has been well appreciated. A comprehensive description of the role of these specialized cells in the peripheral control of inflammation is reviewed elsewhere [7, 9]. Nociceptor neurons as immune cells can detect potentially damaging stimuli, such as pathogens and molecules released from injured tissue, thereby cooperating to induce responses aiming to protect and repair the tissues through inflammation. This mechanism is possible given that nociceptor neuron and immune cells express pattern recognition receptors (PRRs) on their membrane surface or intracellularly [7, 9]. PRRs include several different classes: Toll-like receptors (TLRs), Nod-like receptors, RIG-like receptors, C-type lectin receptors, formylated peptide receptors (FPRs), and scavenger receptors. These receptors recognize pathogen-associated molecular patterns (PAMPs) and damage-associated molecular patterns (DAMPs), which are pathogen conserved structures and molecules released by our necrotic cells [7, 9]. Clinically, bacterial, viral, fungal, and parasitic infections in humans are accompanied by pain or itch, suggesting that distinct types of pathogens can modulate neuronal signaling to potentiate their pathogenesis and/or facilitate their spread to other hosts [9 - 11]. In turn, upon activation, nociceptor neurons control inflammation by releasing neuropeptides [such as calcitonin gene-related peptide (CGRP), vasoactive intestinal polypeptide (VIP), and substance P] that can mediate neurogenic inflammation and modulate the activity of innate and adaptive immune cells [7, 9]. In a mouse model of intraplantar infection by *Staphylococcus aureus*, ablation of nociceptor neurons using Nav1.8-Cre/DTA mice increases neutrophil and monocyte infiltration at the inflammatory site, paw edema, and the weight of popliteal lymph nodes, which are the responsible for draining the footpad. Furthermore, this ablation increases TNF-α production following *S. aureus* infection [12]. This mechanism of limiting the inflammation in an infection context depends on *S. aureus* α-hemolysin, which directly induces calcium influx in nociceptor neurons through disintegrin and metalloproteinase domain-containing protein 10 (ADAM10) receptor that is expressed by sensory neurons. Thus, these activated nociceptor neurons release CGRP, which suppresses macrophages-derived TNF-α production and lymph node hypertrophy, and therefore, limiting the inflammatory response [12]. Other bacterial components are also active. For instance, lipopolysaccharide (LPS) activates TLR4 present in dorsal root ganglion (DRG) sensory neuron triggering a MyD88-dependent signaling pathway. LPS-induced pain is MyD88 dependent and TRIF independent [13]. This MyD88 activation ultimately leads to increase in IL-1β, TNF-α, and COX-2 expression in the DRG in an NF-κB-dependent manner [14]. LPS also increases calcium influx that mediates neurogenic inflammation through activation of TRPA1 channels present in nociceptor neurons without activating TLR4 [15]. Moreover, in a model of sepsis, mice lacking TRPV1 display impairment of phagocytosis and bacterial clearance during septicemia leading to hypotension, hypothermia, and multiple organ damages [16]. These data demonstrate that nociceptor neurons can limit the inflammatory response in a scenario of infection.

Nociceptor neurons also can interact with other resident cells, such as dendritic cells, to regulate cutaneous immune response. For instance, in a model of imiquimod-induced psoriasis, ablation of Nav1.8 and TRPV1 positive sensory neurons ameliorates skin inflammation [17]. Nociceptor neurons interact with dendritic cells, which release IL-23 that activates γδT17 cells. These cells mediate the recruitment of neutrophils and monocytes and thereby worsening cutaneous immune response [17]. Mechanistic details are still required to determine how nociceptor neurons activate dendritic cells.

In terms of other inflammatory diseases, the ablation of the nociceptor neurons by using the Nav1.8-Cre/DTA mice strain [18] or using interference RNA targeting TRPV1 [19] reduce the number of leukocytes in the broncho-alveolar lavage fluid (BALF) in allergic rhinitis and asthma models, suggesting an endogenous role for nociceptor neurons. Moreover, QX-314 (a charged lidocaine derivative molecule) silences nociceptor neurons, which leads to the reduction of the number of infiltrating leukocytes in the BALF, reduction of IL-5 production, and improvement of airway inflammation [18]. IL-5 is one of the main cytokines in asthma. In a cascade of events, IL-5 activates in a calcium-dependent manner Nav1.8-positive nociceptor neurons, which in turn release VIP. Nociceptor neurons-derived VIP activates innate lymphoid cells 2 (ILC2) and culminates in airway inflammatory exacerbation [18]. Therefore, nociceptor neurons play a significant role in the induction of inflammation in airway diseases [18, 19].

Capsaicin was firstly described as a molecule that produces inflammatory pain by activation of TRPV1 receptor present in nociceptive C-fibers [20]. However, long-term use of capsaicin presents anti-inflammatory and analgesic properties due to TRPV1 desensitization [21]. In fact, ablation of gastric sensory neurons reduces the gastroprotective effect of capsaicin, suggesting that these specialized cells possess homeostatic function [21, 22]. Regarding animal models, treatment with capsaicin reduces indomethacin-induced micro bleeding [23] by enhancing gastric protection through stimulation of capsaicin-sensitive sensory neurons [22]. Mechanistically, one of the gastroprotective effects of capsaicin is a consequence of TRPV1 activation of gastric sensory neurons which stimulates CGRP-dependent increase in prostacyclin (PGI_2) production and a decrease in neutrophil recruitment and TNF-α production [21, 23, 24]. Altogether, these data show the importance of nociceptor neurons in the regulation of peripheral inflammation.

BIOLOGY OF THE GLIAL CELLS

Microglia

Microglia represent the resident immune cellular population of the central nervous system (CNS) and their functions include the maintenance of tissue homeostasis, synaptic remodeling, secretion of neurotrophic factors, innate immunity modulation, and adaptive immune activation [25 - 27]. Nowadays, there is an acceptable and rational consensus supporting the idea that in rodents, embryogenic origin and development of microglia is dependent on primitive macrophages progenitors derived from the embryonic yolk sac before the embryonic day 8.5 (E8.5), and not from hematopoietic system. This detection was possible through the use of well-designed study focusing on microglial development that allowed a trustworthy *in vivo* fate mapping of yolk sac-derived cells during embryogenesis [28]. Macrophage progenitor migration from the yolk sac to CNS occurs *via* blood circulation between the days E8.5-E9.5 and these progenitor cells as well as microglia can be found in CNS from day E10.5. Primitive yolk sac-derived microglial progenitor possesses an amoeboid shape and absence of completely formed branched process, while classical microglia can be found in the brain only by postnatal day 28 presents morphology with completely ramified process [29]. This hypothesis is reinforced by other studies, which perform functional settings to evaluate the origin of microglia [30, 31]. Microglia represent approximately 5-20% of all glial cell populations in rodents, depending on the region of CNS [32, 33]. Microglia are currently defined as "macrophages of the CNS", due to their marked resemblance with the traditional leukocyte of the peripheral immune system. In fact, microarray data analyses indicate that microglia are closely related and share common aspects with bone marrow derived and thioglycolate-elicited macrophages [34]. Both of them express markers such as cluster of differentiation (CD)11, CD14, and endothelial growth factor (EGF)-like module-containing mucine-like hormone receptor-like 1 (EMR1, also known as F4/80 in mice), as well as requires interferon regulatory factor 8 (IRF-8), colony-stimulating factor-1 (CFS-1; also known as macrophage colony-stimulating factor, M-CSF) and its receptor (CSF1R), and the transcription factor PU.1 for differentiation and maturation. Additional molecules required for microglial development include CD34, runt-related transcription factor 1 (Runx1), and microRNA (miRNA)-124 [31, 32, 34, 35]. Morphologically, microglia differ from monocyte-derived lineage cells, especially because are composed of many ramified branches, which originate from the cell body and serve to maintain an essential communication with neurons, astrocytes, and oligodendrocytes [32]. In normal CNS, resident microglia population is guaranteed by a self-renewal mechanism presenting a surveillance phenotype that aims the regulation of tissue homeostasis, synaptic remodeling, and secretion of neurotrophic factors [27, 29]. However, during danger or injury of the CNS tissue, the release of DAMPs alter microglia function. DAMPs induce microglia to assume the activated phenotype characterized by changes in gene expression associated with an amoeboid-like format, which coordinates inflammation through the secretion of large quantities of pro-inflammatory mediators [7, 27, 34, 36, 37]. This modification of microglial profile is related to the pathophysiological process of many CNS diseases and behavioral aspects. In fact, spinal cord microglia have been strongly related to the pathogenesis of neural plasticity and consequently neuropathic pain following nerve injury [8]. For instance, after peripheral nerve injury, resting microglia, which are homogeneously distributed in spinal cord ipsilateral dorsal horn and characterized morphologically by small somas with thin-branched process, differentiate into active microglia with hypertrophy and microgliosis. These morphological changes are followed by increase of major histocompatibility complex (MHC) class II proteins, CD14, complement receptor 3 (CR3), cannabinoid receptor subtype 2 (CB_2), C-C motif chemokine receptor 2 (CCR2), C-X3-C motif chemokine receptor 1 (CX_3CR1), TLR2 and TLR4, and ATP receptors $P2X_4$, $P2X_7$, $P2Y_{12}$, and $P2Y_{13}$ [33, 36, 37]. In fact, all these microglial modifications contribute to nerve injury-induced hypersensitivity at spinal level [33].

Microgliosis is one of the most used and reliable feature to determine microglia reactivity and are often evaluated by the expression of CD11b (OX-42) and/or ionized calcium-binding adapter molecule 1 (IBA-1) [32, 36]. These morphological and gene expression alterations prompt reactive microglia to respond to noxious stimuli and modulate the immune response. Noxious stimuli that damage and/or activate first-order neurons induce the secretion of neurotransmitters, chemokines, cytokines, and other mediators that impact on microglia activity in the spinal cord. LPS, a gram-negative bacterial product that acts as an agonist of TLR4 is a well-known potent activator of resting microglia [8, 25, 32, 38 - 40]. After LPS stimulation, cultured microglial cells assume their typical morphology of reactivity and in a short period start to release pro-inflammatory substances including TNF-α, IL-6, and nitric oxide (NO) [25, 32, 39]. In accordance, genetic approaches targeting TLR2 and TLR4 lead to the reductions in spinal cord microglial reactivity and neuropathic pain [41, 42], thus evidencing a prominent role of TLR in the modulation of microglia activation and chronic pain. ATP is one of the molecules released by neurons under depolarization that activates purinergic receptors $P2X_4$, $P2X_7$, $P2Y_{12}$, and $P2Y_{13}$ expressed by microglia [25, 36, 43, 44]. Additionally, spinal cord $P2X_4$ and $P2X_7$ receptors were described as critical components in the pathophysiology of neuropathic pain. The expression of these receptors increase in spinal cord microglia after peripheral nerve injury and pharmacological and genetic approaches targeting these receptors reduces nerve injury-induced pain [32, 37, 45 - 47]. Other purinergic receptors, such as $P2Y_{12}$ and $P2Y_{13}$ possess important role in chronic pain considering that damage to the peripheral nervous system instantaneously leads to their upregulation whilst the blockade of their function has significant implications for the reduction of pain hypersensitivity [36, 48, 49]. ATP acts as a neurotransmitter evoking currents in rat microglia and increasing intracellular calcium-dependent signaling in mouse and human microglia as well as microglia activation *in vivo* in a model of traumatic brain injury [50]. ATP can also activate MAPKs signaling pathway resulting in increased chemotaxis, microgliosis, cytokines, and CatS production [37]. Thus, indicating that ATP and its receptors representing key components in microglial reactive and consequently chronic pain.

As aforementioned, once activated, microglia contribute to the maintenance or initiation of neuroinflammation and central sensitization [25, 27, 36]. It is interesting to mention that under pathological conditions microglia immune functions in CNS depend on the interaction with other immune and non-immune cells. This interaction establishes a complex network that guides neuroplasticity, chronic pain states, and CNS diseases pathogenesis [7, 8, 27, 36, 51]. Microgliosis becomes evident in response to a wide variety of pathological stimuli; for instance, trauma, ischemia, as well as neuronal and/or axonal degeneration. Classical factors responsible for microglial proliferation include granulocyte macrophage colony-stimulating factor (GM-CSF), CSF-1 and its receptor CSF-1R, CD34, neurotrophic factors such as BDNF and neurothophin-3 (NT-3), and cytokines (TNF-α and IL-1β) released by astrocytes and even by recruited microglia. These mediators contribute significantly to microglia differentiation in a PU.1 transcription factor-dependent manner [25, 34 - 36]. Microglia-derived pro-inflammatory mediators further intensify microglia activity and recruitment of other immune cells from peripheral circulation. Nevertheless, microglia may also act as a pro-resolution component, collaborating to the decrease of inflammatory reactions in CNS through the release of anti-inflammatory molecules such as cytokines that drive apoptosis. This dual role of "activated" microglia characterized by distinct phenotypes and it is an important mechanism for CNS homeostasis. Microglia resemble peripheral macrophages encompassing M1 and M2 phenotypes [27, 34, 36]. In fact, M2-like microglia drive resolution of the inflammation, clearance of the resultant debris, and tissue repair [27, 34, 36]. M2-like microglia produce neurotrophic factors (*e.g.* BDNF), expression of arginase-1 (ARG-1) and insulin-degrading enzyme (IDE), anti-inflammatory cytokines such as IL-4 and proteases. These molecules potentiate of phagocytic activity, with almost none or limited damage to the surrounding tissues [27, 34, 36]. In an opposite scenario, M1-like activation is associated with reduction in the release of neurotrophic factors concomitantly with upregulation of pro-inflammatory mediators including cytokines (IL-1β), chemokines, inducible NO synthase (iNOS), and ROS culminating in chronic CNS inflammation, neuronal plasticity, and dysfunction [27, 34, 36].

Other notable functional properties of activated microglia are the capacity to phagocyte cellular debris or necrotic cells and to act as antigen presenting cell in CNS disease [25]. Microglia represent the official phagocyte of the CNS tissue being a determinant component for healthy CNS, but also for development, pathology and tissue repair [32, 52, 53]. Cell death and resultant cellular debris such as nucleic acids, misfolded proteins, and fibrils are efficiently removed through phagocytic activity of activated recruited microglia, and surprisingly, the arrangement of this machinery occurs without triggering an inflammatory response [27, 54, 55]. This "non-inflammatory phagocytosis" mediated by M2-like microglia occurs *via* triggering receptor expressed on myeloid cells-2 (TREM-2), inducing the phosphorylation of the DAP12 protein, which leads to the cytoskeleton reorganization and consequently phagocytosis [27, 35]. There is evidence that TREM-2-dependent signaling downregulates the levels of cytokines with inflammatory/nociceptive role in microglia [25, 35, 56]. The release of proteins related to pathological conditions such as β-amyloid (βA), which occurs in Alzheimer's disease (AD) is also a mechanism known to induce phagocytosis by microglia [25, 34]. In response to bacterial infections, microglia becomes capable of detecting pathogens, orchestrate inflammation and convert to a phagocyte promoting neuroprotection [35]. As previously addressed, ATP is a fundamental molecule for activation of microglia. Damaged cells release ATP and other nucleotides such as uridine-5′-triphosphate (UDP) that interact with the relevant purinergic receptors expressed by microglia $P2Y_6$, $P2Y_{12}$, and $P2X_4$, enabling them to extend their process toward the injury sites, migrate and phagocytosis [32, 34, 35, 56]. In fact, strategies targeting purinergic or TREM-2 receptors compromise the dynamism of microglia to perform their phagocytic activity [35, 57, 58]. Microglia recognize products from gram-positive and gram-negative bacteria as well as viral components and phagocyte pathogens for intracellular killing *via* TLRs [59, 60]. Other important signaling described to induce phagocytosis include the expression of phosphatidylserine present on the surface of apoptotic cells *via* interactions with vitronectin and CD36 receptors in microglia, and the complement receptor CR3 [25, 35, 61 - 64]. Additionally, microglia appear to act as antigen presenting cells (APCs) in the CNS together with other specialized cells like dendritic cells (DC) and macrophages. In a model of experimental autoimmune encephalomyelitis (EAE) microglia increase the expression of classical surface markers of professional APCs such as MHC-II, co-stimulatory molecules B7.1 and B7.2 and cathepsin proteases [25, 65 - 68]. Thus, indicating that microglia can present antigens to T cells in CNS, having thus an important role in modulation of T cells activation.

Astrocytes

Astrocytes, which may also be referred to as astroglia, are the most abundant cell type of glia in the CNS [69]. Although initially considered to be purely structural and supportive components in the CNS, numerous functions have been described over the years. Thus, this helps building the concept that astrocytes are specialized cells that interact with neighboring structures [70]. Astrocytes are involved in several key mechanisms in the nervous system, thus, playing a fundamental role in brain homeostasis [71]. This idea is corroborated by evidence that astrocytes malfunctioning has been associated with the mechanisms of numerous psychiatric or neurological diseases. For instance, AD [72], epilepsy [73], brain tumors [74], multiple sclerosis (MS) [75], autism [73], and depression [76]. In addition, among the several functions described, some studies point to the ability of astrocytes to work as stem cells, influencing neurogenesis. Mature astrocytes, in particular those originated in the subventricular zone and subgranular zone may give rise to new neurons [77 - 79].

The term astrocyte was first published in 1893 by Michael von Lenhonsek (*Lenhossek M. Der feinere Bau des Nervensystems im Lichte neuester Forschung. Fischer's Medicinische Buchhandlung*; Berlin: 1893). Semantically, strocytes means "cell in star format" refering to the morphology of this cell that presents of various processes that extend from the cell body and are responsible for the interaction with other cells or tissues. Several astrocyte subtypes have been described, whose morphology, function and even protein expression may be variable according to their location in the CNS [70, 80]. The first morphological division of astrocytes between two main classes: protoplasmic or fibrous, was suggested by Ramon y Cajal in 1909 (*Histologie du systeme nerveux de l'homme et des vertebres. Maloine,* Paris) and is still applied (Fig. **1**). The same researcher was also responsible for identifying the glial fibrillary acidic protein (GFAP) and characterizing it as the first astrocyte marker, which is still considered a gold standard. The protoplasmic astrocytes are located in the gray matter, whereas in the white matter they are found as fibrous astrocytes (Fig. **1**). However, it was later observed that although these were the two main classes, there is an important heterogeneity between the cells of the astroglia. Other denominations are currently employed to characterize astrocytes locate in specific delimited areas of the CNS. Müller cells found in the retina, Bergmann glia and velate astrocytes in the cerebellum, cortical interlaminar, perivascular astrocytes, tanycytes in periventricular regions and pituocytes in the neurohypophysis [70, 81].

The difference of the glial precursors, as well as the site of which the varied differentiation pathways initiates, can explain this heterogeneity [82]. During fetal development, astrocytes are immature and have high proliferative activity. In humans, the maturity stage is reached about 6 to 12 months after birth, when differentiation reaches the final stage [81, 83]. Cells from the radial glia of the embryonic ventricular zone as well as intermediate progenitors from neonatal subventricular zones give rise to protoplasmic astrocytes, whereas fibrous astrocytes originate mostly from neonatal progenitors of the subventricular zone [79, 82]. Focusing on the spinal cord, the development and distribution of astrocytes in this site are associated with transcription factors expressed by glial progenitor cell [84], and can share components involved in neurogenesis of oligodendrocytes, such as the Ascl1 transcription factor. The expression of Ascl1 progenitor glia cells defines the presence and quantity of protoplasmic astrocytes in the dorsal gray matter and fibrous astrocytes in the white matter of the spinal medulla [85].

The presence or activity of astrocytes in the CNS can be analyzed by the expression of certain proteins by these cells. Although GFAP is the protein most commonly used to study astrocyte activation, other astroglia-like cells may express this marker, generating false-positive results. However these cells are outside the CNS, for instance, keratinocytes and liver cells are also able to express GFAP [79]. The enzyme aldehyde dehydrogenase (AldhL1) and the glutamate transporter GLT-1 are expressed by all astrocytes [82, 86]. These enzymes have also been used as a cellular marker, whereas the calcium-binding protein S100B and the Kir4.1 channel, for example, are considered as astrocyte subtype-specific markers [82, 86].

Astrocytes distribute themselves homogeneously throughout the CNS and possess an anatomical delimitation of territory. Under normal conditions, astrocytes exhibit coupled network conformation and no overlap between their processes [87, 88]. A relevant feature is the presence of gap junctions between the distal ends of the astrocytes, which allow the communication between these cells, changing the permeability to ions and the signaling of calcium [89]. The gap junctions are formed by two opposing hemichannels, which in turn are composed of 6 proteins each, the connexins. Of that, the best known is connexin-43 (Cx43) (Fig. **2**) [90]. Alterations in the expression or activity of the connexins can modulate the communication of the spinal cord gap junctions, for example in response to a pathological stimulus triggering pain and inflammation [91 - 94].

Unlike neuronal cells, astrocytes are not activated electrically, but chemically, in particular by the influx of calcium ions [95]. As regards to the defense and protection of the CNS, astrocytes are part of the composition of the glia limitans barrier and contribute to the formation of the blood-brain barrier [96].

Considering that the processes or extremities of the astrocytes are in direct contact with the cerebral vessels, they can change the diameter of the vessels and

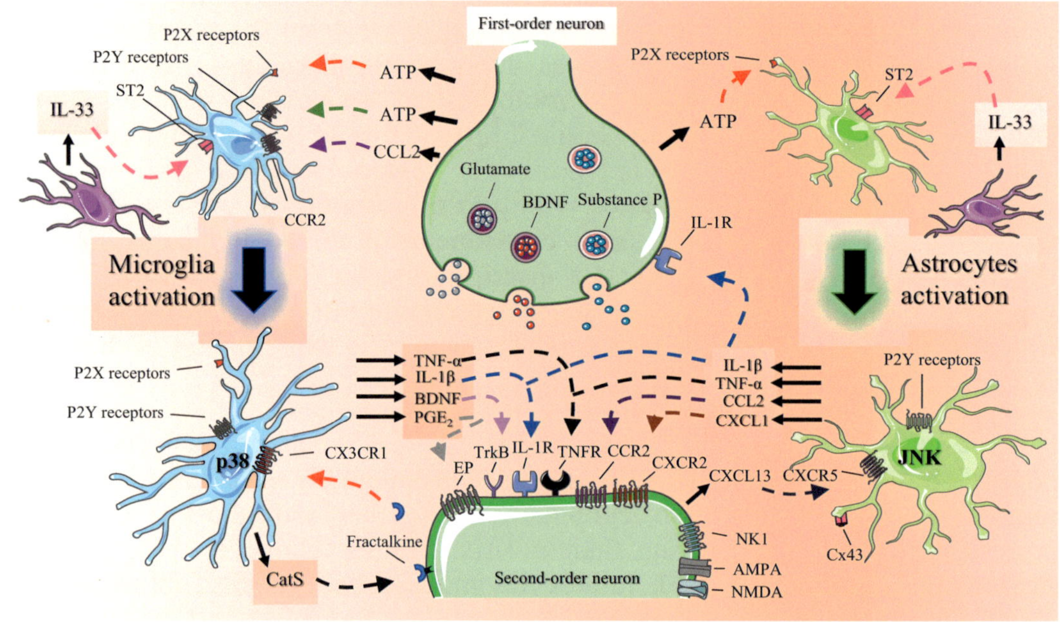

Fig. (2). Interaction between glial cells and nociceptor neurons in chronic pain.
Upon nerve injury, nociceptor neurons release molecules such as ATP (acting on P2X or P2Y receptors), CCL2 (acting on CCR2), fractalkine (CX_3CL1 acting on CX_3CR1), and CXCL13 (acting on CCR5) that can activate both astrocytes and microglia. In turn, glial cells release cytokines (*e.g.* IL-1β, TNF-α, and IL-6), chemokines (*e.g.* CXCL1 and CCL2), growth factors (*e.g.* BDNF), and lipid mediators (*e.g.* PGE_2) that modulate nociceptor activity. The production of these mediators occurs in p38-dependent mechanism (microglia) and JNK-dependent mechanism (astrocytes). For instance, cytokines produced by these cells can enhance the amplitude of AMPA- and glutamate-induced excitatory currents, while only IL-1β also reduces GABA- and glycine-induced inhibitory transmission [143]. BDNF switches the activity of GABA from an inhibitory to an excitatory neurotransmitter [142]. In addition, oligodendrocytes release IL-33 that activates both microglia and astrocytes [130].

consequently, to control the regional blood flow. The influx of calcium in astrocytes induced by neuronal activity leads to the release of mediators such as NO, prostaglandins and other derivatives of arachidonic acid directly into the vessel [97]. The regulation of fluid homeostasis also occurs through this interface, given that the astrocytic processes in contact with the vessels present large amounts of aquaporin-4 water channels [98]. Astrocytes regulate ionic homeostasis through their membrane transporters. These transporters prevent extracellular accumulation of potassium, and modulate the levels of ROS and synaptic neurotransmitters such as gamma-aminobutyric acid (GABA) and glutamate [87, 99]. Excitatory amino acid transporters present in astrocytes are responsible for the reuptake of the excess glutamate in the synaptic space that is metabolized by glutamine synthetase into glutamine. The glutamine is then released *via* astrocytic transporters and recycled by the neurons to the production of new glutamate [100].

In addition to communicating with the vessels, astrocytic processes also maintain contact with neurons and consequently play a major role in synaptic transmission. In the cerebral cortex, the same astrocyte can surround different neurons that are in its domain and participate in several synapses at the same time [101]. This interaction is called the "tripartite synapse" given it involves the pre and postsynaptic regions and the processes of the astrocytes [102]. Modulation of neuronal excitability and consequently of synaptic transmission and plasticity by astrocytes is mainly due to the release of several mediators. For instance, ATP, *D*-serine, and glutamate, which can modulate postsynaptic interneurons or receptors [103 - 105] and by modulating extracellular potassium levels [106]. In turn, the activity of neurons triggers the influx of calcium in the astrocytes, favoring the release of mediators and characterizing a bi-directional signaling pathway between a neuron and astrocytes [95].

Injury and disease of the CNS cause an activation response of the astrocytes, altering their functionality to restrict the possible damage and to re-establish the homeostasis of the nervous tissue. This mechanism comprises molecular, cellular and functional alterations in astrocytes, such as increased expression of GFAP and hypertrophy. Reactive astrogliosis can be modulated by signal transducer and transcriptional activator 3 (STAT3), NF-κB, cyclic adenosine monophosphate (cAMP), cytokines, and ROS [88]. These changes are dependent on the severity, type, and duration of the insult, which can result in both gain and loss of astrocyte functions, and therefore positively or negatively impacting the cells with which they interact [87, 88, 107]. Mild to moderate astrogliosis occurs in the case of infections, and these changes are reversible with the resolution of the inflammatory process. In aggravated cases, when there is severe astrocytic activation making long-term changes to become permanent, there is induction of a maladaptive character. The most serious result may be the formation of a glial scar by astrocytes that undergo excessive proliferation and overlapping of their processes. In this case, reactive astrogliosis reaches the maximum degree of reactivity and scar formation aiming to protect healthy tissue [82].

Once activated, astrocytes respond by producing inflammatory mediators such as chemokines, cytokines and growth factors. Astrocytes also express TLR that upon activation produce several pro-inflammatory mediators, such as ROS, IL-1β, TNF-α, and CCL2 in a MAPK JNK-dependent manner [41, 108]. Indeed, immunohistochemical studies have shown the co-localization of phosphorylated JNK and GFAP in the spinal cord in animals with persistent inflammatory pain

[109] or chronic pain [110, 111] as well as their importance to maintaining the painful state was also demonstrated. In fact, TNF-α-activated astrocytes release CCL2 in a JNK-dependent manner [112]. Mechanistically, it is likely that TNF-α induces CCL2 production by activating an upstream signaling that is dependent on tumor necrosis factor receptor associated factor 6 (TRAF6), which is mainly expressed by astrocytes [113, 114]. TRAF6 activation leads to a downstream activation of astrocyte JNK and consequent CCL2 production [113]. This chemokine acts on the CCR2 receptors present on nociceptor neurons promoting enhanced synaptic transmission and also activating microglia, which contribute to central sensitization and pain maintenance (Fig. **2**) [112, 115].

Oligodendrocytes

When Virchow analyzed the structure of the brain in the 1850s, he observed the presence of other cell types that differed from neurons and astrocytes. However, due to imperfect staining methods, they remained obscure and were only named the "third element" known as microglia [116]. Some decades later, Pío del Río Hortega (1921) applied a staining method involving silver carbonate, thereby shedding new light on the remaining interstitial cells. This technique was the methodological key to identify two distinct elements: the microglia, and the "interfascicular cells" that were later called oligodendroglia [117, 118]. Around 1924 oligodendroglia was confirmed as a variety of neuroglia of ectodermal origin, such as astroglia [117, 119]. After some refinement of the methodology, Del Río-Hortega was able to distinguish four types of oligodendrocytes. Type I cells have a small rounded cell body and generate many different myelin segments on small diameter axons in diverse orientations. Type II cells are similar to type I in size and number, but with fewer and thicker processes than type I and the myelin segments run in parallel to each other. Type II cells are present only in white matter. Type III oligodendrocytes are present in white matter with thick myelinated fibers, like brain stem and spinal cord, and they are also less abundant than types I and II. Type IV oligodendrocytes have a cell body closely opposed to a very large single axon similar to Schwann cells [117, 119, 120]. Therefore, spinal cord and brain contain different subclasses of oligodendrocytes, which derive from multiple sources. In the spinal cord, most of the oligodendrocytes derive from a specialized domain of the ventral ventricular zone, which first gives rise to motor neuron precursors, and then, after the neurogenic/gliogenic switch, to oligodendrocyte precursor cells (OPCs) [120 - 123]. From there, OPCs migrate through all the spinal cord and finally differentiate into white or gray matter oligodendrocytes [124].

The pattern of transcription factor expression in the progenitor domains and the unique spatial organization of the spinal cord into gray matter and white matter make it an ideal setting to elucidate the mechanisms of glial heterogeneity [124]. OPCs express platelet-derived growth-factor receptor-α (PDGFR-α), the transcription factor SOX10 and the proteoglycan NG2 (also known as CSPG4) [124]. These cells maintain proliferative and migratory competence during development and in the adult, and are early responders to injury. Mature oligodendrocytes of the white matter express a variety of myelin markers, including myelin basic protein (MBP), proteolipid protein 1 (PLP1), and adenomatous polyposis coli (APC) protein [124]. In the gray matter, in addition to the myelinating function of mature oligodendrocytes, several proteins have functions to provide trophic support to neurons, consequently survival, such as glial cell line derived neurotrophic factor (GDNF), BDNF, insulin-like growth factor 1 (IGF-1), NT-3, ciliary neurotrophic factor (CNTF), fibroblast growth factor 2 (FGF-2), and enkephalins. These factors enable not only survival but also the growth and differentiation of various types of cells present in the CNS, including neurons [125, 126]. In fact, mature neurons produce low levels of growth factors and neurotrophins, which are mainly produced by OPCs [127], demonstrating that these cells provide trophic support not only to neurons during development but also to the mature nervous system.

A transcription factor that is highly expressed in neural progenitor cells in the developing dorsal horn of the spinal cord is the basic helix-loop-helix (bHLH) factor Ascl1 [122, 127]. In fact, spinal cord oligodendrogenesis dramatically reduces in the white matter in Ascl1 conditionally knockout mice [85]. This loss of OPCs/oligodendrocytes was especially apparent in the dorsal funiculus, a domain where many of the OPCs are likely to be derived from dorsally located Ascl1+ cells [85]. This indicates that the transcription factor Ascl1 controls the distribution of gray matter and white matter OPCs [85].

The morphologic characteristics of the oligodendrocytes can be described as having small cell bodies, with their nucleus filled with significant amounts of chromatin and their cellular extensions filled with cytoplasmic granules. The oligodendrocytes provide multiple axons with myelin sheaths [124, 128], extending processes to as many as 50 axons, and can renew its myelin sheaths in a short time range [128, 129]. Curiously, a large number of granules in the cytosol of oligodendrocytes, reminiscent of secretory glands cells, were also taken as evidence for a function in myelin formation. Myelin insulates the naked axon, a necessary step for optimal signal transduction in the CNS [128].

From an immunological perspective, recent evidence is emerging on the role of oligodendrocytes in the modulation of chronic pain, especially [130 - 132]. Oligodendrocytes actively produce a wide range of immunoregulatory factors, cytokines, ROS, and express receptors for some of these mediators [128, 130 -

132]. For instance, oligodendrocytes express MHC class I molecules and thereby can interact with T cells [133, 134]. *In vitro* data demonstrates that IFN-γ induces the expression of MHC class I expression on oligodendrocytes, supporting the idea that the presence of IFN-γ in demyelinating disorders such as MS may render oligodendrocytes susceptible to MHC class I-dependent cell death [135]. Oligodendrocytes also express TLRs. In fact, spinal cord delivery of zymosan, a TLR2 agonist, promotes cell differentiation and maturation of primary rat oligodendrocytes. Whereas activation with poly-I:C, a TLR3 agonist, reduces survival of the oligodendroglia and drives a less mature phenotype [136]. Oligodendrocytes also express receptors to a wide range of cytokines, such as IL-6, IL-12, and IFN-γ. Expression of these receptors is increased in neurological disorders such as MS and AD [137]. In addition, several chemokine receptors such as CXCR1, CXCR2, and CXCR3 are also expressed on oligodendrocytes at increased levels in MS, stroke, and amyotrophic lateral sclerosis [138].

INTERACTION BETWEEN GLIAL CELLS AND NOCICEPTOR NEURONS IN CHRONIC PAIN

Increased long-lasting discharge of peripheral nociceptors leads to plastic changes in the spinal cord and sensory neurons that modify neuronal phenotype and function in the CNS. These changes are associated with an increase in the excitatory synaptic transmission and decrease in the inhibitory synaptic transmission in the dorsal horn of the spinal cord. These mechanisms play a major role in the increased pain sensation that is experienced in patients with chronic pain. This phenomenon is referred as central sensitization and clearly shows that nociceptor neurons participate of pain processing, rather than being only cells that conduct nervous impulse [139 - 141]. In the contemporary understanding of pain, the mechanism of central sensitization and persistent pathological pain are mediated by complex interactions between sensory neurons and immune cells [7, 8]. Therefore, the neuronal systems are no longer the only player involved in the central sensitization. Rather, a variety of non-neuronal cells, especially glial cells (namely astrocyte, microglia, and oligodendrocyte), might play a major role in the initiation and modulation of the primary afferent nociceptors activity through the release of inflammatory mediators that activate specific receptors expressed by those nociceptors [7, 8]. Importantly, glial cell-derived mediators modulate synaptic transmission at low concentrations. For instance, glial cells cytokines, chemokines, and growth factors affect synaptic activity at nM concentrations whereas neurotransmitters such as glutamate, GABA, and glycine produce synaptic effects at μM range [112, 142, 143]. Given central sensitization has a significant impact on the pain produced by normally innocuous low-threshold afferent inputs (*i.e.* allodynia) and the spread of hypersensitivity to regions beyond the injured tissue (*i.e.* secondary hyperalgesia), in this topic, we describe the role of each glial cell in the modulation of chronic pain.

Microglia

Microglia are resident macrophages within the CNS and constantly perform immune surveillance. This cell type rapidly responds by changing morphology and expression of surface chemokines and cytokines receptors at any sign of disturbance of the peripheral or central nervous system, either by pathogens or damage. These changes prompt microglia to migrate to the spinal cord and proliferate (a phenomenon coined as microgliosis) [144, 145]. Microglia recruitment is mediated by several molecules such as ATP [142, 146], neuregulin-1 [144, 145], CCL2 [147], and fractalkine (CX_3CL1) [148], which also contribute to the polarization of microglia from a resting to a pro-inflammatory state. In fact, after spinal nerve transection, microgliosis have been shown to be partially dependent on fractalkine and ATP given mice lacking CX_3CR1 or $P2Y_{12}$ present reduced mechanical hypersensitivity and microgliosis [149]. Further, the dynamic of microglia proliferation demonstrates that dorsal horn resident microglia are activated and also other set of microglia undergo active cell division after peripheral nerve injury [149]. This indicates that the microgliosis observed in neuropathic pain states might be related not only to activation of microglia but also with increased number of these cells. Activated microglia produce cytokines such as TNF-α and IL-1β [143] and growth factors such as BDNF [142] in a MAPK p38-dependent manner (Fig. **2**) [150]. These cytokines can induce pain and a long-term activation of microglia can contribute to central sensitization [7, 8]. For instance, both TNF-α and IL-1β enhance the amplitude of AMPA- and glutamate-induced excitatory currents, while only IL-1β also reduces GABA- and glycine-induced inhibitory transmission [143]. Other mediators, such as BDNF, released by microglia also contribute to pain signaling. ATP-stimulated microglia releases BDNF that activates spinal lamina I neurons through TrkB receptor [142, 151]. This activation causes an alteration of transmembrane anion gradient through downregulation of the chloride co-transporter KCC2 that switches the activity of approximately 33% of the neurotransmitter GABA from an inhibitory to an excitatory neurotransmitter [142]. Moreover, nociceptor neuron-derived ATP activates the $P2X_7$ receptor in microglia [152] that in turn releases the lysosomal enzyme cathepsin S (CatS). This enzyme cleaves neuronal extracellular membrane-bound fractalkine that activates CX_3CR1 present in microglia triggering the production of IL-1β, TNF-α, and IL-6 in a p38-dependent manner (Fig. **2**) [153, 154]. Further mechanism involving the release of CX_3CL1 from central terminals also includes the activity of matrix metalloproteinases (MMP) 2 and 9 [153], which have a differential contribution in the early and late phase of neuropathic pain [155]. For instance, in the early phase, MMP-9 contributes to neuropathic pain through activation of p38 microglia and IL-1β production [155].

At the late phase, MMP-2 helps in the maintenance of neuropathic pain through activation of astrocytes, IL-1β production, and ERK activation in nociceptor neurons [155].

Upon nerve injury, nociceptor neurons release DAMPs, such as fibronectin, B-defensins, high mobility group box 1 (HMGB1), hyaluronan, and heat shock proteins (HSP) that activate TLR expressed in microglia [41]. For instance, nerve injury and arthritis increase HMGB1 expression in the dorsal horn of the spinal cord [156, 157] and nerve injury also increases the expression of HMGB1 in the sciatic nerve [158]. HMGB1 is expressed by nociceptor neurons, astrocytes, and microglia as observed by the double staining of HMGB1 with NeuN, GFAP, and IBA-1, respectively [157 - 159]. However, it is likely that sensory neurons, but not glial cells, release HMGB1 [159]. This is likely given that upon nerve injury this alarmin remains stored in the nucleus of astrocytes or microglia [159]. Mechanistically, nerve-injury induced HMGB1 activates TLR4 *via* the disulfide bond at carbon 23 and 45 and the free thiol at carbon 106 [160]. This interaction leads to a downstream MyD88-dependent signaling pathway in both astrocytes and microglia that contribute to spinal cord sensitization [156]. Moreover, in models of bone cancer-induced pain and diabetes-induced neuropathic pain, increased spinal cord HMGB1 levels correlates with the development of allodynia and spinal microglia-related $P2X_4$ receptor expression is enhanced by fibronectin [161]. Other molecules, such as CSF1, can be found upregulated in injured DRG and transported to the spinal cord after nerve injury [162]. At the spinal cord, CSF1 activates microglia through CSFR1 that is mainly expressed by these cells. CSF1 induces DAP-12-dependent pain and microgliosis, which is also a relevant mechanism to induce pain [162]. These data indicate that a molecule produced in the periphery upon nerve injury can also activate microglia [162].

Microglia are also involved in recruiting T-lymphocytes to the spinal cord that also plays an important role in neuropathic pain [163, 164]. T-lymphocytes that infiltrate to the spinal cord interact with microglia *via* MHC-II and co-stimulatory molecules, which activate both cells and help to maintain neuropathic pain by releasing pro-inflammatory cytokines including IL-1β, TNF-α, and IL-6 [165].

Microglia play a major role in arthritis as well. In a model of monosodium iodoacetate (MIA)-induced osteoarthritis, phosphorylated p38 (p-p38) is increased seven days after the stimulus, while an increase of phosphorylated ERK1/2 (p-ERK) was observed after 14 days. Importantly, p-p38 mainly co-localizes with OX-42 (microglia marker) and p-ERK with NeuN (neuronal marker). Neither p-ERK nor p-p38 MAPKs co-localized with GFAP staining [166]. This differential activation is consistent with the data showing that microglia activation occurs seven days after stimulus and lasts for 28 days, while astrocytes activation occurs on the 28th day after the stimulus [167]. However, this differential activation of glial cells might be model-specific. In a model of antigen-induced arthritis (AIA) in rats (induced by intradermous injection of CFA) NF-κB p65 co-localizes with NeuN and GFAP, but not with OX-42 in the 14th day after stimulus. This indicates that AIA-induced IL-1β, TNF-α, and IL-6 might be produced by neurons and astrocytes [168]. In collagen-induced arthritis (CIA) model, microglia contribute to the early stages of the disease [169, 170]. In this model, a significant microgliosis occurs in the dorsal horn of the spinal cord 7 days after collagen immunization (7 days before the onset of clinical signs) [169] and remains up-regulated for 18 days after induction, as observed by the increase of IBA-1 and p-p38 expression [154]. The early-phase microgliosis correlates with a time course similar to that of mechanical allodynia and IL-1β production, which occur dependent on the cascade ATP/P2X$_7$/CatS/CX3CR1 [169, 171]. In fact, the pharmacological blockade of spinal CatS reduces the release of the chemokine fractalkine and as consequence microglia-driven mechanical allodynia and the increase of IL-1β in the early phase of CIA [169] (Fig. **2**). Moreover, the release of the pro-nociceptive peptide CGRP from nociceptor central terminals is associated with an increase of p-ERK in lumbar DRGs [170], demonstrating that targeting microglia is an attractive approach. Of note, a significant astrogliosis occur in the dorsal horn of the spinal cord at the late stage (18 days after induction) [154, 169].

Despite the recognized analgesic effects of opioids, a major clinical issue is the fact that the use of opioids can paradoxically induce pain [172]. The underlying mechanism is accepted to involve morphine-induced release of DAMPs, such as HMGB-1 and biglycan [173] that increase the production of spinal cord IL-1β by microglia in a NLRP3-dependent manner as observed by the double staining of NLRP3 and IBA-1 in rats [174]. Furthermore, morphine increases IL-1β mRNA expression *via* TLR4 and increases IL-1β release *via* P2X4 receptor [175]. Altogether, this cascade of events in microglia potentiates morphine-induced hyperalgesia by stimulating IL-1β production in the spinal cord and explains this paradoxical effect [173 - 175].

Astrocytes

Astrocytes express a large number of neurotransmitter receptors and upon elevation of intracellular calcium concentration can release molecules that change neuronal transmission [87]. Furthermore, astrocytes are responsible for the uptake of extracellular glutamate *via* the glutamate transporter-1 (GLT1/EAAT2), which is mainly expressed by these cells [87]. Nerve injury produces a persistent downregulation of these transporters that decrease glutamate uptake and increase excitatory synaptic transmission [87], explaining the contribution of astrocytes in the maintenance of the late-phase neuropathic pain [92]. In terms of mechanisms, TNF-α-activated astrocytes release CXCL1 and contribute to mechanical allodynia through the gap junction Cx43. Importantly, these gap junctions allow the passage of small molecules (less than 1 kD), such as calcium, IP3, cAMP, cGMP, glutamate, glucose, and ATP between glial cells or glial cells and neurons. However, some gap junction channels in glia are not opposed by existing gap junctions in the adjacent glial cells and therefore are called as hemichannels. These gap junctions allow the passage of molecules such as ATP, glutamate, and prostaglandins to the extracellular space, activating other glial cells or neurons [176]. Therefore, astrocytes can modulate neuronal transmission due to the release of molecules such as glutamate and the ion calcium [176]. Both CXCL1 and Cx43 mediate neuronal plasticity given that their inhibition reduces spontaneous excitatory postsynaptic currents (EPSC) in lamina II neurons [92]. Thus, it is likely that targeting CXCL1 is relevant considering that it maintains overexpressed for three weeks after nerve injury and is mainly expressed by astrocytes [92]. Cx43 also mediate chronic hyperalgesia through the release of spinal cord CXCL12, in a model of bone cancer-induced pain in rats [91]. Other chemokine such as CXCL13 also mediates neuropathic pain in a model of spinal nerve ligation [177]. After nerve injury, CXCL13 co-localizes with microtubule-associated protein 2 (MAP2) but not with GFAP or IBA-1, suggesting a neuronal release in the spinal cord, but not by astrocytes or microglia. CXCR5 co-localizes predominantly with GFAP but not with OX-42, suggesting that is mainly expressed by astrocytes (but not microglia). Therefore, CXCL13 released by spinal cord neurons activates astrocytes CXCR5, which leads to the production of CCL2 in an ERK-dependent manner that activates both nociceptor neuron and microglia producing pain (Fig. **2**) [177]. Interestingly, CCL2 co-localizes with substance P and CGRP-positive neurons in both DRG and spinal cord lamina IIo. This indicates CCL2 synthesized in the DRG can be released in central terminals (Fig. **2**) [178]. Mechanistically, CCL2 enhances NDMA-induced current in excitatory nociceptor neurons expressing the vesicular glutamate transporter subtype 2 (VGLUT2). The authors suggest that CCL2 can directly modulate synaptic plasticity in CCR2 in excitatory neurons in the lamina IIo, a mechanism that might contribute to central sensitization in pathological pain [179]. Moreover, a CCL2 antagonist reduces long-term potentiation in C-fibers suggesting a role of CCL2/CCR2 in the maintenance of long-term spinal potentiation [179]. Focusing on the effect of cytokines released in nociceptor neurons, TNF-α from astrocytes increases the inward current induced by activation of AMPA and NMDA receptors as well as their expression on the surface of neurons by changing neuronal excitability and synaptic strength [180, 181]. Moreover, IL-1β through IL-1R induces a downstream activation of Src tyrosine kinase family, which phosphorylates NMDA receptor at positions Tyr416 and Tyr1472 of the NR2A/B subunits [182]. Opening of NMDA receptor channel leads to the influx of calcium and to the increase in the production of PGE_2, which is a molecule involved in nociceptor sensitization (Fig. **2**) [182]. In addition, astrocytes mediate light touch-evoked hypersensitivity, which is an important component of allodynia [183]. Pharmacological inhibition of JNK activation in astrocytes reduces light touch-induced ERK activation in spinal cord lamina I and IIo neurons [183]. These results show an essential intracellular signaling pathways activated in astrocytes necessary to the communication with nociceptor neurons and the consequent allodynia in persistent pain conditions [183].

Oligodendrocytes

The role of oligodendrocytes in chronic pain has just emerged. Oligodendrocytes in the gray matter can be distinguished from those in the white matter on the basis of their level of myelin marker expression [124]. For instance, white matter oligodendrocytes mainly express myelin basic protein (MBP), proteolipid protein 1 (PLP1), and adenomatous polyposis coli (APC) protein. Gray matter oligodendrocytes, on the other hand, express the proteoglycan NG2, platelet-derived growth factor receptor-α (PDGFR-α), and the transcription factor SOX10 [124] which is cross-regulated by OLIG2 transcription factor [184]. In a chronic constrict injury (CCI) model of neuropathic pain, the double staining of OLIG2 with IL-33/citrine reporter mice reveals that oligodendrocytes are the primary source of IL-33, which *via* the ST2 receptor induces astrocyte and microglia activation in the spinal cord [130]. IL-33/ST2 interaction activates intracellular signaling pathways such as phosphatidylinositol 3-kinase (PI3K), mammalian target of rapamycin (mTOR), MAPK, and NF-κB that drive to the production of IL-1β and TNF-α by spinal cord microglia and astrocytes (Fig. **2**) [130]. Although this study focused mainly on the role of IL-33/ST2 signaling in CCI-induced neuropathic pain, it was the first evidence on the participation of spinal cord oligodendrocytes in pain regulation [130]. Also, recent evidence has demonstrated that dorsal root ganglia (DRG) sensory neurons possess ST2 receptor and therefore can be activated by IL-33 in the context of itch [185]. Moreover, in a model of partial sciatic nerve ligation, oligodendrocytes produce high amount of ROS, as observed by the double staining of 4-Hydroxynonen (4-HNE) with OLIG2, and NG2 [132]. In a murine model of HIV-related chronic pain (gp120-induced pain), oligodendrocytes markers of both white and gray matter rapidly increase after injection of gp120 (within 1 h after stimulus) and last for 21 days [131]. However, MBP does not regulate gp120-induced pain given that mechanical allodynia was observed in MBP knockout mice or after siRNA targeting MBP. These data show that MBP and myelination might not be critical for the induction of gp120-induced allodynia, and that the oligodendrocytes of the dorsal horn of the spinal cord mediate chronic pain in mice [131]. Clinically, patients with HIV that develop chronic pain present elevated cell markers of the oligodendrocyte lineage NG2, PDGFR-α, and OLIG2 in the dorsal horn of the spinal cord as evaluated in postmortem spinal cord specimens [131]. It is also interesting to mention that ablation of oligodendrocytes using Cre-recombinase technique targeting myelin oligodendrocyte glycoprotein induces hyperalgesia without early activation of astrocytes or microglia and without T- and B-cell infiltration [186]. Oligodendrocytes ablation induces mechanical and cold hyperalgesia but not heat hyperalgesia or spontaneous pain. These data demonstrate the importance of the endogenous physiological functions of oligodendrocyte in maintaining homeostasis [186]. Therefore, these experimental and clinical data demonstrate the emerging role of oligodendrocytes in chronic pain and that modulation of these cells are a suitable therapeutic approach.

PHARMACOLOGICAL APPROACHES TARGETING SPINAL CORD GLIAL CELLS

Nociceptor neurons are activated by glial cells-derived molecules, which indicates direct modulation of the activity of neurons. Microglia produce pro-inflammatory molecules in a MAPK p38-dependent mechanism, while astrocytes in a JNK-dependent mechanism. These signaling pathways lead to an elevation of intracellular calcium following peripheral nerve injury (Fig. **2**). These MAPKs can also be activated by IL-1β, TNF-α and IL-33, resulting in the activation of various transcription factors (*e.g.* AP-1, c-Jun, c-fos) and to further secretion of IL-1β, TNF-α, IL-6, PGE_2, and BDNF (Fig. **2**). Experimental models demonstrate that drugs targeting glial cells such as pentoxifylline, minocycline, fluorocitrate, and *L*α-aminoadipate (Fig. **3**) are highly effective in attenuating the signs of neuropathic pain [36, 187]. However, clinical data regarding the role of glial cells is less clear [188, 189].

Current regimens for management of neuropathic pain includes the use of tricyclic antidepressants, ion channel-modulating drugs (gabapentin, pregabalin, carbamazepine), and certain anticonvulsants, which often produce undesirable side effects [41]. As such, management of neuropathic pain is a significant challenge for clinicians given that most of these drugs also possess non-satisfactory effect and important side effects. Therefore, glial-cells targeting drugs or strategies aiming at controlling neuron-glia interaction are likely to be highly attractive, and in this scenario, CNS-penetrating drugs could represent a new therapeutic opportunity for the treatment of chronic pain in such cases.

Glial Cell Inhibitors and their Clinical Use

In this section, we describe the mechanisms and effects of the main molecules used as inhibitors of glial activation namely pentoxifylline, α-aminoadipate, fluorocitrate, and minocycline. The clinical use of these molecules is also addressed.

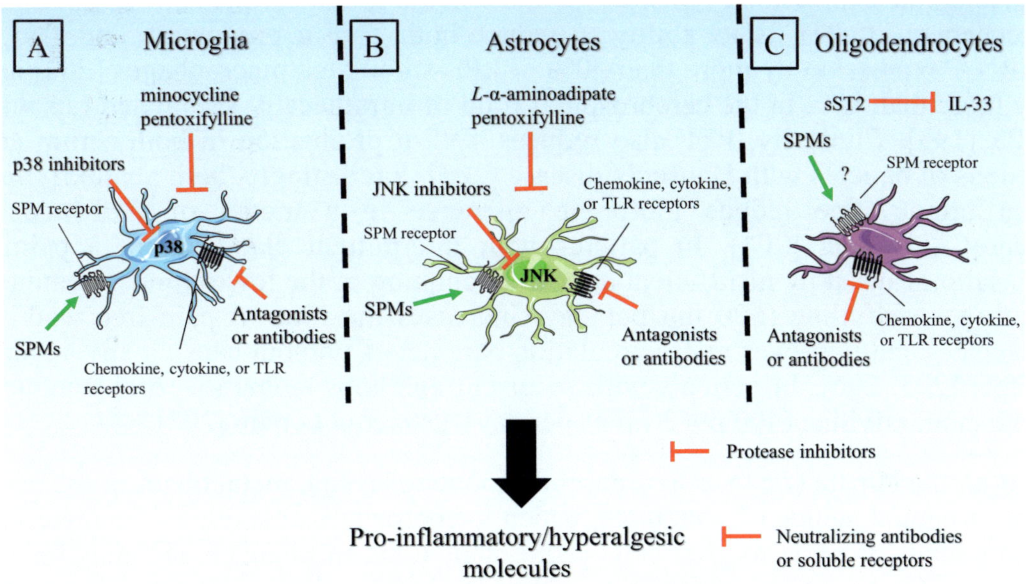

Fig. (3). Targeting glial cells as pharmacological perspectives for the management of chronic pain. Novel therapies targeting glial cell products (*e.g.* antibodies anti-chemokines or anti-cytokines; antibodies anti-CatS or MMPs). (A) Pharmacological perspectives targeting microglia activation [inhibitors of p38 or specialized pro-resolving lipid mediators (SPMs); antagonists of chemokines, cytokines, or TLR receptors]. (B) Pharmacological perspectives targeting astrocytes activation (inhibitors of JNK; SPMs; antagonists of chemokines, cytokines, or TLR receptors). (C) Pharmacological perspectives targeting oligodendrocytes [soluble ST2 receptor; SPMs (remains to be determined whether or not SPMs act on oligodendrocytes); antagonists of chemokines, cytokines, or TLR receptors].

Pentoxifylline (PTF) is an analog of the methylxanthine and a non-selective glial cell inhibitor [190]. PTF reduces both astrocytes and microglia activation in a murine model of neuropathic pain [191, 192]. In fact, PTF inhibits the release of pro-inflammatory mediators, such as TNF-α, IL-1β, IL-6, and PGE_2 from both microglia and astrocytes, and thereby attenuate the pain behavior [190, 193]. Peripheral treatment with PTF has also demonstrated effectiveness in the reduction of overt pain-like behaviors [194] and mechanical hyperalgesia by inhibiting the peripheral release of TNF-α and IL-1β production [195 - 197]. PTF mechanism of action is related to the inhibition of phosphodiesterases, which are intracellular enzymes responsible for cAMP and cGMP degradation [198]. In addition, PTF is a non-specific inhibitor of adenosine receptor [199]. PTF prevents astrocytes proliferation and reduces TNF-α-induced JNK and mTOR activation in cultured astrocytes [200]. *In vitro* data demonstrates that elevation of cAMP levels inhibits mTOR activation [201], thus, the ability of PTF in inhibits phosphodiesterase may account for this effect on mTOR signaling in astrocytes [200]. Furthermore, treatment with PTF reduces glutamatergic activity by reducing the expression of mGlut3, 5, and 7 in the spinal cord [191]. An important mechanism of PTF is its ability to reduce both TNF-α production and TNF-α mRNA expression by more than 50% in LPS-stimulated macrophages [202] and by more than 80% in the cerebrospinal fluid of intrathecally-stimulated rats with LPS [193]. Clinically, PTF also reduces TNF-α production in both serum and lesions of patients with Hansen's disease [203]. Interestingly, both pentoxifylline and minocycline reduce morphine tolerance in a model of CCI-induced neuropathic pain [204]. In patients with intermittent claudication, a painful sensation caused by insufficient arterial circulation in the lower limbs, treatment with pentoxifylline (600 mg per day) increases the time of pain-free walking distances and improves microcirculation parameters without causing any adverse effect [205, 206]. In patients with recurrent aphthous stomatitis, oral treatment with pentoxifylline (400 mg 3 times per day) also reduces pain [207].

L-α-aminoadipate (*L*α-AA) is a natural product of lysine metabolism in the brain and structural analog of glutamate, which in contrast to most other glutamate-like compounds, is toxic to glial cells [208]. This toxic mechanism accounts for the entry of *L*α-AA in astrocytes in a sodium transporter-dependent manner. *L*α-AA influences essential components of astrocytes metabolism, such as enzymes glutamine synthetase and y-glutamylcysteine synthetase [209, 210]. Studies on the stereospecificity of the effects of α-AA have shown that the *L*-isomer has a capacity to induce gliotoxicity [208, 211] whereas the *D*-isomer is a potent antagonist at the NMDA receptor [209]. *L*α-AA has been used to demonstrate the role of astrocytes in neuropathic pain models [130, 183, 190, 212 - 214].

Fluorocitrate is a reversible metabolic inhibitor of astrocytes [190, 215]. Fluorocitrate selectively inhibits the Krebs cycle enzyme aconitase and thereby reducing glutamate uptake, an important energy-dependent molecule for astrocyte function [190, 215]. Fluorocitrate is widely used in neuropathic pain models [130, 190], however, intrathecal fluorocitrate treatment also reduces inflammatory overt pain-like behaviors [216]. Also, rostral ventromedial medulla (RVM) microinjection of fluorocitrate could reverse the glial activation and significantly attenuate mechanical allodynia in a time-dependent manner in cancer-induced bone pain [217].

Minocycline, a tetracycline derivative antibiotic, acts selectively on microglia and its effects include the inhibition of enzymes such as nitric oxide synthase (iNOS) and IL-1 converting enzyme (caspase-1) [218]. Minocycline also inhibits the proliferation of microglial cells and the activation of MAPK p38 [130, 190]. Of note, minocycline has been widely used in neuropathic pain models [130, 190,

191, 219, 220], and it also reduces overt pain-like behaviors [216], ameliorates allergic asthmas, osteoporosis, and atherosclerosis [218]. Moreover, minocycline also prevents microglial activation and is neuroprotective in models of cerebral ischemia [221, 222], Parkinson's disease [223]. Also, RVM microinjection of minocycline could reverse the glial activation and significantly attenuate mechanical allodynia in a time-dependent manner in cancer-induced bone pain [217]. Minocycline can attenuate mechanical allodynia following either acute or persistent sciatic nerve inflammation (sciatic inflammatory neuropathy, SIN) or acute spinal immune activation with intrathecal HIV-1 gp120 and blocked the gp120-induced release of proinflammatory cytokines IL-1β and TNF-α [220]. With respect to its use in the treatment of painful conditions, minocycline has already been investigated in clinical studies. Patients with leprosy nerve function impairment who received oral treatment with 100 mg/day for three months of minocycline improves the sensory and motor function in 81% of cases [224]. In patients with diabetes type 2, minocycline treatment (100 mg per day for up to 6 weeks) reduces neuropathic pain without causing any adverse effect [225]. Minocycline applied topically after third molar surgery (1 mg) significantly reduces the intensity and duration of pain [226, 227]. In patients with recurrent aphthous stomatitis, topical application of minocycline (0.2%) reduces pain [228]. Other studies present controversial results, given that in persistent pain after lumbar discectomy [229] or subacute lumbar radicular pain [230], minocycline appears to have no analgesic effect since did not differ significantly from placebo. When used in patients with neuropathic pain of varied etiologies, minocycline improves the affective dimension of pain, but not its intensity [231]. Given that most rodent studies using minocycline as analgesic performed intrathecal treatment and human studies used oral or venous treatment, pharmacokinetic modulation might improve its analgesic efficacy.

Therefore, in spite of substantial data on the role of glial cells in experimental models of pain, clinical data is still less clear [189]. However, it seems that inhibiting glial cells is a therapeutic approach for, at least, neuropathic pain and some chronic pain conditions as detailed above. Further, it is likely that the development of better pharmacological tools to selective inhibit glial cell and an adequate pharmacokinetic profile is essential to finally achieve a proof-of-concept that inhibiting glial cells is an analgesic approach.

Sexually Dimorphism in Pain

Almost all new analgesic drugs (acting on periphery or CNS) are tested using male rodents. Therefore, the contribution of neuronal-glia interaction in pain processing is well-stablished in male rodents, which may seem a contradiction given that chronic diseases that are followed by chronic pain occur more often in women [188]. Recent evidence using mice of both sexes have shown that microglia are not involved in mediating CCI-induced hypersensitivity in females, suggesting the existence of sexually dimorphic pain processing (Fig. **4**) [219, 232]. Despite CCI induces microgliosis in both male and female mice, intrathecal treatment with minocycline, fluorocitrate, or propentofylline reduces pain in male CD-1 mice and in immunocompromised nude mice (mouse strain lacking T-cell immune response) of both sexes, but not in female CD-1 mice [219]. In male mice, microglia release BDNF that sensitizes nociceptor neurons to produce pain [219]. Moreover, treatment with a MAPK p38 inhibitor reduces pain in male mice, but not in female [219, 233]. Of note, nerve injury-induced pain hypersensitivity induces higher MAPK p38 phosphorylation in males than females [233] and p38 blockage reduces spontaneous EPSC lamina IIo neurons of male mice only [233]. Thus, it is likely that the chronic pain signaling in female mice is related to a microglia-independent mechanism and T-cell-dependent mechanism [219]. In fact, treatment with minocycline in mice lacking Rag1 (lack mature B and T lymphocytes [234]) reduces pain suggesting that in the absence of T-cells, female mice switch to a microglial-dependent mechanism [219]. Supporting this information, adoptive transfer of T-cell to Rag1 knockout mice revert this analgesic effect, female CD-1 mice present higher levels of lymphocytes in the blood than males, and CCI induces an higher T-cell recruitment to the spinal cord in female CD-1 mice than in males [219].

TLR-target therapies, in particular, TLR4, which seems promising to the treatment of neuropathic pain also possess sex dimorphism in the analgesic response [232, 235]. In a model of L5 spinal nerve ligation, male mice lacking TLR2, 3, 4, or 5 presented reduced mechanical hypersensitivity, whereas this analgesic effect was not observed in female mice lacking TLR4 [235]. Therefore, these evidences point to a sexual dimorphism in the regulation of pain in rodents. Using both male and female rodents will be crucial for the discovery of novel mechanisms that underlie sex differences in pain processes. Ultimately, these changes might be meaningful for new strategies for the treatment of chronic pain in women.

Pharmacological Perspectives

Inhibition of glial cells is related to analgesic effect in several experimental models of pain. Nevertheless, clinical data addressing this issue is still unclear. As described in the other topics, glial cells produce several pro-inflammatory mediators (*e.g.* cytokines, chemokines, and growth factors) that depend on the activation of MAPKs JNK (astrocytes) and p38 (microglia). Therefore, in this topic, we provide clinical and pre-clinical evidence of some pharmacological perspectives targeting glial cells activation or glial cells products (Fig. **3**). An exhaustive review of this topic can be found elsewhere [41, 42, 115, 190]. The involvement of MAPKs in pain regulation is widely known. MAPKs are classified into three major families with distinct pathways: ERK, JNK, and p38, which are implicated in the mechanism of chronic and inflammatory pain [42, 115, 190, 236]. Intrathecal delivery of ERK, JNK, or p38 inhibitors reduces the development of allodynia and hyperalgesia in varied pain models [112, 150, 236]. Here, we focus on inhibitors of JNK and p38, considering their higher expression in astrocytes and microglia, respectively [42, 190].

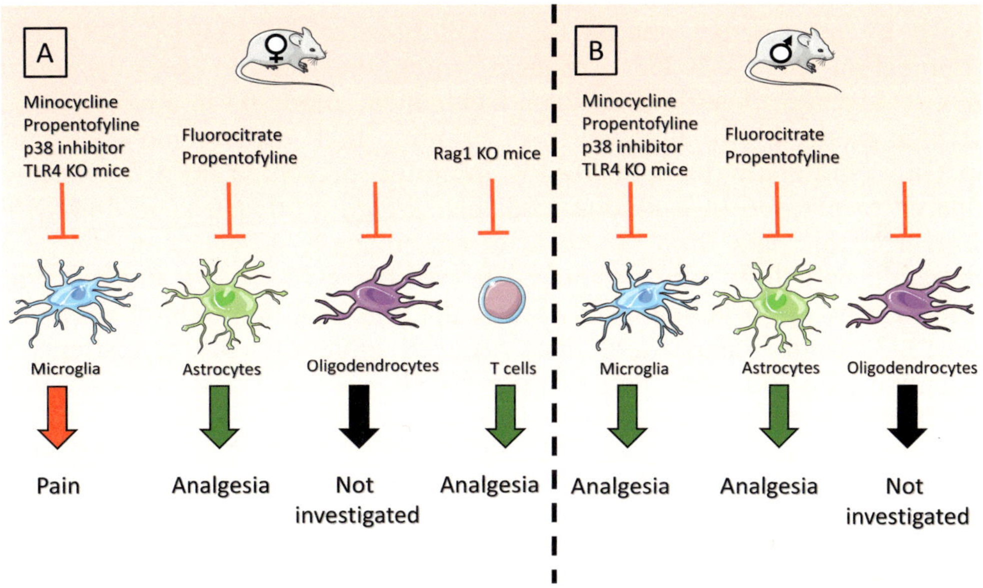

Fig. (4). Sexual dimorphism involving pain regulation in mice.
Chronic pain signaling in female mice is related to a microglia-independent mechanism and a T-cel--dependent mechanism (A). Intrathecal treatment with minocycline (microglia inhibitor), fluorocitrate (astrocyte inhibitor), or propentofylline (non-selective glial cell inhibitor) reduces pain in male (B) but not in female mice (A) [219]. Moreover, treatment with a MAPK p38 inhibitor reduces pain in male mice, but not in female [219, 233]. Male mice lacking TLR2, 3, 4, or 5 presented reduced mechanical hypersensitivity (B), whereas this analgesic effect is not observed in female mice lacking TLR4 (A) [235].

SP600125 is a selective and reversible inhibitor of JNK. It inhibits the expression of proinflammatory/hyperalgesic genes such as COX-2, IFN-γ, TNF-α, and prevents the activation of Jurkat T cells [237]. Intrathecal injection of SP600125 reduces, for instance, granulocyte-colony stimulating factor (G-CSF)-induced hyperalgesia [236], CCI- and IL-33-induced hyperalgesia [130], SNI-induced neuropathic pain [214], and complex regional pain syndrome [110]. Moreover, a proteinase-resistant peptide inhibitor of JNK (D-JNKI-1) ameliorates SNI-induced neuropathic pain [214]. Intrathecal delivery of SP600125 also reduces overt pain-like behaviors, such as abdominal contortions and paw flinches [216].

The p38 MAPK is activated by proinflammatory cytokine and cell stress and play an essential role in the regulation of the inflammatory response, neurodegeneration, and cell death [42, 190]. SB202190 is a highly selective inhibitor of p38 [238]. SB202190 selectively inhibits alpha and beta p38 isoforms and has no effect on JNK and ERK [238]. Intrathecal injection of SB202190 reduces IL-33- [130] and granulocyte-colony stimulating factor (G-CSF)-induced hyperalgesia [236]. Intrathecal delivery of SB202190 also reduces overt pain-like behaviors, such as abdominal contortions and flinches [216]. Importantly, SB202190 increases spontaneous inhibitory postsynaptic current (ISPC), which is reversed by an inactive analog of a p38 blocker (SB202474) [239]. RVM microinjection of SB203580 reduces microglial-derived pro-inflammatory mediators and significantly attenuates mechanical allodynia in a cancer-induced bone pain model [240]. It is worth mentioning that losmapimod (GW856553, from GlaxoSmithKline) a p38 MAPK inhibitor, presented no difference when compared to placebo in a randomized, placebo-controlled trial in 144 patients with neuropathic pain from lumbosacral radiculopathy [241] or in 168 patients neuropathic pain following peripheral nerve injury [242]. On the other hand, another trial with 50 patients shows that the p38 MAPK inhibitor dilmapimod (SB681323, from GlaxoSmithKline) reduced pain intensity in patients with neuropathic pain following nerve injury [243].

Compelling evidence has pointed to the endogenous role of specialized pro-resolving lipid mediators (SPMs) in the regulation of acute inflammatory process [244]. SPMs are divided in those from E-series [if derived from eicosapentaenoic acid (EPA)], D-series [if derived from docosahexaenoic acid (DHA)], or those derived from arachidonic acid [244]. Treatment with isolated SPMs present biological effect in several chronic conditions, such as rheumatic diseases [245] and neuropathic pain [244]. SPMs include molecules such as resolvins (Rv), protectins, and lipoxins (Lx), which are emerging as potential therapies [244]. Isolated RvE1 and RvD1 attenuate pro-inflammatory cytokine release in several animal models of inflammation and pain [246]. For instance, RvE1 and RvD1 inhibit inflammatory and neuropathic pain in mice by suppressing calcium influx in DRG neurons [247 - 249]. At presynaptic sites of spinal cord primary afferent terminals, RvE1 reduces ERK activation, inhibits TNF-α-induced spontaneous EPSC, and attenuates glutamate release [247]. Moreover, intrathecal delivery of LxA4 and RvD1 reduces carrageenan-induced hyperalgesia in rats and TNF-α production in cultured astrocytes [250]. In addition, LxA4 ameliorates neuropathic pain by targeting microglia activation [246]. Interestingly, nociceptor neurons, astrocytes, and microglia express receptors for, LxA4, RvE1, and RvD1 [246, 247, 250].

For centuries cannabis has been worldwide used for medical purpose [251]. With the discovery of CB receptors, increasingly attention has been given to the use of single cannabinoids [cannabidiol or delta-9-tetrahydrocannabinol (THC)] or cannabis as analgesic in varied clinical settings [251]. Experimentally, synthetic CB receptor agonists display safe analgesic profile. For instance, treatment with WIN 55,212-2 (selective CB1 receptor agonist) or JWH-015 (selective CB2 receptor agonist) ameliorate brachial plexus avulsion (BPA)-induced neuropathic pain [252]. In terms of glial cells, treatment with cannabidiol, WIN 55,212-2, and JWH-133 (selective CB2 receptor agonist) reduce microglia activation in a model of AD by reducing calcium influx both *in vitro* and *in vivo.* WIN 55,212-2 was able to reduce the expression of both TNF-α and IL-6 mRNA expression by microglia [253]. The intrathecal treatment with WIN 55,212-2 also reduced astrocytes and microglia activation in a model of paclitaxel-induced neuropathic pain [254]. Interestingly, JWH-015 reduces morphine-induced hyperalgesia by reducing IL-1β, TNF-α, and IL-6 in an Akt- and ERK1/2-dependent manner, indicating that it might be relevant in designing treatments to opioid-induced hyperalgesia [255]. Regarding human data, in a cohort study with 614 patients with different types of chronic pain (neuropathic, MS, HIV *etc.*), the use of cannabidiol products was continued in 76.2% of these patients of whom 64.7% reported an improvement associated with the therapy [256]. In this study, patients were able to choose among infusion or inhalation *via* vaporization of the cannabidiol products [256]. On the other hand, in two different phase III, double-blind, multicenter, randomized, placebo-controlled trials with 399 and 540 patients with cancer pain, treatment with Sativex (nasal spray) showed no difference in reducing self-reported pain when compared to placebo [257]. Thus, clinical data regarding the use of this substance is still controversial. Furthermore, the many side effects due to cannabidiol [258] indicates that better pharmacological approaches would be achieved developing synthetic CB receptor agonists. However, larger and robust clinical trials will determine the efficacy and relevant pharmaceutical formulations containing cannabinoids in clinical settings.

Peripheral and spinal cord production of IL-33 have been implicated in the pathogenesis of different models of pain [130, 259 - 265]. In a model of bone cancer-induced pain, IL-33 presents increased expression in the spinal cord. In this model, IL-33 is produced by astrocytes, but not neurons or microglia, as observed by the double staining with GFAP, but not NeuN or CD11b [259]. Moreover, CCI-induced neuropathic pain also induces the expression of both IL-33 and ST2 mRNA [264, 266] and protein [130] in the spinal cord. The interaction between IL-33 and ST2 leads to the activation of PI3K, mTOR, MAPKs (p38, JNK, and ERK), and NF-kB signaling pathways, which are essential to the production of TNFα and IL-1β by microglial and astrocytes [130]. Furthermore, SNI-induced neuropathic pain or intrathecal injection of IL-33 increase the expression of NMDA receptor (NR1 subunit) in neurons, demonstrating that IL-33/ST2 signaling facilitates pain processing [260]. Importantly, intrathecal treatment with sST2, anti-ST2, or mice lacking ST2 reduce glial cells activation, pro-inflammatory cytokines production, and mechanical hyperalgesia [130, 259, 260].

IL-10 is another cytokine that deserves attention given its immunoregulatory properties [267, 268]. Seminal work demonstrated that intraplantar treatment with IL-10 reduces carrageenan-, bradykinin-, TNF-α, IL-1β, and IL-6-induced hyperalgesia in rats [269]. At spinal cord level, intrathecal administration of an adeno-associated viral encoding IL-10 gene reduces CCI-induced mechanical and thermal hyperalgesia in rats [270, 271]. Moreover, intrathecal delivery of a IL-4/IL-10 fusion protein reduces carrageenan-induced microglia and astrocytes activation [272]. In humans, a phase I study using human recombinant IL-10 in 72 patients with active RA indicated a trend towards clinical improvement [273, 274]. On the other hand, in a multicenter placebo-controlled double-blind, phase II/III study, human recombinant IL-10 (rhIL-10) failed at improving disease activity in 6 patients with RA [275]. Thus, in spite of preclinical data demonstrating the analgesic effect of IL-10 in several experimental models [267, 268, 270, 271], trial with rhIL-10 has been shown some non-satisfactory results [273 - 275]. Despite the lack of effectiveness of IL-10 in clinical trials, strategies aimed at increasing endogenous IL-10 levels seem promising. Burst spinal cord stimulation in patients with failed back surgery syndrome, increases IL-10 serum levels, which correlates with the reduction of back pain score [276]. Thus, larger and robust clinical trials will determine whether or not this cytokine becomes a valuable clinical analgesic approach as it is in animals. It is likely that the difference of route of administration [systemic in humans *versus* locally (intrathecal, for instance) in animals] may account for discrepant effectiveness, and thus, pharmacokinetic and pharmacodynamic studies in humans should also be performed [274]. In addition, seek for novel pharmaceutical formulations may also improve IL-10 efficacy [277, 278].

As mentioned, chemokines possess a fundamental role in the development and maintenance of chronic pain state [115, 187]. Therefore, the development of chemokine antagonists for the management of pain are highly attractive. However, AZD2423 (from AstraZeneca), a CCR2 antagonist that presents potent analgesic effect in neuropathic pain and inflammatory pain models, failed in a randomized, double-blind, placebo-controlled trial in patients with post-traumatic neuralgia [279]. In another trial, BAY 86-5047 (from Bayer) a CCR1 antagonist showed no difference *versus* placebo in a randomized controlled trial in 110 patients with endometriosis-associated pelvic pain [280]. Another compound, RAP-103 (from Rapid Pharmaceuticals) is a mixed CCR2/CCR5 antagonist that inhibits microglia activation and thereby attenuates neuropathic pain [281]. To the moment, this molecule has not been tested in clinical trial. Regarding fractalkine, E6011, a humanized anti-fractalkine monoclonal antibody (from Esai), was well-tolerated and reduced tender and joint swollen when compared to the baseline in a phase 1/2 study with RA patients in Japan [282]. To the date, to our knowledge, there is no placebo-controlled double-blinded study using this drug.

The development of TLR antagonists has also been made by several pharmaceuticals companies to the treatment of a wide range of diseases [41, 283]. Regarding pain, ATNC05 (from Allodynic Therapeutics) is a synergistic mixture of an opioid and TLR4 antagonist for the treatment of different types of chronic pain. ATNC05 reduced pain intensity in phase II randomized, placebo-controlled trial with patients with chronic, neuropathic back, and cervical pain [283].

Thus, it is reasonable to assume that the development of novel therapies targeting glial cell products (*e.g.* antibodies anti-chemokines or anti-cytokines; antibodies anti-CatS or MMPs; antagonists of chemokines, cytokines, or TLR receptors) or therapies targeting signaling pathways (inhibitors of JNK or p38 MAPKs) are likely to be highly attractive (Fig. **3**). However, it worth to mention that a significant difficulty with preclinical models is that the human observer (investigator) may introduce postural changes in the animals that may resemble fear and anxiety, which ultimately may influence the outcome [284, 285]. Conventionally, rodent somatosensory assays involve the application of a stimulus (*e.g.*, something hot, cold, or sharp) by a human investigator to the paws, tail, or abdomen of animals to determine the intensity of the stimulus required for the animal to withdrawal response [286, 287]. The measurement of this withdrawal reflex may reveal changes in sensitivity of the nociceptive system that correspond to aspects of the human experience, such as allodynia or hyperalgesia [287]. However, stimulus-evoked hypersensitivity is only one symptomatic feature found in patients with chronic pain, who more often present with spontaneous ongoing or intermittent pain, that is pain arising in the absence of any peripheral stimulus. Although preclinical models are handy for the discovery of novel targets or mechanism of action of new drugs, they currently lack translational predictive power. In fact, this current poor predictability of preclinical models of pain can imply in higher failure rates of these new drugs in clinical trials resulting in a considerable loss in economic terms to pharmaceutical companies, and more important, results in novel drugs candidate that do not suppress the symptoms of the patients [189, 284]. Nevertheless, it is also very important to highlight that conventional methodologies were and have been used effectively to discover new analgesic drugs and mechanisms of action of already existing drugs. Otherwise, we wouldn't have any new analgesic drug in the clinics or the use of molecules that were not designed to be analgesic (minocycline, for example). Another important point to be addressed is that our tools to measure pain in clinical trials are not totally effective as well [288]. In fact, pain assessment is performed inadequately in many countries, resulting in failures of the management of pain [289]. For instance, a systematic review of methodologies used to measure pain outcomes in clinical trials with patients with low back pain shows that the main methodology used by these studies was the visual analog scale (VAS) [290]. This methodology lacks sensitivity in the measurement of pain in patients with chronic pain [289]. Thus, if an inadequate pain questionnaire is applied, it is hard to determine the efficacy of novel drugs. In corroboration, healthy female individuals reported higher ratings of heat pain than male subjects when using numerical scales (*i.e.* 0-100) [291]. However, these differences disappear when these same individuals rated pain using VAS [291]. These issues have led most analgesics drug development efforts to concentrate in the molecular redesign of already stablished analgesic classes, such as NSAIDs, opioids, tricyclic antidepressants, ion channel- modulating drugs, and certain anticonvulsants, despite their well-known limitations regarding effectiveness, tolerance, and hyperalgesia (in the case of opioids, such as morphine) [174, 189, 285]. An interesting strategy that has been used to drawback opioid dependence and increase opiate efficacy, is the combination of ultra-low doses of an opioid antagonist with an opiate drug [292]. In a phase II randomized, multi-center controlled trial with 360 patients with osteoarthritis, treatment with Oxytrex [oxycodone + ultra-low dose of naltrexone (0.001 mg)] reduced pain intensity when compared to oxycodone alone [293]. Another trial, a phase III randomized, double-blind, multi-center, and placebo-controlled trial with 719 patients with low back pain, Oxytrex reduced the physical dependence (after opiate withdrawal) and increased the analgesic effect of oxycodone [294]. In terms of mechanisms, co-treatment of ultra-low dose of naltrexone (5 ng) with morphine, increases the analgesic effect of this opioid by reducing glial cell activation in rats [295]. Interestingly, low doses of naltrexone ameliorate DSS-induced colitis, suggesting that this drug may also possesses anti-inflammatory effect *per se* [296]. Therefore, association of ultra-low doses of an opioid antagonist with an opiate drug seems as an alternative to reduce opioid physical dependence and to increase opiate analgesic efficacy [292].

CONCLUSIONS

In this chapter, we reviewed the current understanding of the communication between glial cells and sensory neurons. Sensory neurons can regulate the peripheral inflammatory response by releasing neuropeptides such as CGRP, substance P, and VIP that mediate neurogenic inflammation and the activation of innate and adaptive immune cells. Regarding central sensitization, we reviewed that the neuronal systems are no longer the only player involved in this phenomenon. Rather, a variety of non-neuronal cells, especially glial cells (namely astrocyte, microglia, and oligodendrocyte), play a significant role in the initiation and modulation of the primary afferent nociceptors activity (Fig. **1** and **2**). These cells release cytokines (*e.g.* TNF-α, IL-1β, IL-6, and IL-33), growth factors (*e.g.* BDNF), and chemokines (*e.g.* fractalkine, CCL2, and CXCL1) that bind to specific receptors expressed by those nociceptors (Fig. **2**) [7, 8, 115]. Moreover, glial cells have degrees of activation that are related to ionic changes (increase of calcium influx), activation of ion channels (due to phosphorylation by MAPKs, for instance), modulation of expression markers (*e.g.* IBA-1, GFAP, OLIG-2), morphological changes (*e.g.* microgliosis and astrogliosis), and recruitment and proliferation [187, 297]. The understanding of all these molecular changes associated to the emotional component of pain seems a key point to understand the transition of acute to chronic pain. Therefore, although glial cells were considered bystanders in the development of chronic pain, now, these cells are under the spotlight for the scrutiny of novel analgesic drugs (Fig. **3**). A significant challenge for the future is to establish to what extent this immune response initiates or maintains neuropathic pain in human, and thus, whether it is amenable to glial cells-targeting therapies. Furthermore, determining whether or not gender has also influence on pain signaling in humans as has in rodents (Fig. **4**) and continuing addressing the sex bias in pain research (which most of the study are conducted using male animals) will certainly increase the translational relevance of preclinical findings and advance our understanding of chronic pain in women. An important point to keep in mind is that effectively measuring pain in animals is perhaps the most difficult challenge in the field of pain, as the current methodologies mostly detect stimulus-evoked responses from the animal. Stimulus-evoked responses correlate with some aspects of pain, such as withdrawal from a stimulus or learned behavioral avoidance from a potentially painful situation. This type of response is also related to only one symptomatic feature found in chronic pain patients, who more often present with spontaneous ongoing or intermittent pain. Thus, although preclinical models are beneficial for the discovery of novel targets or mechanism of action of new drugs, translational predictive power should be improved to reduce failure rates of clinical trials. Thus, new technologies aimed at evaluating spontaneous rodent behavior (and also potential side effects) and capable of evaluating the reduction of these behaviors in clinically relevant doses may increase productivity of new analgesic drugs. Nevertheless, it also very important to highlight that conventional pre-clinical methodologies were and have been used effectively to discover new analgesic drugs and mechanisms of action of already existing drugs. In addition, our tools to measure pain in humans are not are not totally effective. In summary, advance in both preclinical and clinical phases of the discovery of new analgesic drugs may reduce failure at clinical trials. New developments may be observed in enriched human populations since the animal models also represent enriched populations as observed with several studies using outbred stocks and differential activation of immune cells depending on the model. These elements indicate the need of a wide range of specific treatments for specific conditions. In this sense, an important advance that eventually can be true in the pain field is the individualized treatment as occur in oncology given this take in account the heterogeneity of patients [298, 299]. Further, it is likely that the development of better pharmacological tools to selective inhibit glial cells and an adequate pharmacokinetic profile is essential to finally achieve a proof-of-concept that inhibiting glial cells is an analgesic approach.

CONFLICT OF INTEREST

The authors declare no conflict of interest, financial or otherwise.

ACKNOWLEDGEMENTS

This work was supported by grants from São Paulo Research Foundation under grant agreements 2011/19670-0 (Thematic Project) and 2013/08216-2 (Center for Research in Inflammatory Disease); Coordenadoria de Aperfeiçoamento de Pessoal de Nível Superior (CAPES, Brazil); Conselho Nacional de Desenvolvimento Científico e Tecnológico (CNPq, Brazil); Pesquisa para o Sistema Único de Saúde (PPSUS) funded by Ministério da Ciência, Tecnologia e Inovação (MCTI), Secretaria da Ciência, Tecnologia e Ensino Superior (SETI), Departamento de Ciência e Tecnologia/Ministério da Saúde (DECIT/MS), Financiadora de Estudos e Projetos (FINEP)/SETI (Brazil), Fundação Araucária, Secretaria de Saúde do Estado do Paraná (SESA) and Paraná State Government (Brazil).

REFERENCES

[1] Calati R, Laglaoui Bakhiyi C, Artero S, Ilgen M, Courtet P. The impact of physical pain on suicidal thoughts and behaviors: Meta-analyses. J Psychiatr Res 2015; 71: 16-32. [http://dx.doi.org/10.1016/j.jpsychires.2015.09.004] [PMID: 26522868]

[2] Fishbain DA, Cutler R, Rosomoff HL, Rosomoff RS. Chronic pain-associated depression: antecedent or consequence of chronic pain? A review. Clin J Pain 1997; 13(2): 116-37. [http://dx.doi.org/10.1097/00002508-199706000-00006] [PMID: 9186019]

[3] Moayedi M, Davis KD. Theories of pain: from specificity to gate control. J Neurophysiol 2013; 109(1): 5-12. [http://dx.doi.org/10.1152/jn.00457.2012] [PMID: 23034364]

[4] Koyama T, McHaffie JG, Laurienti PJ, Coghill RC. The subjective experience of pain: where expectations become reality. Proc Natl Acad Sci USA 2005; 102(36): 12950-5. [http://dx.doi.org/10.1073/pnas.0408576102] [PMID: 16150703]

[5] Bushnell MC, Ceko M, Low LA. Cognitive and emotional control of pain and its disruption in chronic pain. Nat Rev Neurosci 2013; 14(7): 502-11. [http://dx.doi.org/10.1038/nrn3516] [PMID: 23719569]

[6] Wiech K, Vandekerckhove J, Zaman J, Tuerlinckx F, Vlaeyen JW, Tracey I. Influence of prior information on pain involves biased perceptual decision-making. Curr Biol 2014; 24(15): R679-81. [http://dx.doi.org/10.1016/j.cub.2014.06.022] [PMID: 25093555]

[7] Pinho-Ribeiro FA, Verri WA Jr, Chiu IM. Nociceptor Sensory Neuron-Immune Interactions in Pain and Inflammation. Trends Immunol 2017; 38(1): 5-19. [http://dx.doi.org/10.1016/j.it.2016.10.001] [PMID: 27793571]

[8] Ji RR, Chamessian A, Zhang YQ. Pain regulation by non-neuronal cells and inflammation. Science 2016; 354(6312): 572-7. [http://dx.doi.org/10.1126/science.aaf8924] [PMID: 27811267]

[9] Talbot S, Foster SL, Woolf CJ. Neuroimmunity: Physiology and Pathology. Annu Rev Immunol 2016; 34: 421-47. [http://dx.doi.org/10.1146/annurev-immunol-041015-055340] [PMID: 26907213]

[10] Chiu IM. Infection, Pain, and Itch. Neurosci Bull In press [PMID: 28144843]

[11] Borghi SM, Fattori V, Conchon-Costa I, Pinge-Filho P, Pavanelli WR, Verri WA Jr. Leishmania infection: painful or painless? Parasitol Res 2017; 116(2): 465-75. [http://dx.doi.org/10.1007/s00436-016-5340-7] [PMID: 27933392]

[12] Chiu IM, Heesters BA, Ghasemlou N, *et al.* Bacteria activate sensory neurons that modulate pain and inflammation. Nature 2013; 501(7465): 52-7. [http://dx.doi.org/10.1038/nature12479] [PMID: 23965627]

[13] Calil IL, Zarpelon AC, Guerrero AT, *et al.* Lipopolysaccharide induces inflammatory hyperalgesia triggering a TLR4/MyD88-dependent cytokine cascade in the mice paw. PLoS One 2014; 9(3): e90013. [http://dx.doi.org/10.1371/journal.pone.0090013] [PMID: 24595131]

[14] Tse KH, Chow KB, Leung WK, Wong YH, Wise H. Lipopolysaccharide differentially modulates expression of cytokines and cyclooxygenases in dorsal root ganglion cells *via* Toll-like receptor-4 dependent pathways. Neuroscience 2014; 267: 241-51. [http://dx.doi.org/10.1016/j.neuroscience.2014.02.041] [PMID: 24607321]

[15] Meseguer V, Alpizar YA, Luis E, *et al.* TRPA1 channels mediate acute neurogenic inflammation and pain produced by bacterial endotoxins. Nat Commun 2014; 5: 3125. [http://dx.doi.org/10.1038/ncomms4125] [PMID: 24445575]

[16] Fernandes ES, Liang L, Smillie SJ, *et al.* TRPV1 deletion enhances local inflammation and accelerates the onset of systemic inflammatory response syndrome. J Immunol 2012; 188(11): 5741-51. [http://dx.doi.org/10.4049/jimmunol.1102147] [PMID: 22547700]

[17] Riol-Blanco L, Ordovas-Montanes J, Perro M, *et al.* Nociceptive sensory neurons drive interleukin-2--mediated psoriasiform skin inflammation. Nature 2014; 510(7503): 157-61. [http://dx.doi.org/10.1038/nature13199] [PMID: 24759321]

[18] Talbot S, Abdulnour RE, Burkett PR, *et al.* Silencing Nociceptor Neurons Reduces Allergic Airway Inflammation. Neuron 2015; 87(2): 341-54. [http://dx.doi.org/10.1016/j.neuron.2015.06.007] [PMID: 26119026]

[19] Rehman R, Bhat YA, Panda L, Mabalirajan U. TRPV1 inhibition attenuates IL-13 mediated asthma features in mice by reducing airway epithelial injury. Int Immunopharmacol 2013; 15(3): 597-605. [http://dx.doi.org/10.1016/j.intimp.2013.02.010] [PMID: 23453702]

[20] Caterina MJ, Schumacher MA, Tominaga M, Rosen TA, Levine JD, Julius D. The capsaicin receptor: a heat-activated ion channel in the pain pathway. Nature 1997; 389(6653): 816-24. [http://dx.doi.org/10.1038/39807] [PMID: 9349813]

[21] Fattori V, Hohmann MS, Rossaneis AC, Pinho-Ribeiro FA, Verri WA. Capsaicin: current

understanding of its mechanisms and therapy of pain and other pre-clinical and clinical uses. Molecules 2016; 21(7): E844.
[http://dx.doi.org/10.3390/molecules21070844] [PMID: 27367653]

[22] Sobue M, Joh T, Oshima T, *et al.* Contribution of capsaicin-sensitive afferent nerves to rapid recovery from ethanol-induced gastric epithelial damage in rats. J Gastroenterol Hepatol 2003; 18(10): 1188-95.
[http://dx.doi.org/10.1046/j.1440-1746.2003.03143.x] [PMID: 12974907]

[23] Mózsik G, Szolcsányi J, Rácz I. Gastroprotection induced by capsaicin in healthy human subjects. World J Gastroenterol 2005; 11(33): 5180-4.
[PMID: 16127749]

[24] Holzer P, Pabst MA. Visceral afferent neurons: role in gastric mucosal protection. News Physiol Sci 1999; 14: 201-6.
[PMID: 11390851]

[25] Garden GA, Möller T. Microglia biology in health and disease. J Neuroimmune Pharmacol 2006; 1(2): 127-37.
[http://dx.doi.org/10.1007/s11481-006-9015-5] [PMID: 18040779]

[26] Ginhoux F, Lim S, Hoeffel G, Low D, Huber T. Origin and differentiation of microglia. Front Cell Neurosci 2013; 7: 45.
[http://dx.doi.org/10.3389/fncel.2013.00045] [PMID: 23616747]

[27] Heneka MT, Kummer MP, Latz E. Innate immune activation in neurodegenerative disease. Nat Rev Immunol 2014; 14(7): 463-77.
[http://dx.doi.org/10.1038/nri3705] [PMID: 24962261]

[28] Ginhoux F, Greter M, Leboeuf M, *et al.* Fate mapping analysis reveals that adult microglia derive from primitive macrophages. Science 2010; 330(6005): 841-5.
[http://dx.doi.org/10.1126/science.1194637] [PMID: 20966214]

[29] Gomez-Nicola D, Perry VH. Microglial dynamics and role in the healthy and diseased brain: a paradigm of functional plasticity. Neuroscientist 2015; 21(2): 169-84.
[http://dx.doi.org/10.1177/1073858414530512] [PMID: 24722525]

[30] Schulz C, Gomez Perdiguero E, Chorro L, *et al.* A lineage of myeloid cells independent of Myb and hematopoietic stem cells. Science 2012; 336(6077): 86-90.
[http://dx.doi.org/10.1126/science.1219179] [PMID: 22442384]

[31] Kierdorf K, Erny D, Goldmann T, *et al.* Microglia emerge from erythromyeloid precursors *via* Pu.1- and Irf8-dependent pathways. Nat Neurosci 2013; 16(3): 273-80.
[http://dx.doi.org/10.1038/nn.3318] [PMID: 23334579]

[32] Kettenmann H, Hanisch UK, Noda M, Verkhratsky A. Physiology of microglia. Physiol Rev 2011; 91(2): 461-553.
[http://dx.doi.org/10.1152/physrev.00011.2010] [PMID: 21527731]

[33] Tsuda M, Inoue K, Salter MW. Neuropathic pain and spinal microglia: a big problem from molecules in "small" glia. Trends Neurosci 2005; 28(2): 101-7.
[http://dx.doi.org/10.1016/j.tins.2004.12.002] [PMID: 15667933]

[34] Saijo K, Glass CK. Microglial cell origin and phenotypes in health and disease. Nat Rev Immunol 2011; 11(11): 775-87.
[http://dx.doi.org/10.1038/nri3086] [PMID: 22025055]

[35] Nayak D, Roth TL, McGavern DB. Microglia development and function. Annu Rev Immunol 2014; 32: 367-402.
[http://dx.doi.org/10.1146/annurev-immunol-032713-120240] [PMID: 24471431]

[36] Grace PM, Hutchinson MR, Maier SF, Watkins LR. Pathological pain and the neuroimmune interface. Nat Rev Immunol 2014; 14(4): 217-31.
[http://dx.doi.org/10.1038/nri3621] [PMID: 24577438]

[37] Inoue K. The function of microglia through purinergic receptors: neuropathic pain and cytokine release. Pharmacol Ther 2006; 109(1-2): 210-26.
[http://dx.doi.org/10.1016/j.pharmthera.2005.07.001] [PMID: 16169595]

[38] Ji RR, Berta T, Nedergaard M. Glia and pain: is chronic pain a gliopathy? Pain 2013; 154 (Suppl. 1): S10-28.
[http://dx.doi.org/10.1016/j.pain.2013.06.022] [PMID: 23792284]

[39] Saijo K, Crotti A, Glass CK. Regulation of microglia activation and deactivation by nuclear receptors. Glia 2013; 61(1): 104-11.
[http://dx.doi.org/10.1002/glia.22423] [PMID: 22987512]

[40] Nicotra L, Loram LC, Watkins LR, Hutchinson MR. Toll-like receptors in chronic pain. Exp Neurol 2012; 234(2): 316-29.
[http://dx.doi.org/10.1016/j.expneurol.2011.09.038] [PMID: 22001158]

[41] Thakur KK, Saini J, Mahajan K, *et al.* Therapeutic implications of toll-like receptors in peripheral neuropathic pain. Pharmacol Res 2017; 115: 224-32.
[http://dx.doi.org/10.1016/j.phrs.2016.11.019] [PMID: 27894923]

[42] Popiolek-Barczyk K, Mika J. Targeting the microglial signaling pathways: New insights in the modulation of neuropathic pain. Curr Med Chem 2016; 23(26): 2908-28.
[http://dx.doi.org/10.2174/0929867323666160607120124] [PMID: 27281131]

[43] Brautigam VM, Frasier C, Nikodemova M, Watters JJ. Purinergic receptor modulation of BV-2 microglial cell activity: potential involvement of p38 MAP kinase and CREB. J Neuroimmunol 2005; 166(1-2): 113-25.
[http://dx.doi.org/10.1016/j.jneuroim.2005.05.012] [PMID: 15979729]

[44] Möller T, Nolte C, Burger R, Verkhratsky A, Kettenmann H. Mechanisms of C5a and C3a complement fragment-induced [Ca2+]i signaling in mouse microglia. J Neurosci 1997; 17(2): 615-24.
[PMID: 8987784]

[45] He WJ, Cui J, Du L, *et al.* Spinal P2X(7) receptor mediates microglia activation-induced neuropathic pain in the sciatic nerve injury rat model. Behav Brain Res 2012; 226(1): 163-70.
[http://dx.doi.org/10.1016/j.bbr.2011.09.015] [PMID: 21933684]

[46] Chu YX, Zhang Y, Zhang YQ, Zhao ZQ. Involvement of microglial P2X7 receptors and downstream signaling pathways in long-term potentiation of spinal nociceptive responses. Brain Behav Immun 2010; 24(7): 1176-89.
[http://dx.doi.org/10.1016/j.bbi.2010.06.001] [PMID: 20554014]

[47] Tsuda M, Shigemoto-Mogami Y, Koizumi S, *et al.* P2X4 receptors induced in spinal microglia gate tactile allodynia after nerve injury. Nature 2003; 424(6950): 778-83.
[http://dx.doi.org/10.1038/nature01786] [PMID: 12917686]

[48] Kobayashi K, Yamanaka H, Fukuoka T, Dai Y, Obata K, Noguchi K. P2Y12 receptor upregulation in activated microglia is a gateway of p38 signaling and neuropathic pain. J Neurosci 2008; 28(11): 2892-902.
[http://dx.doi.org/10.1523/JNEUROSCI.5589-07.2008] [PMID: 18337420]

[49] Tozaki-Saitoh H, Tsuda M, Miyata H, Ueda K, Kohsaka S, Inoue K. P2Y12 receptors in spinal microglia are required for neuropathic pain after peripheral nerve injury. J Neurosci 2008; 28(19): 4949-56.
[http://dx.doi.org/10.1523/JNEUROSCI.0323-08.2008] [PMID: 18463248]

[50] Davalos D, Grutzendler J, Yang G, *et al.* ATP mediates rapid microglial response to local brain injury *in vivo*. Nat Neurosci 2005; 8(6): 752-8.
[http://dx.doi.org/10.1038/nn1472] [PMID: 15895084]

[51] Biber K, Tsuda M, Tozaki-Saitoh H, *et al.* Neuronal CCL21 up-regulates microglia P2X4 expression and initiates neuropathic pain development. EMBO J 2011; 30(9): 1864-73.

[http://dx.doi.org/10.1038/emboj.2011.89] [PMID: 21441897]

[52] Napoli I, Neumann H. Microglial clearance function in health and disease. Neuroscience 2009; 158(3): 1030-8.
[http://dx.doi.org/10.1016/j.neuroscience.2008.06.046] [PMID: 18644426]

[53] Neumann H, Kotter MR, Franklin RJ. Debris clearance by microglia: an essential link between degeneration and regeneration. Brain 2009; 132(Pt 2): 288-95.
[http://dx.doi.org/10.1093/brain/awn109] [PMID: 18567623]

[54] Marín-Teva JL, Dusart I, Colin C, Gervais A, van Rooijen N, Mallat M. Microglia promote the death of developing Purkinje cells. Neuron 2004; 41(4): 535-47.
[http://dx.doi.org/10.1016/S0896-6273(04)00069-8] [PMID: 14980203]

[55] Hristova M, Cuthill D, Zbarsky V, *et al.* Activation and deactivation of periventricular white matter phagocytes during postnatal mouse development. Glia 2010; 58(1): 11-28.
[http://dx.doi.org/10.1002/glia.20896] [PMID: 19544386]

[56] Ransohoff RM, Perry VH. Microglial physiology: unique stimuli, specialized responses. Annu Rev Immunol 2009; 27: 119-45.
[http://dx.doi.org/10.1146/annurev.immunol.021908.132528] [PMID: 19302036]

[57] Takahashi K, Rochford CD, Neumann H. Clearance of apoptotic neurons without inflammation by microglial triggering receptor expressed on myeloid cells-2. J Exp Med 2005; 201(4): 647-57.
[http://dx.doi.org/10.1084/jem.20041611] [PMID: 15728241]

[58] Neher JJ, Neniskyte U, Hornik T, Brown GC. Inhibition of UDP/P2Y6 purinergic signaling prevents phagocytosis of viable neurons by activated microglia *in vitro* and *in vivo*. Glia 2014; 62(9): 1463-75.
[http://dx.doi.org/10.1002/glia.22693] [PMID: 24838858]

[59] Ribes S, Ebert S, Regen T, *et al.* Toll-like receptor stimulation enhances phagocytosis and intracellular killing of nonencapsulated and encapsulated Streptococcus pneumoniae by murine microglia. Infect Immun 2010; 78(2): 865-71.
[http://dx.doi.org/10.1128/IAI.01110-09] [PMID: 19933834]

[60] Takeda K, Kaisho T, Akira S. Toll-like receptors. Annu Rev Immunol 2003; 21: 335-76.
[http://dx.doi.org/10.1146/annurev.immunol.21.120601.141126] [PMID: 12524386]

[61] Witting A, Müller P, Herrmann A, Kettenmann H, Nolte C. Phagocytic clearance of apoptotic neurons by Microglia/Brain macrophages *in vitro*: involvement of lectin-, integrin-, and phosphatidylserine-mediated recognition. J Neurochem 2000; 75(3): 1060-70.
[http://dx.doi.org/10.1046/j.1471-4159.2000.0751060.x] [PMID: 10936187]

[62] Stolzing A, Grune T. Neuronal apoptotic bodies: phagocytosis and degradation by primary microglial cells. FASEB J 2004; 18(6): 743-5.
[PMID: 14766802]

[63] Schafer DP, Lehrman EK, Kautzman AG, *et al.* Microglia sculpt postnatal neural circuits in an activity and complement-dependent manner. Neuron 2012; 74(4): 691-705.
[http://dx.doi.org/10.1016/j.neuron.2012.03.026] [PMID: 22632727]

[64] Stuart LM, Bell SA, Stewart CR, *et al.* CD36 signals to the actin cytoskeleton and regulates microglial migration *via* a p130Cas complex. J Biol Chem 2007; 282(37): 27392-401.
[http://dx.doi.org/10.1074/jbc.M702887200] [PMID: 17623670]

[65] Aloisi F, Serafini B, Adorini L. Glia-T cell dialogue. J Neuroimmunol 2000; 107(2): 111-7.
[http://dx.doi.org/10.1016/S0165-5728(00)00231-9] [PMID: 10854644]

[66] Almolda B, Gonzalez B, Castellano B. Antigen presentation in EAE: role of microglia, macrophages and dendritic cells. Front Biosci (Landmark Ed) 2011; 16: 1157-71.
[http://dx.doi.org/10.2741/3781] [PMID: 21196224]

[67] Byram SC, Carson MJ, DeBoy CA, Serpe CJ, Sanders VM, Jones KJ. CD4-positive T cell-mediated

neuroprotection requires dual compartment antigen presentation. J Neurosci 2004; 24(18): 4333-9. [http://dx.doi.org/10.1523/JNEUROSCI.5276-03.2004] [PMID: 15128847]

[68] Fischer HG, Reichmann G. Brain dendritic cells and macrophages/microglia in central nervous system inflammation. J Immunol 2001; 166(4): 2717-26. [http://dx.doi.org/10.4049/jimmunol.166.4.2717] [PMID: 11160337]

[69] Jäkel S, Dimou L. Glial cells and their function in the adult brain: A journey through the history of their ablation. Front Cell Neurosci 2017; 11: 24. [http://dx.doi.org/10.3389/fncel.2017.00024] [PMID: 28243193]

[70] Ben Haim L, Rowitch DH. Functional diversity of astrocytes in neural circuit regulation. Nat Rev Neurosci 2017; 18(1): 31-41. [http://dx.doi.org/10.1038/nrn.2016.159] [PMID: 27904142]

[71] Parpura V, Verkhratsky A. Astrocytes revisited: concise historic outlook on glutamate homeostasis and signaling. Croat Med J 2012; 53(6): 518-28. [http://dx.doi.org/10.3325/cmj.2012.53.518] [PMID: 23275317]

[72] Acosta C, Anderson HD, Anderson CM. Astrocyte dysfunction in Alzheimer disease. J Neurosci Res In press [PMID: 28467650]

[73] Sicca F, Ambrosini E, Marchese M, *et al.* Gain-of-function defects of astrocytic Kir4.1 channels in children with autism spectrum disorders and epilepsy. Sci Rep 2016; 6: 34325. [http://dx.doi.org/10.1038/srep34325] [PMID: 27677466]

[74] Katz AM, Amankulor NM, Pitter K, Helmy K, Squatrito M, Holland EC. Astrocyte-specific expression patterns associated with the PDGF-induced glioma microenvironment. PLoS One 2012; 7(2): e32453. [http://dx.doi.org/10.1371/journal.pone.0032453] [PMID: 22393407]

[75] John Lin CC, Deneen B. Astrocytes: the missing link in neurologic disease? Semin Pediatr Neurol 2013; 20(4): 236-41. [http://dx.doi.org/10.1016/j.spen.2013.10.004] [PMID: 24365571]

[76] Wang Q, Jie W, Liu JH, Yang JM, Gao TM. An astroglial basis of major depressive disorder? An overview. Glia 2017; 65(8): 1227-50. [http://dx.doi.org/10.1002/glia.23143] [PMID: 28317185]

[77] Song H, Stevens CF, Gage FH. Astroglia induce neurogenesis from adult neural stem cells. Nature 2002; 417(6884): 39-44. [http://dx.doi.org/10.1038/417039a] [PMID: 11986659]

[78] Gengatharan A, Bammann RR, Saghatelyan A. The role of astrocytes in the generation, migration, and integration of new neurons in the adult olfactory bulb. Front Neurosci 2016; 10: 149. [http://dx.doi.org/10.3389/fnins.2016.00149] [PMID: 27092050]

[79] Wang DD, Bordey A. The astrocyte odyssey. Prog Neurobiol 2008; 86(4): 342-67. [PMID: 18948166]

[80] Oberheim NA, Goldman SA, Nedergaard M. Heterogeneity of astrocytic form and function. Methods Mol Biol 2012; 814: 23-45. [http://dx.doi.org/10.1007/978-1-61779-452-0_3] [PMID: 22144298]

[81] Tyzack G, Lakatos A, Patani R. Human stem cell-derived astrocytes: Specification and relevance for neurological disorders. Curr Stem Cell Rep 2016; 2: 236-47. [http://dx.doi.org/10.1007/s40778-016-0049-1] [PMID: 27547709]

[82] Şovrea AS, Boşca AB. Astrocytes reassessment - an evolving concept part one: embryology, biology, morphology and reactivity. J Mol Psychiatry 2013; 1: 18. [http://dx.doi.org/10.1186/2049-9256-1-18] [PMID: 26019866]

[83] Zhang Y, Sloan SA, Clarke LE, *et al.* Purification and characterization of progenitor and mature human astrocytes reveals transcriptional and functional differences with mouse. Neuron 2016; 89(1): 37-53.
[http://dx.doi.org/10.1016/j.neuron.2015.11.013] [PMID: 26687838]

[84] Molofsky AV, Deneen B. Astrocyte development: A Guide for the Perplexed. Glia 2015; 63(8): 1320-9.
[http://dx.doi.org/10.1002/glia.22836] [PMID: 25963996]

[85] Vue TY, Kim EJ, Parras CM, Guillemot F, Johnson JE. Ascl1 controls the number and distribution of astrocytes and oligodendrocytes in the gray matter and white matter of the spinal cord. Development 2014; 141(19): 3721-31.
[http://dx.doi.org/10.1242/dev.105270] [PMID: 25249462]

[86] Higashi K, Fujita A, Inanobe A, *et al.* An inwardly rectifying K(+) channel, Kir4.1, expressed in astrocytes surrounds synapses and blood vessels in brain. Am J Physiol Cell Physiol 2001; 281(3): C922-31.
[PMID: 11502569]

[87] Sofroniew MV, Vinters HV. Astrocytes: biology and pathology. Acta Neuropathol 2010; 119(1): 7-35.
[http://dx.doi.org/10.1007/s00401-009-0619-8] [PMID: 20012068]

[88] Sofroniew MV. Molecular dissection of reactive astrogliosis and glial scar formation. Trends Neurosci 2009; 32(12): 638-47.
[http://dx.doi.org/10.1016/j.tins.2009.08.002] [PMID: 19782411]

[89] Kielian T. Glial connexins and gap junctions in CNS inflammation and disease. J Neurochem 2008; 106(3): 1000-16.
[http://dx.doi.org/10.1111/j.1471-4159.2008.05405.x] [PMID: 18410504]

[90] Nielsen MS, Axelsen LN, Sorgen PL, Verma V, Delmar M, Holstein-Rathlou NH. Gap junctions. Compr Physiol 2012; 2(3): 1981-2035.
[PMID: 23723031]

[91] Hang LH, Li SN, Luo H, *et al.* Connexin 43 mediates CXCL12 production from spinal dorsal horn to maintain bone cancer pain in rats. Neurochem Res 2016; 41(5): 1200-8.
[http://dx.doi.org/10.1007/s11064-015-1815-7] [PMID: 26721509]

[92] Chen G, Park CK, Xie RG, Berta T, Nedergaard M, Ji RR. Connexin-43 induces chemokine release from spinal cord astrocytes to maintain late-phase neuropathic pain in mice. Brain 2014; 137(Pt 8): 2193-209.
[http://dx.doi.org/10.1093/brain/awu140] [PMID: 24919967]

[93] Yoon SY, Robinson CR, Zhang H, Dougherty PM. Spinal astrocyte gap junctions contribute to oxaliplatin-induced mechanical hypersensitivity. J Pain 2013; 14(2): 205-14.
[http://dx.doi.org/10.1016/j.jpain.2012.11.002] [PMID: 23374942]

[94] Choi HS, Roh DH, Yoon SY, *et al.* The role of spinal interleukin-1β and astrocyte connexin 43 in the development of mirror-image pain in an inflammatory pain model. Exp Neurol 2016; 287(Pt 1): 1-13.
[PMID: 27776252]

[95] Perea G, Araque A. GLIA modulates synaptic transmission. Brain Res Brain Res Rev 2010; 63(1-2): 93-102.
[http://dx.doi.org/10.1016/j.brainresrev.2009.10.005] [PMID: 19896978]

[96] Prat A, Biernacki K, Wosik K, Antel JP. Glial cell influence on the human blood-brain barrier. Glia 2001; 36(2): 145-55.
[http://dx.doi.org/10.1002/glia.1104] [PMID: 11596123]

[97] MacVicar BA, Newman EA. Astrocyte regulation of blood flow in the brain. Cold Spring Harb Perspect Biol 2015; 7(5): a020388.
[http://dx.doi.org/10.1101/cshperspect.a020388] [PMID: 25818565]

[98] Tham DK, Joshi B, Moukhles H. Aquaporin-4 cell-surface expression and turnover are regulated by dystroglycan, dynamin, and the extracellular matrix in astrocytes. PLoS One 2016; 11(10): e0165439. [http://dx.doi.org/10.1371/journal.pone.0165439] [PMID: 27788222]

[99] Seifert G, Schilling K, Steinhäuser C. Astrocyte dysfunction in neurological disorders: a molecular perspective. Nat Rev Neurosci 2006; 7(3): 194-206. [http://dx.doi.org/10.1038/nrn1870] [PMID: 16495941]

[100] Robinson MB, Jackson JG. Astroglial glutamate transporters coordinate excitatory signaling and brain energetics. Neurochem Int 2016; 98: 56-71. [http://dx.doi.org/10.1016/j.neuint.2016.03.014] [PMID: 27013346]

[101] Halassa MM, Fellin T, Takano H, Dong JH, Haydon PG. Synaptic islands defined by the territory of a single astrocyte. J Neurosci 2007; 27(24): 6473-7. [http://dx.doi.org/10.1523/JNEUROSCI.1419-07.2007] [PMID: 17567808]

[102] Araque A, Parpura V, Sanzgiri RP, Haydon PG. Tripartite synapses: glia, the unacknowledged partner. Trends Neurosci 1999; 22(5): 208-15. [http://dx.doi.org/10.1016/S0166-2236(98)01349-6] [PMID: 10322493]

[103] Pangrsic T, Potokar M, Stenovec M, *et al.* Exocytotic release of ATP from cultured astrocytes. J Biol Chem 2007; 282(39): 28749-58. [http://dx.doi.org/10.1074/jbc.M700290200] [PMID: 17627942]

[104] Ye ZC, Wyeth MS, Baltan-Tekkok S, Ransom BR. Functional hemichannels in astrocytes: a novel mechanism of glutamate release. J Neurosci 2003; 23(9): 3588-96. [PMID: 12736329]

[105] Ben Achour S, Pascual O. Glia: the many ways to modulate synaptic plasticity. Neurochem Int 2010; 57(4): 440-5. [http://dx.doi.org/10.1016/j.neuint.2010.02.013] [PMID: 20193723]

[106] Bellot-Saez A, Kékesi O, Morley JW, Buskila Y. Astrocytic modulation of neuronal excitability through K(+) spatial buffering. Neurosci Biobehav Rev 2017; 77: 87-97. [http://dx.doi.org/10.1016/j.neubiorev.2017.03.002] [PMID: 28279812]

[107] Pekny M, Pekna M, Messing A, *et al.* Astrocytes: a central element in neurological diseases. Acta Neuropathol 2016; 131(3): 323-45. [http://dx.doi.org/10.1007/s00401-015-1513-1] [PMID: 26671410]

[108] Gorina R, Font-Nieves M, Márquez-Kisinousky L, Santalucia T, Planas AM. Astrocyte TLR4 activation induces a proinflammatory environment through the interplay between MyD88-dependent NFκB signaling, MAPK, and Jak1/Stat1 pathways. Glia 2011; 59(2): 242-55. [http://dx.doi.org/10.1002/glia.21094] [PMID: 21125645]

[109] Gao YJ, Xu ZZ, Liu YC, Wen YR, Decosterd I, Ji RR. The c-Jun N-terminal kinase 1 (JNK1) in spinal astrocytes is required for the maintenance of bilateral mechanical allodynia under a persistent inflammatory pain condition. Pain 2010; 148(2): 309-19. [http://dx.doi.org/10.1016/j.pain.2009.11.017] [PMID: 20022176]

[110] Tian G, Luo X, Tang C, *et al.* Astrocyte contributes to pain development *via* MMP2-JNK1/2 signaling in a mouse model of complex regional pain syndrome. Life Sci 2017; 170: 64-71. [http://dx.doi.org/10.1016/j.lfs.2016.11.030] [PMID: 27919822]

[111] Cao J, Wang JS, Ren XH, Zang WD. Spinal sample showing p-JNK and P38 associated with the pain signaling transduction of glial cell in neuropathic pain. Spinal Cord 2015; 53(2): 92-7. [http://dx.doi.org/10.1038/sc.2014.188] [PMID: 25384402]

[112] Gao YJ, Zhang L, Samad OA, *et al.* JNK-induced MCP-1 production in spinal cord astrocytes contributes to central sensitization and neuropathic pain. J Neurosci 2009; 29(13): 4096-108. [http://dx.doi.org/10.1523/JNEUROSCI.3623-08.2009] [PMID: 19339605]

[113] Lu Y, Jiang BC, Cao DL, *et al.* TRAF6 upregulation in spinal astrocytes maintains neuropathic pain by integrating TNF-α and IL-1β signaling. Pain 2014; 155(12): 2618-29. [http://dx.doi.org/10.1016/j.pain.2014.09.027] [PMID: 25267210]

[114] Lu Y, Cao DL, Jiang BC, Yang T, Gao YJ. MicroRNA-146a-5p attenuates neuropathic pain *via* suppressing TRAF6 signaling in the spinal cord. Brain Behav Immun 2015; 49: 119-29. [http://dx.doi.org/10.1016/j.bbi.2015.04.018] [PMID: 25957028]

[115] Gao YJ, Ji RR. Chemokines, neuronal-glial interactions, and central processing of neuropathic pain. Pharmacol Ther 2010; 126(1): 56-68. [http://dx.doi.org/10.1016/j.pharmthera.2010.01.002] [PMID: 20117131]

[116] García-Marín V, García-López P, Freire M. Cajal's contributions to glia research. Trends Neurosci 2007; 30(9): 479-87. [http://dx.doi.org/10.1016/j.tins.2007.06.008] [PMID: 17765327]

[117] Pérez-Cerdá F, Sánchez-Gómez MV, Matute C. Pío del Río Hortega and the discovery of the oligodendrocytes. Front Neuroanat 2015; 9: 92. [http://dx.doi.org/10.3389/fnana.2015.00092] [PMID: 26217196]

[118] Richardson WD, Kessaris N, Pringle N. Oligodendrocyte wars. Nat Rev Neurosci 2006; 7(1): 11-8. [http://dx.doi.org/10.1038/nrn1826] [PMID: 16371946]

[119] Gill AS, Binder DK. Wilder Penfield, Pio del Rio-Hortega, and the discovery of oligodendroglia. Neurosurgery 2007; 60(5): 940-8. discussion -8.

[120] Lopez Juarez A, He D, Richard Lu Q. Oligodendrocyte progenitor programming and reprogramming: Toward myelin regeneration. Brain Res 2016; 1638(Pt B): 209-20.

[121] Takebayashi H, Nabeshima Y, Yoshida S, Chisaka O, Ikenaka K, Nabeshima Y. The basic helix-loo--helix factor olig2 is essential for the development of motoneuron and oligodendrocyte lineages. Curr Biol 2002; 12(13): 1157-63. [http://dx.doi.org/10.1016/S0960-9822(02)00926-0] [PMID: 12121626]

[122] Zhou Q, Anderson DJ. The bHLH transcription factors OLIG2 and OLIG1 couple neuronal and glial subtype specification. Cell 2002; 109(1): 61-73. [http://dx.doi.org/10.1016/S0092-8674(02)00677-3] [PMID: 11955447]

[123] Lu QR, Sun T, Zhu Z, *et al.* Common developmental requirement for Olig function indicates a motor neuron/oligodendrocyte connection. Cell 2002; 109(1): 75-86. [http://dx.doi.org/10.1016/S0092-8674(02)00678-5] [PMID: 11955448]

[124] Rowitch DH, Kriegstein AR. Developmental genetics of vertebrate glial-cell specification. Nature 2010; 468(7321): 214-22. [http://dx.doi.org/10.1038/nature09611] [PMID: 21068830]

[125] Dougherty KD, Dreyfus CF, Black IB. Brain-derived neurotrophic factor in astrocytes, oligodendrocytes, and microglia/macrophages after spinal cord injury. Neurobiol Dis 2000; 7 (6 Pt B): 574-85. [http://dx.doi.org/10.1006/nbdi.2000.0318] [PMID: 11114257]

[126] Du Y, Dreyfus CF. Oligodendrocytes as providers of growth factors. J Neurosci Res 2002; 68(6): 647-54. [http://dx.doi.org/10.1002/jnr.10245] [PMID: 12111826]

[127] Reynolds J, Logan A, Berry M, Dent RG, Gonzales AM, Toescu EC. Age-dependent changes in Fibroblast growth factor 2 (FGF-2) expression in mouse cerebellar neurons. J Cell Mol Med 2005; 9(2): 398-406. [http://dx.doi.org/10.1111/j.1582-4934.2005.tb00365.x] [PMID: 15963259]

[128] Bradl M, Lassmann H. Oligodendrocytes: biology and pathology. Acta Neuropathol 2010; 119(1): 37-53.

[http://dx.doi.org/10.1007/s00401-009-0601-5] [PMID: 19847447]

[129] McTigue DM, Tripathi RB. The life, death, and replacement of oligodendrocytes in the adult CNS. J Neurochem 2008; 107(1): 1-19. [http://dx.doi.org/10.1111/j.1471-4159.2008.05570.x] [PMID: 18643793]

[130] Zarpelon AC, Rodrigues FC, Lopes AH, *et al.* Spinal cord oligodendrocyte-derived alarmin IL-33 mediates neuropathic pain. FASEB J 2016; 30(1): 54-65. [http://dx.doi.org/10.1096/fj.14-267146] [PMID: 26310268]

[131] Shi Y, Shu J, Liang Z, Yuan S, Tang SJ. EXPRESS: Oligodendrocytes in HIV-associated pain pathogenesis. Mol Pain 2016; 12: 1-7. [http://dx.doi.org/10.1177/1744806916656845] [PMID: 27306410]

[132] Kawaguchi M, Satoh Y, Otsubo Y, Kazama T. Molecular hydrogen attenuates neuropathic pain in mice. PLoS One 2014; 9(6): e100352. [http://dx.doi.org/10.1371/journal.pone.0100352] [PMID: 24941001]

[133] Arnett HA, Hellendall RP, Matsushima GK, *et al.* The protective role of nitric oxide in a neurotoxicant-induced demyelinating model. J Immunol 2002; 168(1): 427-33. [http://dx.doi.org/10.4049/jimmunol.168.1.427] [PMID: 11751989]

[134] Bergsteindottir K, Brennan A, Jessen KR, Mirsky R. In the presence of dexamethasone, gamma interferon induces rat oligodendrocytes to express major histocompatibility complex class II molecules. Proc Natl Acad Sci USA 1992; 89(19): 9054-8. [http://dx.doi.org/10.1073/pnas.89.19.9054] [PMID: 1409602]

[135] Höftberger R, Aboul-Enein F, Brueck W, *et al.* Expression of major histocompatibility complex class I molecules on the different cell types in multiple sclerosis lesions. Brain Pathol 2004; 14(1): 43-50. [http://dx.doi.org/10.1111/j.1750-3639.2004.tb00496.x] [PMID: 14997936]

[136] Bsibsi M, Nomden A, van Noort JM, Baron W. Toll-like receptors 2 and 3 agonists differentially affect oligodendrocyte survival, differentiation, and myelin membrane formation. J Neurosci Res 2012; 90(2): 388-98. [http://dx.doi.org/10.1002/jnr.22767] [PMID: 21971760]

[137] Cannella B, Raine CS. Multiple sclerosis: cytokine receptors on oligodendrocytes predict innate regulation. Ann Neurol 2004; 55(1): 46-57. [http://dx.doi.org/10.1002/ana.10764] [PMID: 14705111]

[138] Omari KM, John GR, Sealfon SC, Raine CS. CXC chemokine receptors on human oligodendrocytes: implications for multiple sclerosis. Brain 2005; 128(Pt 5): 1003-15. [http://dx.doi.org/10.1093/brain/awh479] [PMID: 15774504]

[139] Woolf CJ. Evidence for a central component of post-injury pain hypersensitivity. Nature 1983; 306(5944): 686-8. [http://dx.doi.org/10.1038/306686a0] [PMID: 6656869]

[140] Woolf CJ, Salter MW. Neuronal plasticity: increasing the gain in pain. Science 2000; 288(5472): 1765-9. [http://dx.doi.org/10.1126/science.288.5472.1765] [PMID: 10846153]

[141] Ji RR, Woolf CJ. Neuronal plasticity and signal transduction in nociceptive neurons: implications for the initiation and maintenance of pathological pain. Neurobiol Dis 2001; 8(1): 1-10. [http://dx.doi.org/10.1006/nbdi.2000.0360] [PMID: 11162235]

[142] Coull JA, Beggs S, Boudreau D, *et al.* BDNF from microglia causes the shift in neuronal anion gradient underlying neuropathic pain. Nature 2005; 438(7070): 1017-21. [http://dx.doi.org/10.1038/nature04223] [PMID: 16355225]

[143] Kawasaki Y, Zhang L, Cheng JK, Ji RR. Cytokine mechanisms of central sensitization: distinct and overlapping role of interleukin-1beta, interleukin-6, and tumor necrosis factor-alpha in regulating synaptic and neuronal activity in the superficial spinal cord. J Neurosci 2008; 28(20): 5189-94.

[http://dx.doi.org/10.1523/JNEUROSCI.3338-07.2008] [PMID: 18480275]

[144] Calvo M, Zhu N, Tsantoulas C, *et al.* Neuregulin-ErbB signaling promotes microglial proliferation and chemotaxis contributing to microgliosis and pain after peripheral nerve injury. J Neurosci 2010; 30(15): 5437-50.
[http://dx.doi.org/10.1523/JNEUROSCI.5169-09.2010] [PMID: 20392965]

[145] Calvo M, Zhu N, Grist J, Ma Z, Loeb JA, Bennett DL. Following nerve injury neuregulin-1 drives microglial proliferation and neuropathic pain *via* the MEK/ERK pathway. Glia 2011; 59(4): 554-68.
[http://dx.doi.org/10.1002/glia.21124] [PMID: 21319222]

[146] Tsuda M, Tozaki-Saitoh H, Inoue K. Purinergic system, microglia and neuropathic pain. Curr Opin Pharmacol 2012; 12(1): 74-9.
[http://dx.doi.org/10.1016/j.coph.2011.10.014] [PMID: 22036170]

[147] Zhang J, Shi XQ, Echeverry S, Mogil JS, De Koninck Y, Rivest S. Expression of CCR2 in both resident and bone marrow-derived microglia plays a critical role in neuropathic pain. J Neurosci 2007; 27(45): 12396-406.
[http://dx.doi.org/10.1523/JNEUROSCI.3016-07.2007] [PMID: 17989304]

[148] Verge GM, Milligan ED, Maier SF, Watkins LR, Naeve GS, Foster AC. Fractalkine (CX3CL1) and fractalkine receptor (CX3CR1) distribution in spinal cord and dorsal root ganglia under basal and neuropathic pain conditions. Eur J Neurosci 2004; 20(5): 1150-60.
[http://dx.doi.org/10.1111/j.1460-9568.2004.03593.x] [PMID: 15341587]

[149] Gu N, Peng J, Murugan M, *et al.* Spinal Microgliosis Due to Resident Microglial Proliferation Is Required for Pain Hypersensitivity after Peripheral Nerve Injury. Cell Reports 2016; 16(3): 605-14.
[http://dx.doi.org/10.1016/j.celrep.2016.06.018] [PMID: 27373153]

[150] Jin SX, Zhuang ZY, Woolf CJ, Ji RR. p38 mitogen-activated protein kinase is activated after a spinal nerve ligation in spinal cord microglia and dorsal root ganglion neurons and contributes to the generation of neuropathic pain. J Neurosci 2003; 23(10): 4017-22.
[PMID: 12764087]

[151] Slack SE, Grist J, Mac Q, McMahon SB, Pezet S. TrkB expression and phospho-ERK activation by brain-derived neurotrophic factor in rat spinothalamic tract neurons. J Comp Neurol 2005; 489(1): 59-68.
[http://dx.doi.org/10.1002/cne.20606] [PMID: 15977164]

[152] Inoue K, Tsuda M, Tozaki-Saitoh H. Modification of neuropathic pain sensation through microglial ATP receptors. Purinergic Signal 2007; 3(4): 311-6.
[http://dx.doi.org/10.1007/s11302-007-9071-1] [PMID: 18404444]

[153] Clark AK, Yip PK, Malcangio M. The liberation of fractalkine in the dorsal horn requires microglial cathepsin S. J Neurosci 2009; 29(21): 6945-54.
[http://dx.doi.org/10.1523/JNEUROSCI.0828-09.2009] [PMID: 19474321]

[154] Clark AK, Grist J, Al-Kashi A, Perretti M, Malcangio M. Spinal cathepsin S and fractalkine contribute to chronic pain in the collagen-induced arthritis model. Arthritis Rheum 2012; 64(6): 2038-47.
[http://dx.doi.org/10.1002/art.34351] [PMID: 22213084]

[155] Kawasaki Y, Xu ZZ, Wang X, *et al.* Distinct roles of matrix metalloproteases in the early- and late-phase development of neuropathic pain. Nat Med 2008; 14(3): 331-6.
[http://dx.doi.org/10.1038/nm1723] [PMID: 18264108]

[156] Liu F, Wang Z, Qiu Y, *et al.* Suppression of MyD88-dependent signaling alleviates neuropathic pain induced by peripheral nerve injury in the rat. J Neuroinflammation 2017; 14(1): 70.
[http://dx.doi.org/10.1186/s12974-017-0822-9] [PMID: 28359290]

[157] Agalave NM, Larsson M, Abdelmoaty S, *et al.* Spinal HMGB1 induces TLR4-mediated long-lasting hypersensitivity and glial activation and regulates pain-like behavior in experimental arthritis. Pain 2014; 155(9): 1802-13.

[http://dx.doi.org/10.1016/j.pain.2014.06.007] [PMID: 24954167]

[158] Zhang FF, Morioka N, Harano S, *et al.* Perineural expression of high-mobility group box-1 contributes to long-lasting mechanical hypersensitivity *via* matrix metalloproteinase-9 upregulation in mice with painful peripheral neuropathy. J Neurochem 2015; 136(4): 837-50. [http://dx.doi.org/10.1111/jnc.13434] [PMID: 26578177]

[159] Nakamura Y, Morioka N, Abe H, *et al.* Neuropathic pain in rats with a partial sciatic nerve ligation is alleviated by intravenous injection of monoclonal antibody to high mobility group box-1. PLoS One 2013; 8(8): e73640. [http://dx.doi.org/10.1371/journal.pone.0073640] [PMID: 23991202]

[160] Yang H, Lundbäck P, Ottosson L, *et al.* Redox modification of cysteine residues regulates the cytokine activity of high mobility group box-1 (HMGB1). Mol Med 2012; 18: 250-9. [http://dx.doi.org/10.2119/molmed.2011.00389] [PMID: 22105604]

[161] Tong W, Wang W, Huang J, Ren N, Wu SX, Li YQ. Spinal high-mobility group box 1 contributes to mechanical allodynia in a rat model of bone cancer pain. Biochem Biophys Res Commun 2010; 395(4): 572-6. [http://dx.doi.org/10.1016/j.bbrc.2010.04.086] [PMID: 20399746]

[162] Guan Z, Kuhn JA, Wang X, *et al.* Injured sensory neuron-derived CSF1 induces microglial proliferation and DAP12-dependent pain. Nat Neurosci 2016; 19(1): 94-101. [http://dx.doi.org/10.1038/nn.4189] [PMID: 26642091]

[163] Cao L, DeLeo JA. CNS-infiltrating CD4+ T lymphocytes contribute to murine spinal nerve transection-induced neuropathic pain. Eur J Immunol 2008; 38(2): 448-58. [http://dx.doi.org/10.1002/eji.200737485] [PMID: 18196515]

[164] Costigan M, Moss A, Latremoliere A, *et al.* T-cell infiltration and signaling in the adult dorsal spinal cord is a major contributor to neuropathic pain-like hypersensitivity. J Neurosci 2009; 29(46): 14415-22. [http://dx.doi.org/10.1523/JNEUROSCI.4569-09.2009] [PMID: 19923276]

[165] Grace PM, Rolan PE, Hutchinson MR. Peripheral immune contributions to the maintenance of central glial activation underlying neuropathic pain. Brain Behav Immun 2011; 25(7): 1322-32. [http://dx.doi.org/10.1016/j.bbi.2011.04.003] [PMID: 21496480]

[166] Lee Y, Pai M, Brederson JD, *et al.* Monosodium iodoacetate-induced joint pain is associated with increased phosphorylation of mitogen activated protein kinases in the rat spinal cord. Mol Pain 2011; 7: 39. [http://dx.doi.org/10.1186/1744-8069-7-39] [PMID: 21599960]

[167] Sagar DR, Burston JJ, Hathway GJ, *et al.* The contribution of spinal glial cells to chronic pain behaviour in the monosodium iodoacetate model of osteoarthritic pain. Mol Pain 2011; 7: 88. [http://dx.doi.org/10.1186/1744-8069-7-88] [PMID: 22093915]

[168] Luo JG, Zhao XL, Xu WC, *et al.* Activation of spinal NF-κB/p65 contributes to peripheral inflammation and hyperalgesia in rat adjuvant-induced arthritis. Arthritis Rheumatol 2014; 66(4): 896-906. [http://dx.doi.org/10.1002/art.38328] [PMID: 24757142]

[169] Nieto FR, Clark AK, Grist J, Hathway GJ, Chapman V, Malcangio M. Neuron-immune mechanisms contribute to pain in early stages of arthritis. J Neuroinflammation 2016; 13(1): 96. [http://dx.doi.org/10.1186/s12974-016-0556-0] [PMID: 27130316]

[170] Nieto FR, Clark AK, Grist J, Chapman V, Malcangio M. Calcitonin gene-related peptide-expressing sensory neurons and spinal microglial reactivity contribute to pain states in collagen-induced arthritis. Arthritis Rheumatol 2015; 67(6): 1668-77. [http://dx.doi.org/10.1002/art.39082] [PMID: 25707377]

[171] Clark AK, Wodarski R, Guida F, Sasso O, Malcangio M. Cathepsin S release from primary cultured

microglia is regulated by the P2X7 receptor. Glia 2010; 58(14): 1710-26.
[http://dx.doi.org/10.1002/glia.21042] [PMID: 20629190]

[172] Grace PM, Maier SF, Watkins LR. Opioid-induced central immune signaling: implications for opioid analgesia. Headache 2015; 55(4): 475-89.
[http://dx.doi.org/10.1111/head.12552] [PMID: 25833219]

[173] Grace PM, Strand KA, Galer EL, Rice KC, Maier SF, Watkins LR. Protraction of neuropathic pain by morphine is mediated by spinal damage associated molecular patterns (DAMPs) in male rats. Brain Behav Immun In press
[PMID: 28860068]

[174] Grace PM, Strand KA, Galer EL, *et al.* Morphine paradoxically prolongs neuropathic pain in rats by amplifying spinal NLRP3 inflammasome activation. Proc Natl Acad Sci USA 2016; 113(24): E3441-50.
[http://dx.doi.org/10.1073/pnas.1602070113] [PMID: 27247388]

[175] Liang Y, Chu H, Jiang Y, Yuan L. Morphine enhances IL-1β release through toll-like receptor 4-mediated endocytic pathway in microglia. Purinergic Signal 2016; 12(4): 637-45.
[http://dx.doi.org/10.1007/s11302-016-9525-4] [PMID: 27506813]

[176] Jeon YH, Youn DH. Spinal Gap Junction Channels in Neuropathic Pain. Korean J Pain 2015; 28(4): 231-5.
[http://dx.doi.org/10.3344/kjp.2015.28.4.231] [PMID: 26495077]

[177] Jiang BC, Cao DL, Zhang X, *et al.* CXCL13 drives spinal astrocyte activation and neuropathic pain *via* CXCR5. J Clin Invest 2016; 126(2): 745-61.
[http://dx.doi.org/10.1172/JCI81950] [PMID: 26752644]

[178] Dansereau MA, Gosselin RD, Pohl M, *et al.* Spinal CCL2 pronociceptive action is no longer effective in CCR2 receptor antagonist-treated rats. J Neurochem 2008; 106(2): 757-69.
[http://dx.doi.org/10.1111/j.1471-4159.2008.05429.x] [PMID: 18419759]

[179] Xie RG, Gao YJ, Park CK, *et al.* Spinal CCL2 Promotes Central Sensitization, Long-Term Potentiation, and Inflammatory Pain *via* CCR2: Further Insights into Molecular, Synaptic, and Cellular Mechanisms. Neurosci Bull In press
[PMID: 28265898]

[180] Beattie EC, Stellwagen D, Morishita W, *et al.* Control of synaptic strength by glial TNFalpha. Science 2002; 295(5563): 2282-5.
[http://dx.doi.org/10.1126/science.1067859] [PMID: 11910117]

[181] Stellwagen D, Malenka RC. Synaptic scaling mediated by glial TNF-alpha. Nature 2006; 440(7087): 1054-9.
[http://dx.doi.org/10.1038/nature04671] [PMID: 16547515]

[182] Viviani B, Bartesaghi S, Gardoni F, *et al.* Interleukin-1beta enhances NMDA receptor-mediated intracellular calcium increase through activation of the Src family of kinases. J Neurosci 2003; 23(25): 8692-700.
[PMID: 14507968]

[183] Gao YJ, Ji RR. Light touch induces ERK activation in superficial dorsal horn neurons after inflammation: involvement of spinal astrocytes and JNK signaling in touch-evoked central sensitization and mechanical allodynia. J Neurochem 2010; 115(2): 505-14.
[http://dx.doi.org/10.1111/j.1471-4159.2010.06946.x] [PMID: 20722971]

[184] Liu Z, Hu X, Cai J, *et al.* Induction of oligodendrocyte differentiation by Olig2 and Sox10: evidence for reciprocal interactions and dosage-dependent mechanisms. Dev Biol 2007; 302(2): 683-93.
[http://dx.doi.org/10.1016/j.ydbio.2006.10.007] [PMID: 17098222]

[185] Liu B, Tai Y, Achanta S, *et al.* IL-33/ST2 signaling excites sensory neurons and mediates itch response in a mouse model of poison ivy contact allergy. Proc Natl Acad Sci USA 2016; 113(47):

E7572-9.
[http://dx.doi.org/10.1073/pnas.1606608113] [PMID: 27821781]

[186] Gritsch S, Lu J, Thilemann S, *et al.* Oligodendrocyte ablation triggers central pain independently of innate or adaptive immune responses in mice. Nat Commun 2014; 5: 5472.
[http://dx.doi.org/10.1038/ncomms6472] [PMID: 25434649]

[187] Zhang ZJ, Jiang BC, Gao YJ. Chemokines in neuron-glial cell interaction and pathogenesis of neuropathic pain. Cell Mol Life Sci 2017; 74(18): 3275-91.
[http://dx.doi.org/10.1007/s00018-017-2513-1] [PMID: 28389721]

[188] Mogil JS. Sex differences in pain and pain inhibition: multiple explanations of a controversial phenomenon. Nat Rev Neurosci 2012; 13(12): 859-66.
[http://dx.doi.org/10.1038/nrn3360] [PMID: 23165262]

[189] Yekkirala AS, Roberson DP, Bean BP, Woolf CJ. Breaking barriers to novel analgesic drug development. Nat Rev Drug Discov 2017; 16(8): 545-64.
[http://dx.doi.org/10.1038/nrd.2017.87] [PMID: 28596533]

[190] Mika J, Zychowska M, Popiolek-Barczyk K, Rojewska E, Przewlocka B. Importance of glial activation in neuropathic pain. Eur J Pharmacol 2013; 716(1-3): 106-19.
[http://dx.doi.org/10.1016/j.ejphar.2013.01.072] [PMID: 23500198]

[191] Osikowicz M, Skup M, Mika J, Makuch W, Czarkowska-Bauch J, Przewlocka B. Glial inhibitors influence the mRNA and protein levels of mGlu2/3, 5 and 7 receptors and potentiate the analgesic effects of their ligands in a mouse model of neuropathic pain. Pain 2009; 147(1-3): 175-86.
[http://dx.doi.org/10.1016/j.pain.2009.09.002] [PMID: 19782473]

[192] Mika J, Osikowicz M, Rojewska E, *et al.* Differential activation of spinal microglial and astroglial cells in a mouse model of peripheral neuropathic pain. Eur J Pharmacol 2009; 623(1-3): 65-72.
[http://dx.doi.org/10.1016/j.ejphar.2009.09.030] [PMID: 19766105]

[193] Saito O, Svensson CI, Buczynski MW, *et al.* Spinal glial TLR4-mediated nociception and production of prostaglandin E(2) and TNF. Br J Pharmacol 2010; 160(7): 1754-64.
[http://dx.doi.org/10.1111/j.1476-5381.2010.00811.x] [PMID: 20649577]

[194] Dorazil-Dudzik M, Mika J, Schafer MK, *et al.* The effects of local pentoxifylline and propentofylline treatment on formalin-induced pain and tumor necrosis factor-alpha messenger RNA levels in the inflamed tissue of the rat paw. Anesth Analg 2004; 98(6): 1566-73.
[http://dx.doi.org/10.1213/01.ANE.0000113235.88534.48] [PMID: 15155307]

[195] Vale ML, Benevides VM, Sachs D, *et al.* Antihyperalgesic effect of pentoxifylline on experimental inflammatory pain. Br J Pharmacol 2004; 143(7): 833-44.
[http://dx.doi.org/10.1038/sj.bjp.0705999] [PMID: 15520047]

[196] Carvalho TT, Borghi SM, Pinho-Ribeiro FA, *et al.* Granulocyte-colony stimulating factor (G-CSF- -induced mechanical hyperalgesia in mice: Role for peripheral TNFα, IL-1β and IL-10. Eur J Pharmacol 2015; 749: 62-72.
[http://dx.doi.org/10.1016/j.ejphar.2014.12.023] [PMID: 25584775]

[197] Wei T, Sabsovich I, Guo TZ, *et al.* Pentoxifylline attenuates nociceptive sensitization and cytokine expression in a tibia fracture rat model of complex regional pain syndrome. Eur J Pain 2009; 13(3): 253-62.
[http://dx.doi.org/10.1016/j.ejpain.2008.04.014] [PMID: 18554967]

[198] Ward A, Clissold SP. Pentoxifylline. A review of its pharmacodynamic and pharmacokinetic properties, and its therapeutic efficacy. Drugs 1987; 34(1): 50-97.
[http://dx.doi.org/10.2165/00003495-198734010-00003] [PMID: 3308412]

[199] Ralevic V, Burnstock G. Receptors for purines and pyrimidines. Pharmacol Rev 1998; 50(3): 413-92.
[PMID: 9755289]

[200] Norsted Gregory E, Delaney A, Abdelmoaty S, *et al.* Pentoxifylline and propentofylline prevent

proliferation and activation of the mammalian target of rapamycin and mitogen activated protein kinase in cultured spinal astrocytes. J Neurosci Res 2013; 91(2): 300-12. [http://dx.doi.org/10.1002/jnr.23144] [PMID: 23184810]

[201] Xie J, Ponuwei GA, Moore CE, Willars GB, Tee AR, Herbert TP. cAMP inhibits mammalian target of rapamycin complex-1 and -2 (mTORC1 and 2) by promoting complex dissociation and inhibiting mTOR kinase activity. Cell Signal 2011; 23(12): 1927-35. [http://dx.doi.org/10.1016/j.cellsig.2011.06.025] [PMID: 21763421]

[202] Strieter RM, Remick DG, Ward PA, *et al.* Cellular and molecular regulation of tumor necrosis factor-alpha production by pentoxifylline. Biochem Biophys Res Commun 1988; 155(3): 1230-6. [http://dx.doi.org/10.1016/S0006-291X(88)81271-3] [PMID: 2460096]

[203] Sampaio EP, Moraes MO, Nery JA, Santos AR, Matos HC, Sarno EN. Pentoxifylline decreases *in vivo* and *in vitro* tumour necrosis factor-alpha (TNF-alpha) production in lepromatous leprosy patients with erythema nodosum leprosum (ENL). Clin Exp Immunol 1998; 111(2): 300-8. [http://dx.doi.org/10.1046/j.1365-2249.1998.00510.x] [PMID: 9486396]

[204] Mika J, Wawrzczak-Bargiela A, Osikowicz M, Makuch W, Przewlocka B. Attenuation of morphine tolerance by minocycline and pentoxifylline in naive and neuropathic mice. Brain Behav Immun 2009; 23(1): 75-84. [http://dx.doi.org/10.1016/j.bbi.2008.07.005] [PMID: 18684397]

[205] De Sanctis MT, Cesarone MR, Belcaro G, *et al.* Treatment of intermittent claudication with pentoxifylline: a 12-month, randomized trial--walking distance and microcirculation. Angiology 2002; 53 (Suppl. 1): S7-S12. [PMID: 11865838]

[206] Cesarone MR, Belcaro G, Nicolaides AN, *et al.* Treatment of severe intermittent claudication with pentoxifylline: a 40-week, controlled, randomized trial. Angiology 2002; 53 (Suppl. 1): S1-5. [http://dx.doi.org/10.1177/000331970205300101] [PMID: 11865828]

[207] Thornhill MH, Baccaglini L, Theaker E, Pemberton MN. A randomized, double-blind, placebo-controlled trial of pentoxifylline for the treatment of recurrent aphthous stomatitis. Arch Dermatol 2007; 143(4): 463-70. [http://dx.doi.org/10.1001/archderm.143.4.463] [PMID: 17438178]

[208] Brown DR, Kretzschmar HA. The glio-toxic mechanism of alpha-aminoadipic acid on cultured astrocytes. J Neurocytol 1998; 27(2): 109-18. [http://dx.doi.org/10.1023/A:1006947322342] [PMID: 9609401]

[209] Watkins JC, Krogsgaard-Larsen P, Honoré T. Structure-activity relationships in the development of excitatory amino acid receptor agonists and competitive antagonists. Trends Pharmacol Sci 1990; 11(1): 25-33. [http://dx.doi.org/10.1016/0165-6147(90)90038-A] [PMID: 2155495]

[210] Tsai MJ, Chang YF, Schwarcz R, Brookes N. Characterization of L-alpha-aminoadipic acid transport in cultured rat astrocytes. Brain Res 1996; 741(1-2): 166-73. [http://dx.doi.org/10.1016/S0006-8993(96)00910-9] [PMID: 9001719]

[211] Olney JW, de Gubareff T, Collins JF. Stereospecificity of the gliotoxic and anti-neurotoxic actions of alpha-aminoadipate. Neurosci Lett 1980; 19(3): 277-82. [http://dx.doi.org/10.1016/0304-3940(80)90273-6] [PMID: 7052532]

[212] Khurgel M, Koo AC, Ivy GO. Selective ablation of astrocytes by intracerebral injections of alpha-aminoadipate. Glia 1996; 16(4): 351-8. [http://dx.doi.org/10.1002/(SICI)1098-1136(199604)16:4<351::AID-GLIA7>3.0.CO;2-2] [PMID: 8721675]

[213] Bridges RJ, Hatalski CG, Shim SN, *et al.* Gliotoxic actions of excitatory amino acids. Neuropharmacology 1992; 31(9): 899-907. [http://dx.doi.org/10.1016/0028-3908(92)90128-C] [PMID: 1436396]

[214] Zhuang ZY, Wen YR, Zhang DR, *et al.* A peptide c-Jun N-terminal kinase (JNK) inhibitor blocks mechanical allodynia after spinal nerve ligation: respective roles of JNK activation in primary sensory neurons and spinal astrocytes for neuropathic pain development and maintenance. J Neurosci 2006; 26(13): 3551-60.
[http://dx.doi.org/10.1523/JNEUROSCI.5290-05.2006] [PMID: 16571763]

[215] Hassel B, Paulsen RE, Johnsen A, Fonnum F. Selective inhibition of glial cell metabolism *in vivo* by fluorocitrate. Brain Res 1992; 576(1): 120-4.
[http://dx.doi.org/10.1016/0006-8993(92)90616-H] [PMID: 1515906]

[216] Pavao-de-Souza GF, Zarpelon AC, Tedeschi GC, *et al.* Acetic acid- and phenyl-p-benzoquino-e-induced overt pain-like behavior depends on spinal activation of MAP kinases, PI(3)K and microglia in mice. Pharmacol Biochem Behav 2012; 101(3): 320-8.
[http://dx.doi.org/10.1016/j.pbb.2012.01.018] [PMID: 22306747]

[217] Mao-Ying QL, Wang XW, Yang CJ, *et al.* Robust spinal neuroinflammation mediates mechanical allodynia in Walker 256 induced bone cancer rats. Mol Brain 2012; 5: 16.
[http://dx.doi.org/10.1186/1756-6606-5-16] [PMID: 22607655]

[218] Garrido-Mesa N, Zarzuelo A, Gálvez J. Minocycline: far beyond an antibiotic. Br J Pharmacol 2013; 169(2): 337-52.
[http://dx.doi.org/10.1111/bph.12139] [PMID: 23441623]

[219] Sorge RE, Mapplebeck JC, Rosen S, *et al.* Different immune cells mediate mechanical pain hypersensitivity in male and female mice. Nat Neurosci 2015; 18(8): 1081-3.
[http://dx.doi.org/10.1038/nn.4053] [PMID: 26120961]

[220] Ledeboer A, Sloane EM, Milligan ED, *et al.* Minocycline attenuates mechanical allodynia and proinflammatory cytokine expression in rat models of pain facilitation. Pain 2005; 115(1-2): 71-83.
[http://dx.doi.org/10.1016/j.pain.2005.02.009] [PMID: 15836971]

[221] Yrjänheikki J, Keinänen R, Pellikka M, Hökfelt T, Koistinaho J. Tetracyclines inhibit microglial activation and are neuroprotective in global brain ischemia. Proc Natl Acad Sci USA 1998; 95(26): 15769-74.
[http://dx.doi.org/10.1073/pnas.95.26.15769] [PMID: 9861045]

[222] Yrjänheikki J, Tikka T, Keinänen R, Goldsteins G, Chan PH, Koistinaho J. A tetracycline derivative, minocycline, reduces inflammation and protects against focal cerebral ischemia with a wide therapeutic window. Proc Natl Acad Sci USA 1999; 96(23): 13496-500.
[http://dx.doi.org/10.1073/pnas.96.23.13496] [PMID: 10557349]

[223] Du Y, Ma Z, Lin S, *et al.* Minocycline prevents nigrostriatal dopaminergic neurodegeneration in the MPTP model of Parkinson's disease. Proc Natl Acad Sci USA 2001; 98(25): 14669-74.
[http://dx.doi.org/10.1073/pnas.251341998] [PMID: 11724929]

[224] Narang T. Arshdeep, Dogra S. Minocycline in leprosy patients with recent onset clinical nerve function impairment. Dermatol Ther (Heidelb) 2017; 30(1)

[225] Syngle A, Verma I, Krishan P, Garg N, Syngle V. Minocycline improves peripheral and autonomic neuropathy in type 2 diabetes: MIND study. Neurol Sci 2014; 35(7): 1067-73.
[http://dx.doi.org/10.1007/s10072-014-1647-2] [PMID: 24497205]

[226] Gelesko S, Long L, Faulk J, Phillips C, Dicus C, White RP Jr. Cryotherapy and topical minocycline as adjunctive measures to control pain after third molar surgery: an exploratory study. J Oral Maxillofac Surg 2011; 69(11): e324-32.
[http://dx.doi.org/10.1016/j.joms.2011.03.059] [PMID: 21802812]

[227] Stavropoulos MF, Shugars DA, Phillips C, Conrad SM, Fleuchaus PT, White RP Jr. Impact of topical minocycline with third molar surgery on clinical recovery and health-related quality of life outcomes. J Oral Maxillofac Surg 2006; 64(7): 1059-65.
[http://dx.doi.org/10.1016/j.joms.2006.03.007] [PMID: 16781338]

[228] Gorsky M, Epstein J, Raviv A, Yaniv R, Truelove E. Topical minocycline for managing symptoms of recurrent aphthous stomatitis. Spec Care Dentist 2008; 28(1): 27-31. [http://dx.doi.org/10.1111/j.1754-4505.2008.00006.x] [PMID: 18271771]

[229] Martinez V, Szekely B, Lemarié J, *et al.* The efficacy of a glial inhibitor, minocycline, for preventing persistent pain after lumbar discectomy: a randomized, double-blind, controlled study. Pain 2013; 154(8): 1197-203. [http://dx.doi.org/10.1016/j.pain.2013.03.028] [PMID: 23706627]

[230] Vanelderen P, Van Zundert J, Kozicz T, *et al.* Effect of minocycline on lumbar radicular neuropathic pain: a randomized, placebo-controlled, double-blind clinical trial with amitriptyline as a comparator. Anesthesiology 2015; 122(2): 399-406. [http://dx.doi.org/10.1097/ALN.0000000000000508] [PMID: 25373391]

[231] Sumitani M, Ueda H, Hozumi J, *et al.* Minocycline does not decrease intensity of neuropathic pain intensity, but does improve its affective dimension. J Pain Palliat Care Pharmacother 2016; 30(1): 31-5. [PMID: 25700217]

[232] Sorge RE, LaCroix-Fralish ML, Tuttle AH, *et al.* Spinal cord Toll-like receptor 4 mediates inflammatory and neuropathic hypersensitivity in male but not female mice. J Neurosci 2011; 31(43): 15450-4. [http://dx.doi.org/10.1523/JNEUROSCI.3859-11.2011] [PMID: 22031891]

[233] Taves S, Berta T, Liu DL, *et al.* Spinal inhibition of p38 MAP kinase reduces inflammatory and neuropathic pain in male but not female mice: Sex-dependent microglial signaling in the spinal cord. Brain Behav Immun 2016; 55: 70-81. [http://dx.doi.org/10.1016/j.bbi.2015.10.006] [PMID: 26472019]

[234] Mombaerts P, Iacomini J, Johnson RS, Herrup K, Tonegawa S, Papaioannou VE. RAG-1-deficient mice have no mature B and T lymphocytes. Cell 1992; 68(5): 869-77. [http://dx.doi.org/10.1016/0092-8674(92)90030-G] [PMID: 1547488]

[235] Stokes JA, Cheung J, Eddinger K, Corr M, Yaksh TL. Toll-like receptor signaling adapter proteins govern spread of neuropathic pain and recovery following nerve injury in male mice. J Neuroinflammation 2013; 10: 148. [http://dx.doi.org/10.1186/1742-2094-10-148] [PMID: 24321498]

[236] Carvalho TT, Flauzino T, Otaguiri ES, *et al.* Granulocyte-colony stimulating factor (G-CSF) induces mechanical hyperalgesia *via* spinal activation of MAP kinases and PI3K in mice. Pharmacol Biochem Behav 2011; 98(2): 188-95. [http://dx.doi.org/10.1016/j.pbb.2010.12.027] [PMID: 21236293]

[237] Bennett BL, Sasaki DT, Murray BW, *et al.* SP600125, an anthrapyrazolone inhibitor of Jun N-terminal kinase. Proc Natl Acad Sci USA 2001; 98(24): 13681-6. [http://dx.doi.org/10.1073/pnas.251194298] [PMID: 11717429]

[238] Manthey CL, Wang SW, Kinney SD, Yao Z. SB202190, a selective inhibitor of p38 mitogen-activated protein kinase, is a powerful regulator of LPS-induced mRNAs in monocytes. J Leukoc Biol 1998; 64(3): 409-17. [PMID: 9738669]

[239] Zhang H, Nei H, Dougherty PM. A p38 mitogen-activated protein kinase-dependent mechanism of disinhibition in spinal synaptic transmission induced by tumor necrosis factor-alpha. J Neurosci 2010; 30(38): 12844-55. [http://dx.doi.org/10.1523/JNEUROSCI.2437-10.2010] [PMID: 20861388]

[240] Liu X, Bu H, Liu C, *et al.* Inhibition of glial activation in rostral ventromedial medulla attenuates mechanical allodynia in a rat model of cancer-induced bone pain. J Huazhong Univ Sci Technolog Med Sci 2012; 32(2): 291-8. [http://dx.doi.org/10.1007/s11596-012-0051-5] [PMID: 22528236]

[241] Ostenfeld T, Krishen A, Lai RY, *et al.* A randomized, placebo-controlled trial of the analgesic efficacy and safety of the p38 MAP kinase inhibitor, losmapimod, in patients with neuropathic pain from lumbosacral radiculopathy. Clin J Pain 2015; 31(4): 283-93. [http://dx.doi.org/10.1097/AJP.0000000000000122] [PMID: 25751578]

[242] Ostenfeld T, Krishen A, Lai RY, *et al.* Analgesic efficacy and safety of the novel p38 MAP kinase inhibitor, losmapimod, in patients with neuropathic pain following peripheral nerve injury: a double-blind, placebo-controlled study. Eur J Pain 2013; 17(6): 844-57. [http://dx.doi.org/10.1002/j.1532-2149.2012.00256.x] [PMID: 23239139]

[243] Anand P, Shenoy R, Palmer JE, *et al.* Clinical trial of the p38 MAP kinase inhibitor dilmapimod in neuropathic pain following nerve injury. Eur J Pain 2011; 15(10): 1040-8. [http://dx.doi.org/10.1016/j.ejpain.2011.04.005] [PMID: 21576029]

[244] Serhan CN, Chiang N, Dalli J, Levy BD. Lipid mediators in the resolution of inflammation. Cold Spring Harb Perspect Biol 2014; 7(2): a016311. [http://dx.doi.org/10.1101/cshperspect.a016311] [PMID: 25359497]

[245] Fattori V, Amaral FA, Verri WA Jr. Neutrophils and arthritis: Role in disease and pharmacological perspectives. Pharmacol Res 2016; 112: 84-98. [http://dx.doi.org/10.1016/j.phrs.2016.01.027] [PMID: 26826283]

[246] Martini AC, Berta T, Forner S, *et al.* Lipoxin A4 inhibits microglial activation and reduces neuroinflammation and neuropathic pain after spinal cord hemisection. J Neuroinflammation 2016; 13(1): 75. [http://dx.doi.org/10.1186/s12974-016-0540-8] [PMID: 27059991]

[247] Xu ZZ, Zhang L, Liu T, Park JY, Berta T, Yang R, *et al.* Resolvins RvE1 and RvD1 attenuate inflammatory pain *via* central and peripheral actions. Nat Med 2010; 16(5): 592-7. 1p following 7 [http://dx.doi.org/10.1038/nm.2123]

[248] Bang S, Yoo S, Yang TJ, Cho H, Kim YG, Hwang SW. Resolvin D1 attenuates activation of sensory transient receptor potential channels leading to multiple anti-nociception. Br J Pharmacol 2010; 161(3): 707-20. [http://dx.doi.org/10.1111/j.1476-5381.2010.00909.x] [PMID: 20880407]

[249] Xu ZZ, Berta T, Ji RR. Resolvin E1 inhibits neuropathic pain and spinal cord microglial activation following peripheral nerve injury. J Neuroimmune Pharmacol 2013; 8(1): 37-41. [http://dx.doi.org/10.1007/s11481-012-9394-8] [PMID: 22878925]

[250] Abdelmoaty S, Wigerblad G, Bas DB, *et al.* Spinal actions of lipoxin A4 and 17(R)-resolvin D1 attenuate inflammation-induced mechanical hypersensitivity and spinal TNF release. PLoS One 2013; 8(9): e75543. [http://dx.doi.org/10.1371/journal.pone.0075543] [PMID: 24086560]

[251] Hill KP, Palastro MD, Johnson B, Ditre JW. Cannabis and Pain: A Clinical Review. Cannabis Cannabinoid Res 2017; 2(1): 96-104. [http://dx.doi.org/10.1089/can.2017.0017] [PMID: 28861509]

[252] Paszcuk AF, Dutra RC, da Silva KA, Quintão NL, Campos MM, Calixto JB. Cannabinoid agonists inhibit neuropathic pain induced by brachial plexus avulsion in mice by affecting glial cells and MAP kinases. PLoS One 2011; 6(9): e24034. [http://dx.doi.org/10.1371/journal.pone.0024034] [PMID: 21931637]

[253] Martín-Moreno AM, Reigada D, Ramírez BG, *et al.* Cannabidiol and other cannabinoids reduce microglial activation *in vitro* and *in vivo*: relevance to Alzheimer's disease. Mol Pharmacol 2011; 79(6): 964-73. [http://dx.doi.org/10.1124/mol.111.071290] [PMID: 21350020]

[254] Burgos E, Gómez-Nicola D, Pascual D, Martín MI, Nieto-Sampedro M, Goicoechea C. Cannabinoid agonist WIN 55,212-2 prevents the development of paclitaxel-induced peripheral neuropathy in rats.

Possible involvement of spinal glial cells. Eur J Pharmacol 2012; 682(1-3): 62-72. [http://dx.doi.org/10.1016/j.ejphar.2012.02.008] [PMID: 22374260]

[255] Merighi S, Gessi S, Varani K, Fazzi D, Mirandola P, Borea PA. Cannabinoid CB(2) receptor attenuates morphine-induced inflammatory responses in activated microglial cells. Br J Pharmacol 2012; 166(8): 2371-85. [http://dx.doi.org/10.1111/j.1476-5381.2012.01948.x] [PMID: 22428664]

[256] Fanelli G, De Carolis G, Leonardi C, *et al.* Cannabis and intractable chronic pain: an explorative retrospective analysis of Italian cohort of 614 patients. J Pain Res 2017; 10: 1217-24. [http://dx.doi.org/10.2147/JPR.S132814] [PMID: 28579820]

[257] Fallon MT, Albert Lux E, McQuade R, *et al.* Sativex oromucosal spray as adjunctive therapy in advanced cancer patients with chronic pain unalleviated by optimized opioid therapy: two double-blind, randomized, placebo-controlled phase 3 studies. Br J Pain 2017; 11(3): 119-33. [http://dx.doi.org/10.1177/2049463717710042] [PMID: 28785408]

[258] Blake A, Wan BA, Malek L, *et al.* A selective review of medical cannabis in cancer pain management. Ann Palliat Med In press [PMID: 28866904]

[259] Zhao J, Zhang H, Liu SB, *et al.* Spinal interleukin-33 and its receptor ST2 contribute to bone cancer-induced pain in mice. Neuroscience 2013; 253: 172-82. [http://dx.doi.org/10.1016/j.neuroscience.2013.08.026] [PMID: 23988433]

[260] Liu S, Mi WL, Li Q, *et al.* Spinal IL-33/ST2 signaling contributes to neuropathic pain *via* neuronal CaMKII-CREB and astroglial JAK2-STAT3 cascades in mice. Anesthesiology 2015; 123(5): 1154-69. [http://dx.doi.org/10.1097/ALN.0000000000000850] [PMID: 26352378]

[261] Zarpelon AC, Cunha TM, Alves-Filho JC, *et al.* IL-33/ST2 signalling contributes to carrageenin-induced innate inflammation and inflammatory pain: role of cytokines, endothelin-1 and prostaglandin E2. Br J Pharmacol 2013; 169(1): 90-101. [http://dx.doi.org/10.1111/bph.12110] [PMID: 23347081]

[262] Verri WA Jr, Guerrero AT, Fukada SY, *et al.* IL-33 mediates antigen-induced cutaneous and articular hypernociception in mice. Proc Natl Acad Sci USA 2008; 105(7): 2723-8. [http://dx.doi.org/10.1073/pnas.0712116105] [PMID: 18250323]

[263] Verri WA Jr, Souto FO, Vieira SM, *et al.* IL-33 induces neutrophil migration in rheumatoid arthritis and is a target of anti-TNF therapy. Ann Rheum Dis 2010; 69(9): 1697-703. [http://dx.doi.org/10.1136/ard.2009.122655] [PMID: 20472598]

[264] Bertozzi MM, Rossaneis AC, Fattori V, *et al.* Diosmin reduces chronic constriction injury-induced neuropathic pain in mice. Chem Biol Interact 2017; 273: 180-9. [http://dx.doi.org/10.1016/j.cbi.2017.06.014] [PMID: 28625489]

[265] Magro DA, Hohmann MS, Mizokami SS, *et al.* An interleukin-33/ST2 signaling deficiency reduces overt pain-like behaviors in mice. Braz J Med Biol Res 2013; 46(7): 601-6. [http://dx.doi.org/10.1590/1414-431X20132894] [PMID: 23903682]

[266] Longhi-Balbinot DT, Rossaneis AC, Pinho-Ribeiro FA, *et al.* The nitroxyl donor, Angeli's salt, reduces chronic constriction injury-induced neuropathic pain. Chem Biol Interact 2016; 256: 1-8. [http://dx.doi.org/10.1016/j.cbi.2016.06.009] [PMID: 27287419]

[267] Verri WA Jr, Cunha TM, Parada CA, Poole S, Cunha FQ, Ferreira SH. Hypernociceptive role of cytokines and chemokines: targets for analgesic drug development? Pharmacol Ther 2006; 112(1): 116-38. [http://dx.doi.org/10.1016/j.pharmthera.2006.04.001] [PMID: 16730375]

[268] Kwilasz AJ, Grace PM, Serbedzija P, Maier SF, Watkins LR. The therapeutic potential of interleukin-10 in neuroimmune diseases. Neuropharmacology 2015; 96(Pt A): 55-69. [http://dx.doi.org/10.1016/j.neuropharm.2014.10.020]

[269] Poole S, Cunha FQ, Selkirk S, Lorenzetti BB, Ferreira SH. Cytokine-mediated inflammatory hyperalgesia limited by interleukin-10. Br J Pharmacol 1995; 115(4): 684-8. [http://dx.doi.org/10.1111/j.1476-5381.1995.tb14987.x] [PMID: 7582491]

[270] Milligan ED, Sloane EM, Langer SJ, *et al.* Controlling neuropathic pain by adeno-associated virus driven production of the anti-inflammatory cytokine, interleukin-10. Mol Pain 2005; 1: 9. [http://dx.doi.org/10.1186/1744-8069-1-9] [PMID: 15813997]

[271] Milligan ED, Sloane EM, Langer SJ, *et al.* Repeated intrathecal injections of plasmid DNA encoding interleukin-10 produce prolonged reversal of neuropathic pain. Pain 2006; 126(1-3): 294-308. [http://dx.doi.org/10.1016/j.pain.2006.07.009] [PMID: 16949747]

[272] Eijkelkamp N, Steen-Louws C, Hartgring SA, *et al.* IL4-10 Fusion Protein Is a Novel Drug to Treat Persistent Inflammatory Pain. J Neurosci 2016; 36(28): 7353-63. [http://dx.doi.org/10.1523/JNEUROSCI.0092-16.2016] [PMID: 27413147]

[273] St Clair EW. Interleukin 10 treatment for rheumatoid arthritis. Ann Rheum Dis 1999; 58 (Suppl. 1): I99-I102. [http://dx.doi.org/10.1136/ard.58.2008.i99] [PMID: 10577984]

[274] Dumont FJ. Therapeutic potential of IL-10 and its viral homologues: an update. Expert Opin Ther Pat 2003; 13(10): 1551-77.

[275] van Roon J, Wijngaarden S, Lafeber FP, Damen C, van de Winkel J, Bijlsma JW. Interleukin 10 treatment of patients with rheumatoid arthritis enhances Fc gamma receptor expression on monocytes and responsiveness to immune complex stimulation. J Rheumatol 2003; 30(4): 648-51. [PMID: 12672180]

[276] Kinfe TM, Muhammad S, Link C, Roeske S, Chaudhry SR, Yearwood TL. Burst spinal cord stimulation increases peripheral antineuroinflammatory interleukin 10 levels in failed back surgery syndrome patients with predominant back pain. Neuromodulation 2017; 20(4): 322-30. [http://dx.doi.org/10.1111/ner.12586] [PMID: 28194840]

[277] Soderquist RG, Milligan ED, Harrison JA, *et al.* PEGylation of interleukin-10 for the mitigation of enhanced pain states. J Biomed Mater Res A 2010; 93(3): 1169-79. [PMID: 19768789]

[278] Soderquist RG, Sloane EM, Loram LC, *et al.* Release of plasmid DNA-encoding IL-10 from PLGA microparticles facilitates long-term reversal of neuropathic pain following a single intrathecal administration. Pharm Res 2010; 27(5): 841-54. [http://dx.doi.org/10.1007/s11095-010-0077-y] [PMID: 20224990]

[279] Kalliomäki J, Attal N, Jonzon B, *et al.* AZD2423 PTN Study Group. A randomized, double-blind, placebo-controlled trial of a chemokine receptor 2 (CCR2) antagonist in posttraumatic neuralgia. Pain 2013; 154(5): 761-7. [http://dx.doi.org/10.1016/j.pain.2013.02.003] [PMID: 23523116]

[280] Trummer D, Walzer A, Groettrup-Wolfers E, Schmitz H. Efficacy, safety and tolerability of the CCR1 antagonist BAY 86-5047 for the treatment of endometriosis-associated pelvic pain: a randomized controlled trial. Acta Obstet Gynecol Scand 2017; 96(6): 694-701. [http://dx.doi.org/10.1111/aogs.13105] [PMID: 28168715]

[281] Padi SS, Shi XQ, Zhao YQ, *et al.* Attenuation of rodent neuropathic pain by an orally active peptide, RAP-103, which potently blocks CCR2- and CCR5-mediated monocyte chemotaxis and inflammation. Pain 2012; 153(1): 95-106. [http://dx.doi.org/10.1016/j.pain.2011.09.022] [PMID: 22033364]

[282] Tanaka Y, Takeuchi T, Umehara H, *et al.* Safety, pharmacokinetics, and efficacy of E6011, an antifractalkine monoclonal antibody, in a first-in-patient phase 1/2 study on rheumatoid arthritis. Mod Rheumatol 2017; 1-8. [PMID: 28681650]

[283] Patra MC, Choi S. Recent progress in the development of Toll-like receptor (TLR) antagonists. Expert Opin Ther Pat 2016; 26(6): 719-30.

[284] Andrews NA, Latrémolière A, Basbaum AI, *et al.* Ensuring transparency and minimization of methodologic bias in preclinical pain research: PPRECISE considerations. Pain 2016; 157(4): 901-9. [http://dx.doi.org/10.1097/j.pain.0000000000000458] [PMID: 26683237]

[285] Clark JD. Preclinical pain research: Can we do better? Anesthesiology 2016; 125(5): 846-9. [http://dx.doi.org/10.1097/ALN.0000000000001340] [PMID: 27575448]

[286] Laird JM, Martinez-Caro L, Garcia-Nicas E, Cervero F. A new model of visceral pain and referred hyperalgesia in the mouse. Pain 2001; 92(3): 335-42. [http://dx.doi.org/10.1016/S0304-3959(01)00275-5] [PMID: 11376906]

[287] Le Bars D, Gozariu M, Cadden SW. Animal models of nociception. Pharmacol Rev 2001; 53(4): 597-652. [PMID: 11734620]

[288] Grimmer-Somers K, Vipond N, Kumar S, Hall G. A review and critique of assessment instruments for patients with persistent pain. J Pain Res 2009; 2: 21-47. [http://dx.doi.org/10.2147/JPR.S4949] [PMID: 21197292]

[289] Breivik H, Borchgrevink PC, Allen SM, *et al.* Assessment of pain. Br J Anaesth 2008; 101(1): 17-24. [http://dx.doi.org/10.1093/bja/aen103] [PMID: 18487245]

[290] Froud R, Patel S, Rajendran D, *et al.* A systematic review of outcome measures use, analytical approaches, reporting methods, and publication volume by year in low back pain trials published between 1980 and 2012: Respice, adspice, et prospice. PLoS One 2016; 11(10): e0164573. [http://dx.doi.org/10.1371/journal.pone.0164573] [PMID: 27776141]

[291] Price DD, Patel R, Robinson ME, Staud R. Characteristics of electronic visual analogue and numerical scales for ratings of experimental pain in healthy subjects and fibromyalgia patients. Pain 2008; 140(1): 158-66. [http://dx.doi.org/10.1016/j.pain.2008.07.028] [PMID: 18786761]

[292] Burns LH, Leri F, Olmstead MC. Ultra-low-dose naltrexone decreases dependence and addictive properties of opioids.Opiate Receptors and Antagonists: From Bench to Clinic. Totowa, NJ: Humana Press 2009; pp. 247-61. [http://dx.doi.org/10.1007/978-1-59745-197-0_13]

[293] Chindalore VL, Craven RA, Yu KP, Butera PG, Burns LH, Friedmann N. Adding ultralow-dose naltrexone to oxycodone enhances and prolongs analgesia: a randomized, controlled trial of Oxytrex. J Pain 2005; 6(6): 392-9. [http://dx.doi.org/10.1016/j.jpain.2005.01.356] [PMID: 15943961]

[294] Webster LR, Butera PG, Moran LV, Wu N, Burns LH, Friedmann N. Oxytrex minimizes physical dependence while providing effective analgesia: a randomized controlled trial in low back pain. J Pain 2006; 7(12): 937-46. [http://dx.doi.org/10.1016/j.jpain.2006.05.005] [PMID: 17157780]

[295] Mattioli TA, Milne B, Cahill CM. Ultra-low dose naltrexone attenuates chronic morphine-induced gliosis in rats. Mol Pain 2010; 6: 22. [http://dx.doi.org/10.1186/1744-8069-6-22] [PMID: 20398374]

[296] Matters GL, Harms JF, McGovern C, *et al.* The opioid antagonist naltrexone improves murine inflammatory bowel disease. J Immunotoxicol 2008; 5(2): 179-87. [http://dx.doi.org/10.1080/15476910802131469] [PMID: 18569389]

[297] Ji RR, Xu ZZ, Gao YJ. Emerging targets in neuroinflammation-driven chronic pain. Nat Rev Drug Discov 2014; 13(7): 533-48. [http://dx.doi.org/10.1038/nrd4334] [PMID: 24948120]

[298] Gonzalez-Angulo AM, Hennessy BT, Mills GB. Future of personalized medicine in oncology: a systems biology approach. J Clin Oncol 2010; 28(16): 2777-83.
[http://dx.doi.org/10.1200/JCO.2009.27.0777] [PMID: 20406928]

[299] Schilsky RL. Personalized medicine in oncology: the future is now. Nat Rev Drug Discov 2010; 9(5): 363-6.
[http://dx.doi.org/10.1038/nrd3181] [PMID: 20431568]

CHAPTER 5

Cholinesterase Inhibitors

Pamela E. Potter* and **Laszlo Kerecsen**

Department of Pharmacology, Arizona College of Osteopathic Medicine, Midwestern University, Glendale, Arizona, USA

Abstract: Inhibitors of the acetylcholinesterase enzyme were first described in the latter part of the 19th century. Some of these inhibitors also inhibit the butyryl-cholinesterase enzyme. Therapeutic uses of the cholinesterase inhibitors include ophthalmology, anesthesia, myasthenia gravis, muscarinic antagonist overdose and Alzheimer's disease. Many pesticides act by inhibiting cholinesterase, with the potential for accidental or deliberate poisoning. Cholinesterase inhibitors were also developed as nerve agents for chemical warfare.

This chapter describes the discovery and early studies on the effects and mechanism of action of cholinesterase inhibitors. Subsequent development led to the discovery of a large and varied group of cholinesterase inhibitors. These drugs will be discussed with regard to their therapeutic uses and clinical considerations. Finally, concerns regarding cholinesterase inhibitor toxicity when used as pesticides and nerve agents will be discussed.

Keywords: Acetylcholinesterase, Acetylcholine, Alzheimer's disease, Atropine, Butyrylcholinesterase, Donepezil, Edrophonium, Galantamine, Glaucoma, Myasthenia gravis, Neostigmine, Nerve agent, Organophosphate, Physostigmine, Pesticide, Pralidoxime, Pyridostigmine, Rivastigmine.

INTRODUCTION

History and Development of Cholinesterase Inhibitors

Physostigmine was first isolated in 1864 from the *Physostigma venenosum* Barbour plant. It was also called eserine, from the name for the African Calabar bean (or ordeal bean), éseré [1 - 3]. The history of scientific studies of the effects of this extract, which date from the 1860's, is outlined in the review by Karczmar [4]. Physiological effects that were observed included miosis, salivation, bradycardia, and skeletal muscle twitches [4]. It was remarked very early that the

* **Corresponding author Pamela E. Potter:** Department of Pharmacology, Arizona College of Osteopathic Medicine, Midwestern University, Glendale, Arizona, USA; Tel: 623-572-3391; Fax: 623-572-3648; E-mail: ppotte@midwestern.edu

miotic effect of physostigmine might be beneficial in the eye [2, 5]. Subsequently, it was determined that physostigmine exerted a muscarinic effect on the smooth muscle of the iris, and that the effect required an intact presynaptic nerve terminal [6]. Further investigation confirmed that physostigmine and neostigmine produced both miosis and stimulation of the intestine, both of which were antagonized by atropine [7 - 9]. Studies of the effects of physostigmine on skeletal muscle demonstrated stimulation followed by paralysis, but also the ability to reverse curare-induced paralysis [10]. Antagonism of the effects of curare at the neuromuscular junction was noted [9]. Since these effects resembled those of acetylcholine (ACh), the drugs were thought to cause accumulation of ACh [11], through inhibition of acetylcholinesterase (AChE; EC3.1.1.7) [12, 13].

Subsequent studies described the irreversible inhibition of AChE by di-isopropylfluorophosphate (DFP) and other organophosphates as distinct from the reversible effects of physostigmine [14 - 21]. Today, of course a great deal is known about the mechanism by which the cholinesterase inhibitors exert their effects [1]. Cholinesterase inhibitors act by prolonging the effects of ACh released from the nerve terminal, to stimulate both muscarinic and nicotinic receptors, and overdose or poisoning with these compounds leads to skeletal muscle paralysis due to desensitization of nicotinic receptors. Thus the observed pharmacological effects of cholinesterase inhibitors can be very complex.

The chemical structure of physostigmine was soon elucidated [22], and analogues such as neostigmine were subsequently developed [7]. Neostigmine was introduced in 1931 as a gastrointestinal stimulant [1]. Several excellent reviews on the history and development of these compounds have been published [2, 4, 23].

There are two major cholinesterase enzymes: AChE and butyrylcholinesterase (BChE; AC 3.1.1.8), sometimes referred to as "pseudocholinesterase". AChE is found in erythrocytes and in the synaptic cleft of peripheral and central cholinergic neurons, where it acts to terminate the effect of released ACh [24, 25]. BChE is found in the liver and circulates in the blood, where it hydrolyzes drugs such as succinylcholine, and is also found in the brain, where it may play a role in modulating cholinergic transmission and development of the CNS [25, 26]. Some inhibitors are highly specific for AChE, while others inhibit the action of both enzymes.

AChE has two active sites- an anionic site and a positively charged, catalytic, esteratic site [1, 25, 27]. The positively charged quaternary nitrogen of ACh is drawn to the anionic site, while the ester lines up with the hydroxyl group on a serine residue of the enzyme at the esteratic site (Fig. **1**). An intermediate compound is formed, then choline is released, leaving the acetyl group on the enzyme, from which it is rapidly and spontaneously hydrolyzed to acetate, and the enzyme is reactivated. Cholinesterase inhibitors bind to the enzyme in a similar fashion to produce enzyme inhibition. For example, with physostigmine or neostigmine, the positively charged nitrogen is attracted to the anionic site, and the carbamate group forms a covalent bond with the esteratic site (Fig. **1**). The carbamate inhibitors, such as neostigmine, pyridostigmine and physostigmine, are hydrolyzed slowly from the enzymes, which defines their duration of action, usually about 2-4 hours [12, 13, 25, 28, 29]. Thus physostigmine, neostigmine, and pyridostigmine are considered reversible inhibitors [30]. Edrophonium undergoes rapid and weak electrostatic binding to the anionic site (Fig. **1**), which is very short lived. Edrophonium has a very short duration of action, approximately 10 minutes following a single dose [27, 29, 31]. This makes edrophonium a very short-acting reversible inhibitor. AChE inhibitors in common clinical use are shown in Table **1**.

Table 1. Properties of some therapeutic acetylcholinesterase inhibitors.

Drug	Brand name (s)	Class/Type of Binding	Duration	CNS Effect	Uses
Physostigmine	Eserine	Carbamate, reversible	0.5-2 hr	Yes	Treatment of atropine poisoning, glaucoma
Neostigmine	Prostigmin	Carbamate, reversible	0.5-4 hr	No	Reversal of NMJ blockade, myasthenia gravis
Pyridostigmine	Mestinon, Regonol	Carbamate, reversible	4-6 hr	No	Reversal of NMJ blockade, myasthenia gravis, prevention of organophosphate poisoning
Ambenonium	Mytelase	Carbamate, reversible	3-8 hr	No	Reversal of NMJ blockade, myasthenia gravis
Tacrine	Cognex	Pyridine, reversible	4-6 hr	Yes	Alzheimer's disease (discontinued)
Donepezil	Aricept	Piperidine, non-covalent, reversible	> 6hr	Yes	Alzheimer's disease
Galantamine	Reminyl, Razadyne	Tertiary alkaloid, reversible	>6 hr	Yes	Alzheimer's disease
Rivastigmine	Exelon	Carbamate, pseudo-irreversible	10-12 hr	Yes	Alzheimer's disease

(Table 1) contd.....

Drug	Brand name (s)	Class/Type of Binding	Duration	CNS Effect	Uses
Edrophonium	Tensilon	Electrostatic, rapidly reversible	5-15 min	No	Diagnosis of myasthenia gravis, reversal of NMJ blockade
Echothiophate	Phospholine	Organophosphate, irreversible	> 24 hr	N/A (topical)	Glaucoma

Irreversible inhibitors, such as the organophosphates, bind to the esteratic site and phosphorylate the enzyme [3, 18, 20, 21, 25]. This bond might be irreversible, or may very slowly hydrolyze, depending on the chemical structure of the drug. However, as shown in Fig. (**1**), over a matter of minutes or a few hours, one alkyl group dissociates, and this "aging" renders the bond much more stable, and generally irreversible [29, 32]. The very reactive oxime, 2-PAM (pralidoxime), which is a strong nucleophile, is used therapeutically to bind to organophosphates, and can reactivate the enzyme if given prior to the "aging" process [33, 34]. Interactions of the different types of cholinesterase inhibitors are shown in Fig. (**1**). Some examples of carbamate and organophosphate compounds used as pesticides and nerve agents are shown in Table **2**.

Table 2. Pesticides and nerve gases.

Compound	Brand Name	Type of Binding	Relative Human Toxicity*	Comments
Carbaryl	Sevin	Carbamate	Low	Widely used
Propoxur	Baygon	Carbamate	High	Restricted from indoor use
Carbofuran	Furadan	Carbamate	High	Banned in crops for human consumption
Aldicarb	Temik	Carbamate	High	Use in US agriculture phased out by 2017
Malathion	Chemathion	Organophosphate	Low	Widely used
Parathion	Folidol	Organophosphate	Very high	Use banned due to toxicity
Terbufos	Contraven	Organophosphate	Very high	Use in agriculture restricted
Chlorpyrifos	Dursban	Organophosphate	Moderate	Not for residential use, wide use, many brands

(Table 2) contd.....

Compound	Brand Name	Type of Binding	Relative Human Toxicity*	Comments
Dimethoate	Afidox	Organophosphate	Moderate	Widely used in agriculture, many brand names
DFP (di-isopropylfluorophosphate)		Organophosphate	High	Experimental use (serine protease inhibitor)
Sarin		Organophosphate	Very high	Nerve gas used by terrorists in Japan
Soman		Organophosphate	Very high	Nerve gas, chemical weapon
Tabun		Organophosphate	Very high	Nerve gas, chemical weapon
VX		Organophosphate	Very high	Nerve gas, chemical weapon

* Toxicity data from [223]

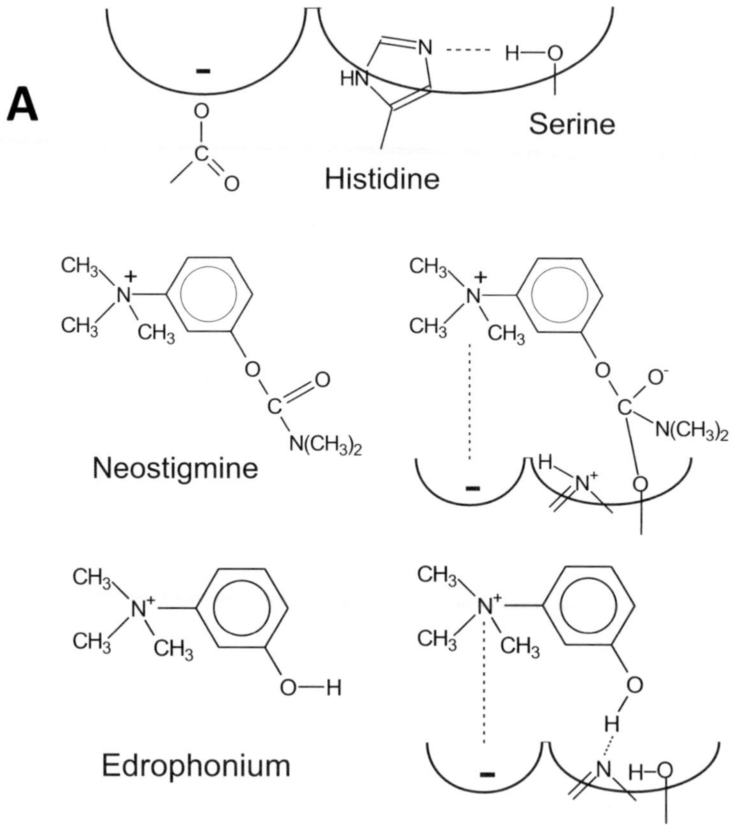

Fig. 1 contd.....

B

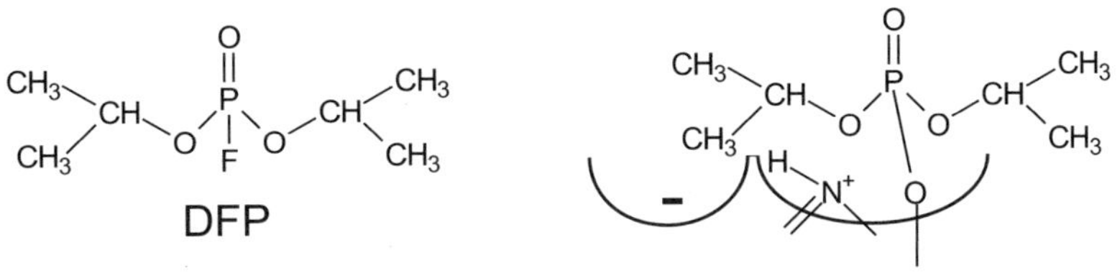

C

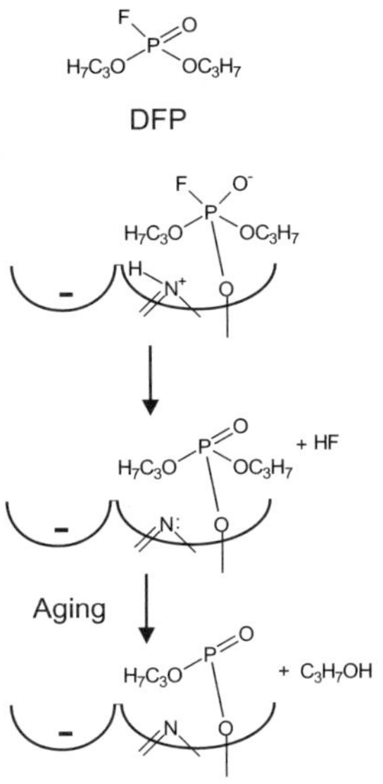

Fig. (1). Interaction of cholinesterase inhibitors with AChE
A: Neostigmine is drawn to the anionic site of AChE. It binds to and acetylates the serine OH at the esteratic site.
B: Edrophonium interacts with AChE by electrostatic binding which is rapidly reversible.
C: DFP (di-isopropylfluorophosphate) phosphorylates the serine OH at the esteratic site. At this point, the enzyme can be reactivated if a strong nucleophile such as pralidoxime bind to the organophosphate. If aging occurs, the leaving group, in this case an isopropyl group, dissociates and the phosphorylation becomes irreversible, inactivating the enzyme.

BChE was first described in the blood in 1932, where it was shown to catalyze the hydrolysis of both choline and non-choline esters [26, 35, 36]. Not surprisingly, BChE is less efficient than AChE for hydrolysis of ACh, but much more efficient for hydrolysis of butyrylcholine [26, 37]. BChE hydrolyzes succinylcholine and also is involved in metabolism of carbamates such as physostigmine, as well as organophosphate cholinesterase inhibitors [26, 37]. The active site of BChE is shown in Fig. (**2**). Similar to AChE, a serine residue is important for catalytic activity; serine 266, histidine 466 and glutamic acid 353 comprise a triad of amino acids at the catalytic site. There is an anionic site that lines up with the quaternary nitrogen group, and an acyl site that lines up with the ester group. A number of inhibitors of BChE are currently being developed, some of which are highly selective [38]. These will be discussed in more detail below.

THERAPEUTIC TARGETS AND USES

Ophthalmology

Physostigmine was first suggested as a useful agent in ophthalmology in 1877 [5, 23], and ophthalmology remains the major use of this drug today. It constricts the pupil and decreases intraocular pressure, making it useful for treatment of glaucoma, particularly narrow angle glaucoma. However, since it is a tertiary amine, it may be absorbed through the nasal membranes, leading to systemic effects. Side effects due to systemic absorption include excessive salivation and abdominal discomfort due to increased activation of muscarinic receptors [39, 40]. Echothiophate, a quaternary organophosphate cholinesterase inhibitor which has minimal systemic absorption, was introduced in 1959 [41]. As this compound is an irreversible cholinesterase inhibitor, it has a very long duration of action, making it useful when a rapid and long-acting reduction of intraocular pressure is needed [42]. However, long-lasting effects of echothiophate include a tendency to increase formation of cataracts [43]. In addition, since muscarinic agonists and cholinesterase inhibitors have significant effects on vision, they are generally drugs of last choice, used primarily for treatment of refractory glaucoma [44].

The Neuromuscular Junction

AChE inhibitors act by increasing the duration of action of ACh in the synaptic cleft. This is particularly important at the neuromuscular junction, which has a high concentration of nicotinic receptors. Stimulation of these receptors with nicotinic agonists results in rapid desensitization of the receptors and blockade of neuromuscular transmission. Administration of an optimum dose of a cholinesterase inhibitor, in contrast, can strengthen neuromuscular transmission without producing blockade. Thus, cholinesterase inhibitors are used to reverse the effects of blockade with non-depolarizing neuromuscular blocking agents, or to strengthen neuromuscular transmission in myasthenia gravis.

Reversal of Neuromuscular blockade

Curare was historically used in arrow poisons to produce paralysis of skeletal muscle transmission [45]. Curare and d-tubocurarine were originally used as neuromuscular blocking agents in general anesthesia, but they exerted significant side effects [46]. The modern non-depolarizing neuromuscular blocking agents such as cisatracurium, rocuronium and vecuronium are less toxic and widely used in anesthesia [47]. Because these drugs are competitive antagonists at the neuromuscular junction, cholinesterase inhibitors can reverse their actions by increasing the ACh concentration in the synaptic cleft sufficiently to compete for nicotinic receptor binding. Reversal of curare-induced neuromuscular blockade by physostigmine was observed during early studies of the cholinesterase inhibitors [10]. Subsequently, the ability of other cholinesterase inhibitors, such as neostigmine, pyridostigmine, and edrophonium, to reverse neuromuscular blockade was described and characterized [48 - 51]. Use of cholinesterase inhibitors to reverse neuromuscular blockade has been standard practice in surgical procedures since the 1950s. Neostigmine and edrophonium are widely used [52]. Neostigmine has a similar duration of action as physostigmine, but as a quaternary ammonium compound, it does not cross the blood brain barrier so causes fewer side effects [1]. Pyridostigmine is very similar to neostigmine, but with a longer duration of action [53]. Edrophonium has a very short duration of action, and is rapidly eliminated by the kidney [1, 27].

Side effects of cholinesterase inhibitors for reversal of neuromuscular blockade are an issue. Bradycardia, excessive salivation, and increases in gastrointestinal activity may occur due to enhanced muscarinic stimulation [27, 54 - 56]. Muscarinic receptor blockers such as glycopyrrolate and atropine are frequently added to prevent muscarinic effects while allowing nicotinic stimulation to remain intact [27, 57, 58]. However, adding a muscarinic antagonist does carry the risk of causing tachycardia, dry mouth, and rarely, delirium [59 - 61]. Fortunately, when given at appropriate therapeutic doses, these side effects are rare. Other concerns that have been raised about using cholinesterase inhibitors to reverse neuromuscular blockade include the risk of inducing weakness, especially in patients with myasthenia gravis, but this appears to occur mainly when too high a dose of cholinesterase inhibitor is used, or if the drug is given when the effects of the non-depolarizing neuromuscular blocking have nearly worn off [27, 55].

Sugammadex (Briodon®), which is not a cholinesterase inhibitor, has been introduced for reversal of blockade produced by rocuronium and vecuronium. Since this compound acts by directly binding to the neuromuscular blocking agent, rather than inhibiting cholinesterase, it does not produce cholinergic side effects [47, 52, 62]. It has been used for several years in Europe, and received FDA approval for use in the United States in December of 2015.

Myasthenia Gravis

Myasthenia gravis is characterized by progressive weakness of skeletal muscles and/or the eyelids and extraocular muscles [63 - 66]. Weakness results from development of antibodies to nicotinic receptors at the neuromuscular junction [65 - 67]. Diagnostic testing for myasthenia gravis includes measurement of antibodies to the nicotinic acetylcholine receptor, and one arm of treatment focuses on immunosuppression with corticosteroids and other immunosuppressant drugs. The other arm of treatment aims at improving muscle strength. Reports that application of physostigmine and neostigmine increased the strength of neuromuscular transmission [68] led to the development of cholinesterase inhibitors as treatment for myasthenia gravis [69, 70]. Administration of a cholinesterase inhibitor will result in an increase in muscle strength in a patient with myasthenia gravis, and this approach is still used today for definitive diagnosis. Neostigmine was initially used for treatment as well as diagnosis [71 - 75]. Edrophonium has a very short duration of action, which has made it useful in the diagnosis of the disease, since its effects last only about 10 minutes [66, 76]. The short duration of action is helpful, since, although unlikely, bradycardia and other effects of excessive cholinergic stimulation may occur [66, 77, 78]. Neostigmine is poorly absorbed orally and has a relatively short duration of action (about 2 hours). Pyridostigmine is somewhat better absorbed, has a longer duration of action, and is thought to produce fewer side effects than neostigmine [70, 79]. For these reasons, pyridostigmine is the treatment of first choice for myasthenia gravis [66, 80].

Side effects due to cholinergic stimulation include salivation, abdominal cramping and diarrhea, nausea, sweating, bradycardia, miosis and muscle twitches [66]. The majority of muscarinic side effects can be prevented by treating with selective anticholinergic agents such as atropine or glycopyrrolate. Since neostigmine, pyridostigmine and edrophonium are quaternary ammonium compounds, they do not cross the blood brain barrier and their effects are limited to the periphery [81].

The Central Nervous System

Treatment of Alzheimer's Disease

Alzheimer's disease (AD) is characterized by severe short term memory loss and cognitive impairment. Pathological hallmarks of the disease are the presence of amyloid plaques and tau containing neurofibrillary tangles. The cognitive dysfunction and memory loss are considered a consequence of a massive loss of cholinergic neurons [82 - 85], and the "cholinergic hypothesis" has thus far provided the primary target for treating AD [86].

Initial attempts to improve cholinergic function involved administration of choline or lecithin, a source of choline, analogous to the use of L-dopa in Parkinson's disease, with the hope of increasing ACh in the cholinergic neurons that remained. Unfortunately, choline is not rate-limiting in the synthesis of acetylcholine, and although many clinical trials were conducted, neither treatment provided significant improvement [87 - 92]. Arecoline, a non-selective tertiary muscarinic agonist known to enhance learning [93], was combined with physostigmine in AD patients [94]. There was very little improvement and the dose was difficult to optimize. The authors concluded that "neither physostigmine nor arecoline offer a practical therapy for Alzheimer disease" [94]. Nevertheless, many subsequent studies of the effect of physostigmine in AD were conducted, but improvement in memory was modest at best [95 - 98]. Physostigmine appears to have a "U-shaped" dose response curve, which means that it will be ineffective if the dose is either too high or too low [99]. These studies did suggest that cholinesterase inhibitor therapy should work, if there were drugs that were more lipid soluble, which would increase the ratio of CNS to peripheral effects, and that had better pharmacodynamic properties.

In the early 1990s tacrine (tetrahydroaminoacridine), was introduced [100, 101]. It had more favorable pharmacokinetics than physostigmine, with good CNS penetration, and, like physostigmine, caused inhibition of both AChE and BChE [102]. Tacrine was also thought to have some activity as a muscarinic receptor agonist, which would further enhance its effects [103]. It was effective in some AD patients at improving memory and cognition, and was the first drug to be approved specifically for treatment of AD. Unfortunately, it has a poor adverse effect profile, similar to that of physostigmine. Both drugs caused adverse cardiac effects and gastrointestinal overactivity related to peripheral muscarinic receptor activation by ACh [101, 104]. Worse yet, tacrine at full therapeutic levels produced hepatotoxicity, indicated by increases in serum aminotransferase levels, in nearly 50% of patients [101, 104]. Since it was the only drug at that time with any effectiveness in AD, tacrine was used in up to 300,000 patients until newer drugs became available [104]. It was withdrawn from the US market in 2013.

The next generation of cholinesterase inhibitors for treatment of AD was developed to maximize CNS effects [104, 105]. Donepezil was introduced in the late 1990s [106 - 108]. Donepezil is a piperidine derivative that forms weak ionic bonds with AChE, for which it is highly selective [109]. The bond is reversible, but the drug has a long half-life, up to 70 hrs [109]. Donepezil has a much better side effect profile than tacrine, with far less peripheral cholinergic stimulation, and no hepatotoxicity [106 - 108]. Blood brain barrier penetration is excellent, favoring central over peripheral effects [105]. Treatment with donepezil has been reported to cause improvement in memory and cognition in about 80% of patients for at least two years if treatment is instituted in early stages of the disease [110], when there are still some remaining cholinergic neurons.

Rivastigmine was introduced in 1998, and galantamine followed in 2001. Galantamine, a phenanthrene tertiary alkaloid, binds reversibly and selectively to AChE with weak ionic bonds, and also causes some stimulation of nicotinic receptors [102, 109]. It is possible that the stimulation of nicotinic receptors contributes to the beneficial effect in AD [111, 112]. Rivastigmine is a carbamate that forms a long-lasting bond to AChE, lasting up to 10 hours, so is classified a pseudo-irreversible inhibitor, and it also causes some inhibition of BChE [109]. It has been suggested that inhibition of BChE could be beneficial in treatment of AD [113, 114], and newer multifunctional drugs designed to inhibit AChE, BChE and/or other targets will be discussed below. However, in spite of varying selectivity for AChE and BChE, there does not seem to be convincing evidence of the superiority of one of these three drugs over the others.

Both rivastigmine and galantamine have more side effects than donepezil, in particular a higher incidence of nausea, vomiting and diarrhea [115, 116]. All of these cholinesterase inhibitors come in oral preparations, and rivastigmine is also available for administration as a transdermal patch, which may provide a more uniform drug concentration. These three cholinesterase inhibitors have become the dominant drugs for current treatment of AD, and are effective in the majority of patients. Combination of cholinesterase inhibitors with memantine (Namenda®), an inhibitor of NMDA glutamate receptors appears to enhance the beneficial effects of both drugs [117]. A combination product, Namzaric®, which combines memantine with donepezil, is now available [118].

While the cholinesterase inhibitors have been widely used for several years of treatment in AD side effects can be quite problematic in some patients [119]. Nausea and diarrhea are the most common side effects, as well as vomiting, particularly with galantamine and rivastigmine, due to increased levels of peripheral ACh stimulating muscarinic receptors [115, 116]. Although rare, bradycardia and syncope may occur in some patients [120 - 122], and this can lead to falls and hip fractures [123]. In spite of these cardiac concerns, there is evidence that the increase in vagal tone in AD patients treated with cholinesterase inhibitors decreases overall cardiovascular mortality [124]. Elderly patients have a higher incidence of overactive bladder, and this may be worsened by treatment cholinesterase inhibitors [125]. Overactive bladder in the elderly is frequently treated with muscarinic receptor blockers such as tolterodine (Detrol®) that have little blood brain barrier penetration, and this combination is used in AD patients. This might not be very beneficial, as anticholinergic drugs, including tolterodine, have been associated with an increased risk of AD and may worsen symptoms in patients with dementia [126 - 128]. Some peripheral side effects, especially nausea and vomiting, may be reduced by using rivastigmine patches to provide sustained drug delivery which avoid peaks and troughs in drug concentration

[129]. However, use of skin patches can increase the incidence of skin irritation and itching, which can be of particular concern in an elderly population.

Drug interactions with cholinesterase inhibitors in patients being treated for AD must also be considered, as this is an elderly population who may also have additional significant health challenges. Antipsychotic drugs, gastrointestinal drugs, and antihypertensive drugs appear to have the highest incidence of serious drug interactions with cholinesterase inhibitors [130]. Many antipsychotics block muscarinic receptors in the brain, and drugs that increase or decrease gastrointestinal motility often act by either stimulating or blocking muscarinic receptors. This could potentially reduce the beneficial central effects of cholinesterase inhibitors, or might exacerbate their peripheral side effects. Beta blockers and verapamil, both of which decrease heart rate, will increase the risk of bradycardia in patients taking cholinesterase inhibitors due to combination with ACh-mediated slowing of the heart.

Many AD patients suffer from agitation, delusions and hallucinations [131]. While the use of cholinesterase inhibitors may reduce these symptoms [132 - 134], symptoms persist in some patients. Use of both typical and atypical antipsychotic drugs has been associated with an increased risk of mortality in AD patients [135, 136], and drug interactions are problematic. Based on these interactions and concerns, alternate therapies are being considered [137].

In theory, treatment of AD with cholinesterase inhibitors could decrease β-amyloid deposition and slow the progression of AD. Amyloid precursor protein (APP) is processed in the brain by one of two primary mechanisms. Cleavage of APP by β-secretase followed by γ-secretase leads to production of sAPPβ and neurotoxic β-amyloid, which accumulates in amyloid plaques and is considered to be neurotoxic [138]. In contrast, normal processing leads to production of sAPPα, which is considered neuroprotective and neurotrophic [138, 139]. Stimulation with M1 muscarinic receptor agonists increased secretion of sAPPα and decreased production of β-amyloid in cell culture [140]. Rivastigmine had the same effect in primary neuronal cultures [141]. Muscarinic agonists also reduce accumulation of β-amyloid in animals following selective central cholinergic lesions [142, 143]. Treatment with donepezil reduced mitochondrial accumulation of β-amyloid and reduced mitochondrial dysfunction in transgenic mice [144]. Donepezil also protected against β-amyloid toxicity in animal models of AD [145 - 147], and decreased learning and memory deficits in these models [148]. It is thought that interaction of the peripheral anionic site of AChE augments neurotoxicity in AD through induction of β-amyloid aggregation, and that by preventing this cascade, cholinesterase inhibitors could have a disease-modifying effect [149 - 151].

Although *in vitro* and animal studies have been encouraging, there is considerable controversy about how beneficial cholinesterase inhibitor treatment is over the long term. Some authors claim that cholinesterase inhibitors lack a disease-modifying effect [152, 153], and others have found no significant changes in CSF β-amyloid or tau six months to a year following initiation of treatment [152, 154, 155]. Some authors feel that cholinesterase inhibitor treatment is even detrimental. One study indicated that treatment led to increased tau accumulation [156], but it might be argued that these patients probably survived longer than those who were not treated, and thus the progression of pathology was worse, given that this is a progressive disease. Two trials showed greater cognitive decline in patients with mild cognitive impairment (MCI) or AD who were treated with a cholinesterase inhibitor compared to those who were not [157, 158].

On the other hand, treatment with cholinesterase inhibitors has been shown to delay the need for placement into nursing homes by at least one year [159 - 161]. This delay could result from an improvement in symptoms, allowing the patients to live at home longer, but it could also represent a slowing of the pathology of the disease. The effect of cholinesterase inhibitors in patients with MCI, considered by many to be a possible precursor to AD, suggests that treatment can in fact be beneficial. In a number of studies, cholinesterase inhibitor treatment decreased the progression from MCI to AD, especially in women [162 - 165]. In contrast, several meta-analyses concluded that cholinesterase inhibitor treatment had no effect on conversion from MCI to AD [153, 166 - 168]. There are three alleles of the APO E gene, and those with APO E4 are at higher risk of developing AD [169]. These meta-analyses did not address the proportion of patients in the trials who were APOE E4 positive, as this can influence the degree of neuritic plaque formation, the amount of β-amyloid deposition, and the rate at which the disease progresses [170, 171], so the results have been skewed by that factor. Since cholinesterase inhibitor treatment alleviates symptoms in AD patients, it may be difficult to establish a definitive end point where a patient converts from MCI to AD.

There are numerous factors which affect the likelihood that a patient will respond to treatment with cholinesterase inhibitors, and it is difficult to perform studies that take these all into account [172]. Other problems with these studies are varying means of assessing cognitive function and endpoints, making it difficult to compare one study to another. Also, a lot of studies were conducted at a time before diagnostic markers such as amyloid-PET or CSF levels of amyloid were available, and the study populations may have contained many patients who had dementia from causes other than AD. Nevertheless, many neurologists favor the use of cholinesterase inhibitors in patients with MCI [173], and overall analysis indicates that cholinesterase inhibitor treatment is effective and relatively safe [174].

Another treatment strategy focuses on the development of multifunctional cholinesterase inhibitors, which affect multiple targets. One of these targets is BChE. AChE levels in the brain are decreased in AD, whereas BChE increases as the disease progresses, and BChE is associated with β-amyloid in neuritic plaques [175, 176]. Tacrine, the first cholinesterase inhibitor used in AD, inhibits both AChE and BChE, and decreases levels of β-amyloid [177]. Selective BChE inhibitors, such as cymserine analogues, were shown to enhance learning in aged rats, decrease β-amyloid toxicity, and decrease β-amyloid levels both in rodents and in cell culture [113, 178, 179]. Knowledge of structure activity relationships is driving the development of other selective inhibitors of BChE [38].

While tacrine failed as a therapeutic agent due to liver toxicity, it was multifunctional to a degree in that it inhibited both AChE and BChE, and may have had muscarinic agonist effect [180 - 182]. The development of tacrine analogues which are less likely to be hepatoxic has recently been reviewed [183]. One of these analogues was quite selective for BChE and caused a significant decrease in aggregation of β-amyloid [184]. Other derivatives in this group, although less potent inhibitors of AChE and BChE, were even more effective at decreasing aggregation of β-amyloid [184]. An isoindoline-1,3-dione derivative also inhibits BChE and AChE, and decreases β-amyloid [185]. In addition to inhibition of AChE, BChE and β-amyloid aggregation, some tacrine analogues also inhibit NMDA receptors, thus having a potential neuroprotective effect. Still others are antioxidants, or exert other protective effects in the brain [183]. Other potential drugs, including a benzochromenopryimidinimine compound, have been shown to exhibit anticholinesterase activity, decrease β-amyloid aggregation and act as antioxidants [186].

Tacrine-coumarin hybrids have also shown to be slightly more selective for inhibition of AChE than BChE, to decrease aggregation of β-amyloid, and to inhibit the enzyme β-secretase, which is involved in the abnormal processing of APP to β-amyloid [187]. A benzamide-isoquinoline derivative also inhibited AChE, BChE, β-amyloid aggregation, and β-secretase [188].

Other targets for multifunctional cholinesterases include blockade of NMDA receptors, mimicking in one compound the combination of donepezil and memantine. Carbacrine, a tacrine derivative, was shown to be a very potent inhibitor of AChE, inhibited aggregation of β-amyloid, and was more efficacious than memantine as an NMDA receptor antagonist [149]. Modification of this analogue produced memegal, which was more potent at the NMDA receptor, had antioxidant activity, and was shown to be neuroprotective [149]. Many of these new multifunctional compounds have not yet been studied extensively in animals or in clinical trials in humans, but it is clear that development of multifunctional cholinesterase inhibitors represents a promising approach to development of more effective treatments for AD. Such multifunctional drugs could potentially both treat the symptoms of AD by increasing ACh, and slow the progression of the disease by preventing the formation and deposition of β-amyloid.

Treatment of Muscarinic Antagonist Poisoning

Because physostigmine is a tertiary amine, it has significant CNS effects [95, 189, 190]. Poisoning with muscarinic antagonists such as atropine or scopolamine produces toxicity that includes tachycardia, increased body temperature, decreased bowel activity, agitation and delirium. While the peripheral symptoms can be controlled by administration of a muscarinic agonist, the CNS symptoms cannot, as there is a lack of effective centrally acting muscarinic agonists. Thus, physostigmine, because of its entry into the CNS, is used to treat poisoning with muscarinic receptor antagonists [81, 191, 192].

Schizophrenia

Drugs which activate muscarinic or nicotinic receptors may improve symptoms of schizophrenia [193, 194]. There is a decrease in both muscarinic and nicotinic receptors in schizophrenia, which may contribute to the cognitive disorders seen in the disease [195 - 198]. Levels of activity of both choline acetyltransferase and AChE, markers for cholinergic nerve terminals, are decreased in the prefrontal cortex in schizophrenia [199]. M1 muscarinic receptor stimulation increases release of dopamine in the prefrontal cortex, an area where dopamine is decreased in schizophrenia [200], and decreases dopamine release in areas where overactivity may contribute to psychosis [201 - 204]. The M1/M4 preferring agonist, xanomeline, has a positive effect in schizophrenia [205]. The role of nicotinic receptors in schizophrenia is unknown, but smoking is very common among people with schizophrenia and may represent an attempt to alleviate their symptoms [206, 207]. Thus, cholinesterase inhibitors have been suggested as possible treatment options for schizophrenia [208, 209].

PESTICIDES AND NERVE AGENTS

Many compounds that were developed as pesticides inhibit cholinesterase, as AChE is important for function in the nervous system of insects [210 - 212]. The first reported work on organophosphate pesticides was in 1854, with the synthesis of tetraethylpyrophosphate (TEPP) by Clermont [2, 213]. Clermont tasted the compound and survived, which was fortunate for him as TEPP is extremely toxic.

Synthetic phosphates and phosphonates, as well as esters of phosphoric acid, were synthesized in the early part of the 20th century [214, 215]. Lange and Kreuger in Germany synthesized a number of compounds in this class during the 1930s [216, 217]. Lange left Germany and later settled in the United States, but his work inspired Gerhard Schrader, at IG Farben in Germany, to continue and extend these studies during the 1930s to produce new and more toxic pesticides including parathion, and subsequently, to develop the "nerve gases", which may be more accurately termed nerve agents [213].

Pesticides

More than 50 carbamate cholinesterase inhibitors have been developed as pesticides [218], and organophosphates are also widely used for this purpose [219]. Selective toxicity of these pesticides takes advantage of different rates of activation of some cholinesterase inhibitors in insects compared to humans [220, 221], but poisoning is common with these compounds [222, 223]. Poisoning may be accidental or intentional, and in the years from 2002 to 2006, 30,000 exposures to organophosphates and 14,000 exposures to carbamates were recorded in the US, with about 20 fatalities during this time [213]. The incidence of poisoning in rural parts of Asia, where 200,000 deaths occur per year, is far higher [213]. Cholinesterase inhibitors have been used intentionally in both suicides and homicides [213]. Carbamate pesticides also accumulate in ground water [218], where they may cause human and animal exposure. Organophosphates and carbamates are used in pet collars and powders to control fleas, but may cause poisoning from overdose [224]. Toxicity of these products determines their uses to a great degree. Those considered of "low toxicity" can be sold for household use, whereas those with higher toxicity are used only by licensed pest control specialists. Given their wide use, exposure of farm workers to organophosphates is problematic [219], making it important to develop methods to monitor the health effects of exposure to these compounds [225]. The use of these compounds in agriculture is highly regulated in North America, depending on the level of toxicity and the rate at which the compounds are degraded and lose activity, but may not be as well regulated world-wide. Both acute poisoning and the effects of long-term low level exposure from environmental or work-related sources continue to be problematic with these compounds [226 - 228].

Nerve Agents

The history of the nerve agents arose from the early work with pesticides. Schrader, who synthesized more than 2000 compounds [229], observed the toxic effect or organophosphates in mammals. The first highly toxic organophosphate to be synthesized was tabun in 1936 [230]. Since it made several laboratory personnel very ill following a spill of a small amount, its significant toxicity and potential as a military weapon was recognized [231]. Synthesis of sarin and soman followed shortly thereafter, and all patents pertaining to these compounds were soon declared secret by the German War Ministry [232]. Extensive production and development of tabun and sarin were carried out during World War II in Germany. While often termed "nerve gases", these compounds are all liquids, but are frequently delivered in a vaporized form. For reasons that are not altogether clear, none of them were used as weapons during the war. Following World War II, these compounds were found and designated by NATO in order of their synthesis as GA, GB, and GD [233].

The British were attempting to develop nerve gases during this same time period. DFP was synthesized by McCombie and Saunders [234 - 236], but it was neither as potent nor as toxic as the German compounds. Nevertheless, DFP caused substantial toxicity, in particular difficulty with breathing [234]. In an attempt to replace DDT as a pesticide, the British subsequently synthesized VX, which is more toxic than the other agents in this class, and unlike the others, does not vaporize easily, but is a heavy, dense, liquid [231, 237]. Organophosphates normally break down quite rapidly to inactive compounds, but since VX is much less volatile, it may persist on surfaces for hours to weeks [238]. A similar compound, designated VR or Russian VX, which was developed in Russia, is highly toxic, and may be even more persistent in the environment than VX [239]. Exposure to most of these agents is usually by inhalation, but VX, due to is oily consistency, may be absorbed through the skin. The symptoms of poisoning vary depending on the route of exposure. Inhalation preferentially affects the eyes, salivation and respiratory function. Absorption through the skin will cause sweating and muscle fasiculations at the site of entry, with gastrointestinal symptoms developing over time [230, 231].

A leak of VX in the US resulted in the death of 6000 sheep in 1968 [230], and a year later production of nerve gases in the US was halted [231], although small stockpiles of sarin, tabun and VX were maintained [240]. In 1997, the Chemical Weapons Convention called for the destruction of most of the nerve gases on a worldwide basis, and as of 2016, 90% have been eliminated (http://www.cwc.gov/; https://www.opcw.org/news-publications/publications/facts-and- figu-res/#c1920). The only recorded use of nerve agents in warfare was during the Iraq-Iran war in the mid-1980s. In combination with sulfur mustard compounds, it is thought that use of tabun and sarin led to approximately 45,000 casualties in that conflict [241]. It has also been reported that there was some exposure of military personnel to sarin in 1991 during the Gulf War, after an Iraqi chemical weapons facility was destroyed [231]. Sarin was used in two terrorist attacks in

Japan in 1994 and 1995, affecting a total of over 5000 people, 19 of whom died [242, 243].

Toxicity and Treatment of Poisoning

Exposure to organophosphates is usually through inhalation. Symptoms include difficulty breathing and increased bronchial secretions, miosis, blurred vision, tearing of the eyes, and headache, salivation, bradycardia, and increased gastrointestinal activity due to muscarinic receptor stimulation [223, 238, 244 - 246]. Nicotinic receptor stimulation followed by blockade produces skeletal muscle contraction following by receptor desensitization and paralysis [238, 246]. Since organophosphates are generally very lipid soluble and enter the brain easily, they produce CNS toxicity. CNS symptoms depend on the severity of poisoning and the agent used. Moderate exposure results in anxiety, irritability, memory impairment, slurred speech, headache, blurred vision, depression and dizziness [213, 238]. Confusion, lethargy and loss of consciousness may develop with more severe poisoning [213, 238, 244, 245]. Seizures may occur, and are more likely with nerve agents than with pesticide organophosphates [213, 247]. Seizures are treated with benzodiazepines [231]. CNS effects of the carbamates that get into the brain are similar to those of organophosphates, but generally less severe and of shorter duration [213]. If the patient survives exposure, long-term effects may include memory impairment [248, 249].

The most dramatic acute, high dose exposure to a nerve agent occurred in the 1995 sarin attack in the Tokyo, Japan subway. About 5000 people were poisoned, of whom 11 died. The victims who survived were studied at various times up to ten years following the incident. There was a high incidence of post-traumatic stress disorder along with increases in depression and poor performance on memory tasks [250 - 252] in these survivors. The mechanism producing these long-term CNS effects is not known [250].

Long-term poisoning with organophosphate pesticides is also reported to result in impairment of memory and concentration, depression, and psychosis [244, 253]. A study in banana farmers who worked with pesticides found that those exposed to chronic low levels of organophosphates suffered depression [254]. Other studies of long-term low-level organophosphate exposure have provided variable results, ranging from no effect to increased anxiety, impaired cognition, or psychiatric disturbances [255, 256]. Higher level chronic exposure has been shown to result in numerous central effects similar to those with acute exposures, such as headache, anxiety, insomnia, depression, and occasional psychotic behavior [226, 231, 243, 245, 257 - 259].

It was known relatively early that the toxicity of the organophosphates resulted from irreversible inhibition of AChE [260]. Subsequent reports described the toxicity of DFP, TEPP, paraoxon, sarin and tabun in detail [261 - 264]. Since many of the effects of poisoning resembled parasympathetic activation (Table **3**), muscarinic antagonists, in particular atropine, were used for treatment, both for organophosphate [265 - 268] and for carbamate toxicity [269, 270]. While scopolamine would be better than atropine at blocking central nervous system effects of nerve agents, atropine produces fewer side effects [231]. Today atropine is one of the mainstays of treatment of cholinesterase poisoning, and it is effective at blocking the parasympathetic symptoms of AChE inhibition.

Table 3. Cholinesterase inhibitor toxicity.

Affected Area	**Severity**		
	Mild	**Moderate**	**Severe**
Eyes, Nose and Mouth	Miosis, blurred vision, eye pain, tearing, headache, rhinorrhea, salivation	Continued symptoms	Copious salivation
Respiratory	Bronchoconstriction and wheezing	Dyspnea, bronchorrhea, wheezing	Severe airway restriction, apnea
Skin	Sweating with local exposure	Sweating	
Cardiac		Mild arrhythmias	Life-threatening arrhythmias
Gastrointestinal		Nausea, vomiting, abdominal cramps, diarrhea	
Neuromuscular Junction		Facisculations, mild weakness	Flaccid paralysis
CNS		Irritability, anxiety, memory impairment, slurred speech	Seizures, loss of consciousness

Before organophosphates undergo “aging”, they can be removed from the cholinesterase enzyme with strong nucleophiles such as pralidoxime, which reactivates AChE [271]. The positively charged nitrogen in pralidoxime is attracted to the negative charges at the anionic site of cholinesterase. This proximity to the organophosphate bound to the AChE enzyme provides an opportunity for the nucleophile to attack the phosphate bond, and draw the organophosphate away from AChE, liberating the enzyme [272 - 274]. Current standards of treatment for organophosphate poisoning include administration of atropine and pralidoxime, along with benzodiazepines [223, 238, 246]. Although its use in carbamate poisoning has been controversial, pralidoxime has been shown to reactivate AChE after poisoning with some carbamates other than carbaryl [275], and it appears that it may be useful in these cases as well [34, 276].

Prophylaxis

Pyridostigmine is provided to military personnel deemed at risk of nerve agent exposure [277]. Reversible carbamate AChE inhibitors compete with organophosphates for binding to AChE, and have been shown in many studies to reduce the toxicity and improve survival following organophosphate poisoning [278 - 282]. This approach has also been suggested for prophylaxis against poisoning with pesticides [283]. Pyridostigmine is the only drug currently approved in the US for this use.

SUMMARY

There is a wide variety of cholinesterase inhibitors available. The effects of some are beneficial for several different disease states and for reversal of the actions of certain drugs, some are useful and reasonably well tolerated as pesticides, and others, especially the nerve agents, produce severe toxicity. The mechanism by which these compounds inhibit AChE is shown in Fig. (**1**), and inhibition of BChE is shown in Fig. (**2**). An overview of the compounds used therapeutically is shown in Table **1**. Selected pesticides and nerve agents are summarized in Table **2**. The effects of cholinesterase poisoning and agents used for treatment or prevention of poisoning are summarized in Table **3**. New cholinesterase inhibitors, some of which address multiple targets, continue to be developed.

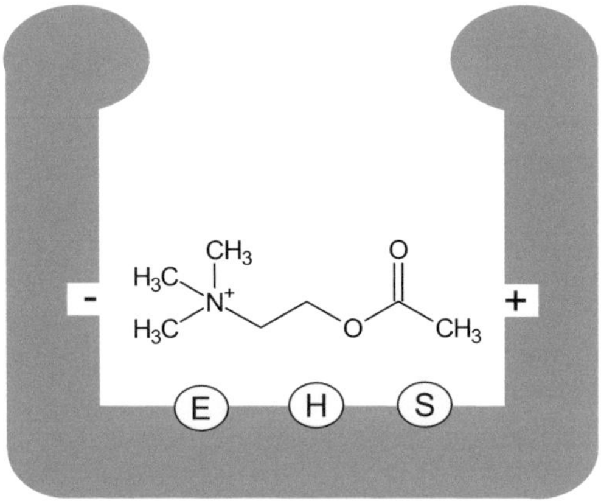

Fig. (2). Interaction of butyrylcholine with BChE
Butyrylcholine is drawn into the active site of the enzyme, which consists of the amino acids serine (S), histidine (H) and glutamate (E). The acyl portion of butyrylcholine is drawn to the acyl site, and the quaternary ammonium is drawn to the anionic site. Hydrolysis of ACh and other esters occurs in a similar fashion.

Butyrylcholine is drawn into the active site of the enzyme, which consists of the amino acids serine (S), histidine (H) and glutamate (E). The acyl portion of butyrylcholine is drawn to the acyl site, and the quaternary ammonium is drawn to the anionic site. Hydrolysis of ACh and other esters occurs in a similar fashion.

CONFLICT OF INTEREST

The authors declare no conflict of interest, financial or otherwise.

ACKNOWLEDGEMENTS

Declared none.

REFERENCES

[1] Taylor P. Anticholinesterase Agents.Goodman & Gilman's pharmacological basis of therapeutics. 12th ed., New York: McGraw-Hill 2011.

[2] Holmstedt B. Cholinesterase inhibitors: an introduction.Cholinest-erases and Cholinesterase Inhibitors. London: Martin Dunitz 2000; pp. 1-8.

[3] Holmstedt B. Cholinesterase inhibitors, an introduction.Cholinesterases and Anticholinesterase Agents Hanbuch der Experimentallen Pharmakologie 15. Berlin: Springer-Verlag 1963; pp. 428-85. [http://dx.doi.org/10.1007/978-3-642-99875-1_9]

[4] Karczmar A. History of the research with anticholinesterase agents.Anticholinesterase Agents, International Encyclopedia of Pharmacology and Therapeutics 1. Oxford: Pergamon Press 1970.

[5] Laqueur 1. Ueber Atropin und Physostigmin in ihre Wirkung auf den intraocularen Druck. . Albrecht von Graefes Archiv fur klinische und experimentelle Ophthalmologie Albrecht von Graefe's archive for clinical and experimental ophthalmology. 1877; 23: 149-76.

[6] Anderson HK. The paralysis of involuntary muscle: Part III. On the action of pilocarpine, physostigmine, and atropine upon the paralysed iris. J Physiol 1905; 33(4-5): 414-38. [http://dx.doi.org/10.1113/jphysiol.1905.sp001129] [PMID: 16992820]

[7] Stedman E. Studies on the relationship between chemical constitution and physiological action: Part I. position isomerism in relation to the miotic activity of some synthetic urethanes. Biochem J 1926; 20(4): 719-34. [http://dx.doi.org/10.1042/bj0200719] [PMID: 16743713]

[8] Stedman E. Studies on the relationship between chemical constitution and physiological action: Part II. The miotic activity of urethanes derived from the isomeric hydroxybenzyldimethylamines. Biochem J 1929; 23(1): 17-24. [http://dx.doi.org/10.1042/bj0230017] [PMID: 16744184]

[9] Aeschlimann JA, Reinert M. The pharmacological action of some analogues of physostigmine. J Pharmacol Exp Ther 1931; 43(3): 413-44.

[10] Langley JN, Kato T. The physiological action of physostigmine and its action on denervated skeletal muscle. J Physiol 1915; 49(5): 410-31. [http://dx.doi.org/10.1113/jphysiol.1915.sp001718] [PMID: 16993304]

[11] Stewart WC. Accumulation of acetylcholine in brain and blood of animals poisoned with cholinesterase inhibitors. Br J Pharmacol Chemother 1952; 7(2): 270-6. [http://dx.doi.org/10.1111/j.1476-5381.1952.tb01322.x] [PMID: 14954125]

[12] Goldstein A. The mechanism of enzyme-inhibitor-substrate reactions: Illustrated by the

cholinesterase-physostigmine-acetylcholine system. J Gen Physiol 1944; 27(6): 529-80. [http://dx.doi.org/10.1085/jgp.27.6.529] [PMID: 19873399]

[13] Straus OH, Goldstein A. Technical assistance of Frank L. Plachte. Zone behavior of enzymes: Illustrated by the effect of dissociation constant and dilution on the system cholinesterase-physostigmine. J Gen Physiol 1943; 26(6): 559-85. [http://dx.doi.org/10.1085/jgp.26.6.559] [PMID: 19873367]

[14] Koelle GB. Protection of cholinesterase against irreversible inactivation by di-isopropyl fluorophosphate *in vitro*. J Pharmacol Exp Ther 1946; 88(3): 232-7. [PMID: 20274546]

[15] Koelle GB, Gilman A. The relationship between cholinesterase inhibition and the pharmacological action of di-isopropyl fluorophosphate (DFP). J Pharmacol Exp Ther 1946; 87(4) (Suppl.): 421-34. [PMID: 20279263]

[16] Bodansky O, Mazur A. Mechanism of *in vitro* and *in vivo* inhibition of cholinesterase activity by diisopropyl fluorophosphate. Fed Proc 1946; 5(1 Pt 2): 123. [PMID: 21066635]

[17] Mazur A, Bodansky O. The mechanism of *in vitro* and *in vivo* inhibition of cholinesterase activity by diisopropyl fluorophosphate. J Biol Chem 1946; 163: 261-76. [PMID: 21023648]

[18] Hobbiger F. Inhibition of cholinesterases by irreversible inhibitors *in vitro* and *in vivo*. Br J Pharmacol Chemother 1951; 6(1): 21-30. [http://dx.doi.org/10.1111/j.1476-5381.1951.tb00616.x] [PMID: 14821298]

[19] Aldridge WN, Davies DR. Determination of cholinesterase activity in human blood. BMJ 1952; 1(4765): 945-7. [http://dx.doi.org/10.1136/bmj.1.4765.945] [PMID: 14916207]

[20] Aldridge WN, Davison AN. The inhibition of erythrocyte cholinesterase by tri-esters of phosphoric acid. II. Diethyl p-nitrophenyl thionphosphate (E605) and analogues. Biochem J 1952; 52(4): 663-71. [http://dx.doi.org/10.1042/bj0520663] [PMID: 13018298]

[21] Aldridge WN, Davison AN. The inhibition of erythrocyte cholinesterase by tri-esters of phosphoric acid. I. Diethyl p nitrophenyl phosphate (E600) and analogues. Biochem J 1952; 51(1): 62-70. [http://dx.doi.org/10.1042/bj0510062] [PMID: 14944533]

[22] Stedman E, Barger G. XLII.-Physostigmine (eserine). Part III. J Chem Soc Trans 1925; 127(0): 247-58. [http://dx.doi.org/10.1039/CT9252700247]

[23] Holmstedt B. The ordeal bean of Old Calabar: the pageant of Physostigma venenosum in medicine.1972. [http://dx.doi.org/10.4159/harvard.9780674865266.c12]

[24] Sperling F, Karczmar AG, *et al.* The effects of di-isopropyl fluorophosphate and physostigmine on the sympathetic ganglia. Fed Proc 1947; 6(1): 373. [PMID: 20343782]

[25] Taylor JS. Anticholinesterase agents.Goodman and gilman's the pharmacological basis of therapeutics. 7th ed. New York: MacMillan 1985; pp. 110-29.

[26] Darvesh S, Hopkins DA, Geula C. Neurobiology of butyrylcholinesterase. Nat Rev Neurosci 2003; 4(2): 131-8. [http://dx.doi.org/10.1038/nrn1035] [PMID: 12563284]

[27] Caldwell JE. Clinical limitations of acetylcholinesterase antagonists. J Crit Care 2009; 24(1): 21-8. [http://dx.doi.org/10.1016/j.jcrc.2008.08.003] [PMID: 19272535]

[28] Wilson IB, Hatch MA, Ginsburg S. Carbamylation of acetvlcholinesterase. J Biol Chem 1960; 235:

2312-5.
[PMID: 13845075]

[29] Koelle GB. Pharmacology of organophosphates. J Appl Toxicol 1994; 14(2): 105-9.
[http://dx.doi.org/10.1002/jat.2550140211] [PMID: 8027504]

[30] Darvesh S, Darvesh KV, McDonald RS, *et al.* Carbamates with differential mechanism of inhibition toward acetylcholinesterase and butyrylcholinesterase. J Med Chem 2008; 51(14): 4200-12.
[http://dx.doi.org/10.1021/jm8002075] [PMID: 18570368]

[31] Mooser G, Sigman DS. Ligand binding properties of acetylcholinesterase determined with fluorescent probes. Biochemistry 1974; 13(11): 2299-307.
[http://dx.doi.org/10.1021/bi00708a010] [PMID: 4857568]

[32] Hobbiger F. Pharmacology of anticholinesterase drugs.Neuromuscular Junction Handbuch der Experimentallen Pharmakologie 42. Berlin: Springer-Verlag 1976; pp. 921-88.

[33] Hobbiger F. Protection against the lethal effects of organophosphates by pyridine-2-aldoxime methiodide. Br J Pharmacol Chemother 1957; 12(4): 438-46.
[http://dx.doi.org/10.1111/j.1476-5381.1957.tb00162.x] [PMID: 13489171]

[34] Howland M. Pralidoxime.Goldfrank's toxicologic emergencies. New York: McGraw Hill Medical 2011; pp. 1467-72.

[35] Stedman E, Stedman E, Easson LH. Choline-esterase. An enzyme present in the blood-serum of the horse. Biochem J 1932; 26(6): 2056-66.
[http://dx.doi.org/10.1042/bj0262056] [PMID: 16745037]

[36] Mendel B, Rudney H. Studies on cholinesterase: 1. Cholinesterase and pseudo-cholinesterase. Biochem J 1943; 37(1): 59-63.
[http://dx.doi.org/10.1042/bj0370059] [PMID: 16747599]

[37] Silver A. The biology of cholinesterases. Amsterdam New York: North-Holland Pub. Co.;American Elsevier Pub. Co 1974; p. 596.

[38] Dighe SN, Deora GS, De la Mora E, *et al.* Discovery and structure-activity relationships of a highly selective butyrylcholinesterase inhibitor by structure-based virtual screening. J Med Chem 2016; 59(16): 7683-9.
[http://dx.doi.org/10.1021/acs.jmedchem.6b00356] [PMID: 27405689]

[39] Becker B, Ballin N. Glaucoma. Annu Rev Med 1966; 17(1): 235-42.
[http://dx.doi.org/10.1146/annurev.me.17.020166.001315] [PMID: 5327158]

[40] Bartlett JD, Jaanus SD. Clinical ocular pharmacology. 5th ed. St. Louis, Mo.: Butterworth-Heinemann/Elsevier; 2008. xvi, 793 p.

[41] Becker B, Pyle GC, Drews RC. The tonographic effects of echothiophate (phospholine) iodide: reversal by pyridine-2-aldoxine methiodide (P2AM). Am J Ophthalmol 1959; 47(5 Pt 1): 635-40.
[http://dx.doi.org/10.1016/S0002-9394(14)78187-5] [PMID: 13649819]

[42] Fisher R, Smith R, Wheeler C. Comparison between the tonographic effects of pilocarpine and echothiophate iodide in glaucoma simplex. Br J Ophthalmol 1965; 49(7): 369-73.
[http://dx.doi.org/10.1136/bjo.49.7.369] [PMID: 5829767]

[43] Thoft RA. Incidence of lens changes in patients treated with echothiophate iodide. Arch Ophthalmol 1968; 80(3): 317-20.
[http://dx.doi.org/10.1001/archopht.1968.00980050319004] [PMID: 5670686]

[44] Schmidt KG, Horowitz Y, Buckman G, Segev E, Levinger E, Geyer O. Lowering of IOP by echothiophate iodide in pseudophakic eyes with glaucoma. Curr Eye Res 2010; 35(8): 698-702.
[http://dx.doi.org/10.3109/02713681003794076] [PMID: 20673046]

[45] Lee MR. Curare: the South American arrow poison. J R Coll Physicians Edinb 2005; 35(1): 83-92.
[PMID: 15825249]

[46] Griffith H, Johnson GE. The use of curare in general anesthesia. Anesthesiology 1942; 3(4): 418-20. [http://dx.doi.org/10.1097/00000542-194207000-00006]

[47] Nicholson WT, Sprung J, Jankowski CJ. Sugammadex: a novel agent for the reversal of neuromuscular blockade. Pharmacotherapy 2007; 27(8): 1181-8. [http://dx.doi.org/10.1592/phco.27.8.1181] [PMID: 17655516]

[48] Hobbiger F. The mechanism of anticurare action of certain neostigmine analogues. Br J Pharmacol Chemother 1952; 7(2): 223-36. [http://dx.doi.org/10.1111/j.1476-5381.1952.tb01317.x] [PMID: 14954120]

[49] Smith CM, Cohen HL, Pelikan EW, Unna KR. Mode of action of antagonists to curare. J Pharmacol Exp Ther 1952; 105(4): 391-9. [PMID: 14955768]

[50] Nastuk WL, Alexander JT. The action of 3-hydroxyphenyldimethylethyl-ammonium (tensilon) on neuromuscular transmission in the frog. J Pharmacol Exp Ther 1954; 111(3): 302-28. [PMID: 13175111]

[51] Katz B, Thesleff S. The interaction between edrophonium (tensilon) and acetylcholine at the motor end-plate. Br J Pharmacol Chemother 1957; 12(2): 260-4. [http://dx.doi.org/10.1111/j.1476-5381.1957.tb00131.x] [PMID: 13446384]

[52] Srivastava A, Hunter JM. Reversal of neuromuscular block. Br J Anaesth 2009; 103(1): 115-29. [http://dx.doi.org/10.1093/bja/aep093] [PMID: 19468024]

[53] Miller RD. Antagonism of neuromuscular blockade. Anesthesiology 1976; 44(4): 318-29. [http://dx.doi.org/10.1097/00000542-197604000-00010] [PMID: 769606]

[54] Clutton RE, Boyd C, Flora R, Payne J, McGrath CJ. Autonomic and cardiovascular effects of neuromuscular blockade antagonism in the dog. Vet Surg 1992; 21(1): 68-75. [http://dx.doi.org/10.1111/j.1532-950X.1992.tb00015.x] [PMID: 1580060]

[55] Bevan DR, Donati F, Kopman AF. Reversal of neuromuscular blockade. Anesthesiology 1992; 77(4): 785-805. [http://dx.doi.org/10.1097/00000542-199210000-00025] [PMID: 1416176]

[56] Stein L, Wise CD. Release of norepinephrine from hypothalamus and amygdala by rewarding medial forebrain bundle stimulation and amphetamine. J Comp Physiol Psychol 1969; 67(2): 189-98. [http://dx.doi.org/10.1037/h0026767] [PMID: 4306672]

[57] Azar I, Pham AN, Karambelkar DJ, Lear E. The heart rate following edrophonium-atropine and edrophonium-glycopyrrolate mixtures. Anesthesiology 1983; 59(2): 139-41. [http://dx.doi.org/10.1097/00000542-198308000-00013] [PMID: 6869871]

[58] Naguib M, Gomaa M. Atropine-neostigmine mixture: a dose-response study. Can J Anaesth 1989; 36(4): 412-7. [http://dx.doi.org/10.1007/BF03005340] [PMID: 2758540]

[59] Cooper MJ, Abinader EG. Atropine-induced ventricular fibrillation: case report and review of the literature. Am Heart J 1979; 97(2): 225-8. [http://dx.doi.org/10.1016/0002-8703(79)90360-0] [PMID: 760453]

[60] Wolff MS, Kleinberg I. The effect of ammonium glycopyrrolate (Robinul)-induced xerostomia on oral mucosal wetness and flow of gingival crevicular fluid in humans. Arch Oral Biol 1999; 44(2): 97-102. [http://dx.doi.org/10.1016/S0003-9969(98)00113-7] [PMID: 10206327]

[61] Bellani AE, Rodolà F, Cannelli G, Barbi S. Intravenous premedication with atropine and postanesthetic delirium. Report of two cases. Riv Eur Sci Med Farmacol 1991; 13(3-4): 137-9. [PMID: 1821049]

[62] Abad-Gurumeta A, Ripollés-Melchor J, Casans-Francés R, *et al.* A systematic review of sugammadex vs neostigmine for reversal of neuromuscular blockade. Anaesthesia 2015; 70(12): 1441-52.

[http://dx.doi.org/10.1111/anae.13277] [PMID: 26558858]

[63] Drachman DB. Myasthenia gravis (second of two parts). N Engl J Med 1978; 298(4): 186-93. [http://dx.doi.org/10.1056/NEJM197801262980404] [PMID: 339085]

[64] Drachman DB. Myasthenia gravis (first of two parts). N Engl J Med 1978; 298(3): 136-42. [http://dx.doi.org/10.1056/NEJM197801192980305] [PMID: 201840]

[65] Juel VC, Massey JM. Myasthenia gravis 2007.http://www.ncbi.nlm.nih.gov/pubmed/17986328 [http://dx.doi.org/10.1186/1750-1172-2-44]

[66] Kothari MJ. Myasthenia gravis. J Am Osteopath Assoc 2004; 104(9): 377-84. [PMID: 15452103]

[67] Lindstrom J, Dau P. Biology of myasthenia gravis. Annu Rev Pharmacol Toxicol 1980; 20: 337-62. [http://dx.doi.org/10.1146/annurev.pa.20.040180.002005] [PMID: 6992700]

[68] Eccles JC, MacFARLANE WV. Actions of anti-cholinesterases on endplate potential of frog muscle. J Neurophysiol 1949; 12(1): 59-80. [PMID: 18122899]

[69] Mehndiratta MM, Pandey S, Kuntzer T. Acetylcholinesterase inhibitor treatment for myasthenia gravis. Cochrane Database Syst Rev 2011; 2(2): CD006986. [PMID: 21328290]

[70] Riggs JE. Pharmacologic enhancement of neuromuscular transmission in myasthenia gravis. Clin Neuropharmacol 1982; 5(3): 277-92. [http://dx.doi.org/10.1097/00002826-198205030-00003] [PMID: 6288236]

[71] Walker MB. Case showing the Effect of Prostigmin on Myasthenia Gravis. Proc R Soc Med 1935; 28(6): 759-61. [PMID: 19990268]

[72] Walker MB. Treatment of myasthenia gravis with physostigmine. Lancet 1934; 223(5779): 1200-1. [http://dx.doi.org/10.1016/S0140-6736(00)94294-6]

[73] Pritchard EA. The use of "Prostigmin" in the treatment of myasthenia gravis. Lancet 1935; 225(5817): 432-4. [http://dx.doi.org/10.1016/S0140-6736(00)57094-9]

[74] Rowland LP. Prostigmine-responsiveness and the diagnosis of myasthenia gravis. Neurology 1955; 5(9): 612-23. [http://dx.doi.org/10.1212/WNL.5.9.612] [PMID: 13253829]

[75] Hutchinson EC, Matthews WB. The intra-arterial injection of neostigmine as a diagnostic test in myasthenia gravis. J Neurol Neurosurg Psychiatry 1953; 16(1): 47-8. [http://dx.doi.org/10.1136/jnnp.16.1.47] [PMID: 13023440]

[76] Osserman KE, Kaplan LI. Rapid diagnostic test for myasthenia gravis: increased muscle strength, without fasciculations, after intravenous administration of edrophonium (tensilon) chloride. J Am Med Assoc 1952; 150(4): 265-8. [http://dx.doi.org/10.1001/jama.1952.03680040007002] [PMID: 14955435]

[77] Van Dyk HJ, Florence L. The Tensilon test. A safe office procedure. Ophthalmology 1980; 87(3): 210-2. [http://dx.doi.org/10.1016/S0161-6420(80)35252-4] [PMID: 7422259]

[78] Ludwig S, Bristow G. Hazards of edrophonium. Anesthesiology 1979; 51(6): 567. [http://dx.doi.org/10.1097/00000542-197912000-00022] [PMID: 517789]

[79] Osserman KE. Progress report on mestinon bromide (pyridostigmine bromide). Am J Med 1955; 19(5): 737-9. [http://dx.doi.org/10.1016/S0002-9343(55)80018-6] [PMID: 13268474]

[80] Kumar V, Kaminski HJ. Treatment of myasthenia gravis. Curr Neurol Neurosci Rep 2011; 11(1): 89-96.
[http://dx.doi.org/10.1007/s11910-010-0151-1] [PMID: 20927659]

[81] Pappano AJ. Cholinoceptor-activating and cholinesterase-inhibiting drugs.Basic & clinical pharmacology. 9th ed. New York: Lange Medical Books/McGraw Hill 2004; pp. 95-111.

[82] Bowen DM, Smith CB, White P, Davison AN. Neurotransmitter-related enzymes and indices of hypoxia in senile dementia and other abiotrophies. Brain 1976; 99(3): 459-96.
[http://dx.doi.org/10.1093/brain/99.3.459] [PMID: 11871]

[83] Davies P, Maloney AJ. Selective loss of central cholinergic neurons in Alzheimer's disease. Lancet 1976; 2(8000): 1403.
[http://dx.doi.org/10.1016/S0140-6736(76)91936-X] [PMID: 63862]

[84] Perry EK, Gibson PH, Blessed G, Perry RH, Tomlinson BE. Neurotransmitter enzyme abnormalities in senile dementia. Choline acetyltransferase and glutamic acid decarboxylase activities in necropsy brain tissue. J Neurol Sci 1977; 34(2): 247-65.
[http://dx.doi.org/10.1016/0022-510X(77)90073-9] [PMID: 144789]

[85] Whitehouse PJ, Price DL, Struble RG, Clark AW, Coyle JT, Delon MR. Alzheimer's disease and senile dementia: loss of neurons in the basal forebrain. Science 1982; 215(4537): 1237-9.
[http://dx.doi.org/10.1126/science.7058341] [PMID: 7058341]

[86] Bartus RT, Dean RL III, Beer B, Lippa AS. The cholinergic hypothesis of geriatric memory dysfunction. Science 1982; 217(4558): 408-14.
[http://dx.doi.org/10.1126/science.7046051] [PMID: 7046051]

[87] Etienne P, Dastoor D, Gauthier S, Ludwick R, Collier B. Alzheimer disease: lack of effect of lecithin treatment for 3 months. Neurology 1981; 31(12): 1552-4.
[http://dx.doi.org/10.1212/WNL.31.12.1552] [PMID: 7198209]

[88] Fisman M, Merskey H, Helmes E, McCready J, Colhoun EH, Rylett BJ. Double blind study of lecithin in patients with Alzheimer's disease. Can J Psychiatry 1981; 26(6): 426-8.
[http://dx.doi.org/10.1177/070674378102600608] [PMID: 7028239]

[89] Little A, Levy R, Chuaqui-Kidd P, Hand D. A double-blind, placebo controlled trial of high-dose lecithin in Alzheimer's disease. J Neurol Neurosurg Psychiatry 1985; 48(8): 736-42.
[http://dx.doi.org/10.1136/jnnp.48.8.736] [PMID: 3897460]

[90] Vroulis GA, Smith RC, Brinkman S, Schoolar J, Gordon J. The effects of lecithin on memory in patients with senile dementia of the Alzheimer's type [proceedings]. Psychopharmacol Bull 1981; 17(1): 127-8. [proceedings].
[PMID: 7232644]

[91] Boyd WD, Graham-White J, Blackwood G, Glen I, McQueen J. Clinical effects of choline in Alzheimer senile dementia. Lancet 1977; 2(8040): 711.
[http://dx.doi.org/10.1016/S0140-6736(77)90517-7] [PMID: 71516]

[92] Etienne P, Gauthier S, Johnson G, *et al.* Clinical effects of choline in Alzheimer's disease. Lancet 1978; 1(8062): 508-9.
[http://dx.doi.org/10.1016/S0140-6736(78)90180-0] [PMID: 76060]

[93] Sitaram N, Weingartner H, Gillin JC. Human serial learning: enhancement with arecholine and choline impairment with scopolamine. Science 1978; 201(4352): 274-6.
[http://dx.doi.org/10.1126/science.351808] [PMID: 351808]

[94] Christie JE, Shering A, Ferguson J, Glen AI. Physostigmine and arecoline: effects of intravenous infusions in Alzheimer presenile dementia. Br J Psychiatry 1981; 138(1): 46-50.
[http://dx.doi.org/10.1192/bjp.138.1.46] [PMID: 7023592]

[95] Mohs RC, Davis BM, Johns CA, *et al.* Oral physostigmine treatment of patients with Alzheimer's

disease. Am J Psychiatry 1985; 142(1): 28-33.
[http://dx.doi.org/10.1176/ajp.142.1.28] [PMID: 3881051]

[96] Schwartz AS, Kohlstaedt EV. Physostigmine effects in Alzheimer's disease: relationship to dementia severity. Life Sci 1986; 38(11): 1021-8.
[http://dx.doi.org/10.1016/0024-3205(86)90236-5] [PMID: 3512944]

[97] Thal LJ, Masur DM, Blau AD, Fuld PA, Klauber MR. Chronic oral physostigmine without lecithin improves memory in Alzheimer's disease. J Am Geriatr Soc 1989; 37(1): 42-8.
[http://dx.doi.org/10.1111/j.1532-5415.1989.tb01567.x] [PMID: 2642499]

[98] Stern Y, Sano M, Mayeux R. Effects of oral physostigmine in Alzheimer's disease. Ann Neurol 1987; 22(3): 306-10.
[http://dx.doi.org/10.1002/ana.410220305] [PMID: 3674795]

[99] Collerton D. Cholinergic function and intellectual decline in Alzheimer's disease. Neuroscience 1986; 19(1): 1-28.
[http://dx.doi.org/10.1016/0306-4522(86)90002-3] [PMID: 3537837]

[100] Davis KL, Thal LJ, Gamzu ER, *et al.* A double-blind, placebo-controlled multicenter study of tacrine for Alzheimer's disease. N Engl J Med 1992; 327(18): 1253-9.
[http://dx.doi.org/10.1056/NEJM199210293271801] [PMID: 1406817]

[101] Knapp MJ, Knopman DS, Solomon PR, Pendlebury WW, Davis CS, Gracon SI. A 30-week randomized controlled trial of high-dose tacrine in patients with Alzheimer's disease. JAMA 1994; 271(13): 985-91.
[http://dx.doi.org/10.1001/jama.1994.03510370037029] [PMID: 8139083]

[102] Lilienfeld S. Galantamine--a novel cholinergic drug with a unique dual mode of action for the treatment of patients with Alzheimer's disease. CNS Drug Rev 2002; 8(2): 159-76.
[http://dx.doi.org/10.1111/j.1527-3458.2002.tb00221.x] [PMID: 12177686]

[103] Freeman SE, Dawson RM. Tacrine: a pharmacological review. Prog Neurobiol 1991; 36(4): 257-77.
[http://dx.doi.org/10.1016/0301-0082(91)90002-I] [PMID: 1714613]

[104] Francis PT, Palmer AM, Snape M, Wilcock GK. The cholinergic hypothesis of Alzheimer's disease: a review of progress. J Neurol Neurosurg Psychiatry 1999; 66(2): 137-47.
[http://dx.doi.org/10.1136/jnnp.66.2.137] [PMID: 10071091]

[105] Sugimoto H, Yamanishi Y, Iimura Y, Kawakami Y. Donepezil hydrochloride (E2020) and other acetylcholinesterase inhibitors. Curr Med Chem 2000; 7(3): 303-39.
[http://dx.doi.org/10.2174/0929867003375191] [PMID: 10637367]

[106] Rogers SL, Friedhoff LT. The efficacy and safety of donepezil in patients with Alzheimer's disease: results of a US Multicentre, Randomized, Double-Blind, Placebo-Controlled Trial. Dementia 1996; 7(6): 293-303.
[PMID: 8915035]

[107] Rogers SL, Doody RS, Mohs RC, Friedhoff LT. Donepezil improves cognition and global function in Alzheimer disease: a 15-week, double-blind, placebo-controlled study. Arch Intern Med 1998; 158(9): 1021-31.
[http://dx.doi.org/10.1001/archinte.158.9.1021] [PMID: 9588436]

[108] Rogers SL, Farlow MR, Doody RS, Mohs R, Friedhoff LT. A 24-week, double-blind, placebo-controlled trial of donepezil in patients with Alzheimer's disease. Neurology 1998; 50(1): 136-45.
[http://dx.doi.org/10.1212/WNL.50.1.136] [PMID: 9443470]

[109] Hogan DB, Patterson C. Progress in clinical neurosciences: Treatment of Alzheimer's disease and other dementias--review and comparison of the cholinesterase inhibitors. Can J Neurol Sci 2002; 29(4): 306-14.
[http://dx.doi.org/10.1017/S031716710000216X] [PMID: 12463485]

[110] Rogers SL, Friedhoff LT. Long-term efficacy and safety of donepezil in the treatment of Alzheimer's

disease: an interim analysis of the results of a US multicentre open label extension study. Eur Neuropsychopharmacol 1998; 8(1): 67-75.
[http://dx.doi.org/10.1016/S0924-977X(97)00079-5] [PMID: 9452942]

[111] Maelicke A, Samochocki M, Jostock R, *et al.* Allosteric sensitization of nicotinic receptors by galantamine, a new treatment strategy for Alzheimer's disease. Biol Psychiatry 2001; 49(3): 279-88.
[http://dx.doi.org/10.1016/S0006-3223(00)01109-4] [PMID: 11230879]

[112] Samochocki M, Höffle A, Fehrenbacher A, *et al.* Galantamine is an allosterically potentiating ligand of neuronal nicotinic but not of muscarinic acetylcholine receptors. J Pharmacol Exp Ther 2003; 305(3): 1024-36.
[http://dx.doi.org/10.1124/jpet.102.045773] [PMID: 12649296]

[113] Greig NH, Utsuki T, Ingram DK, *et al.* Selective butyrylcholinesterase inhibition elevates brain acetylcholine, augments learning and lowers Alzheimer beta-amyloid peptide in rodent. Proc Natl Acad Sci USA 2005; 102(47): 17213-8.
[http://dx.doi.org/10.1073/pnas.0508575102] [PMID: 16275899]

[114] Ballard CG. Advances in the treatment of Alzheimer's disease: benefits of dual cholinesterase inhibition. Eur Neurol 2002; 47(1): 64-70.
[http://dx.doi.org/10.1159/000047952] [PMID: 11803198]

[115] Lockhart IA, Mitchell SA, Kelly S. Safety and tolerability of donepezil, rivastigmine and galantamine for patients with Alzheimer's disease: systematic review of the 'real-world' evidence. Dement Geriatr Cogn Disord 2009; 28(5): 389-403.
[http://dx.doi.org/10.1159/000255578] [PMID: 19893314]

[116] Fuschillo C, Ascoli E, Franzese G, *et al.* Alzheimer's disease and acetylcholinesterase inhibitor agents: a two-year longitudinal study. Arch Gerontol Geriatr Suppl 2004; (9): 187-94.
[http://dx.doi.org/10.1016/j.archger.2004.04.026] [PMID: 15207413]

[117] Atri A, Shaughnessy LW, Locascio JJ, Growdon JH. Long-term course and effectiveness of combination therapy in Alzheimer disease. Alzheimer Dis Assoc Disord 2008; 22(3): 209-21.
[http://dx.doi.org/10.1097/WAD.0b013e31816653bc] [PMID: 18580597]

[118] Owen RT. Memantine and donepezil: a fixed drug combination for the treatment of moderate to severe Alzheimer's dementia. Drugs Today (Barc) 2016; 52(4): 239-48.
[PMID: 27252988]

[119] Wong CW. Pharmacotherapy for dementia: A practical approach to the use of cholinesterase inhibitors and memantine. Drugs Aging 2016; 33(7): 451-60.
[http://dx.doi.org/10.1007/s40266-016-0372-3] [PMID: 27154396]

[120] Gill SS, Anderson GM, Fischer HD, *et al.* Syncope and its consequences in patients with dementia receiving cholinesterase inhibitors: a population-based cohort study. Arch Intern Med 2009; 169(9): 867-73.
[http://dx.doi.org/10.1001/archinternmed.2009.43] [PMID: 19433698]

[121] Hernandez RK, Farwell W, Cantor MD, Lawler EV. Cholinesterase inhibitors and incidence of bradycardia in patients with dementia in the veterans affairs new England healthcare system. J Am Geriatr Soc 2009; 57(11): 1997-2003.
[http://dx.doi.org/10.1111/j.1532-5415.2009.02488.x] [PMID: 19793162]

[122] Park-Wyllie LY, Mamdani MM, Li P, Gill SS, Laupacis A, Juurlink DN. Cholinesterase inhibitors and hospitalization for bradycardia: a population-based study. PLoS Med 2009; 6(9): e1000157.
[http://dx.doi.org/10.1371/journal.pmed.1000157] [PMID: 19787032]

[123] Kim DH, Brown RT, Ding EL, Kiel DP, Berry SD. Dementia medications and risk of falls, syncope, and related adverse events: meta-analysis of randomized controlled trials. J Am Geriatr Soc 2011; 59(6): 1019-31.
[http://dx.doi.org/10.1111/j.1532-5415.2011.03450.x] [PMID: 21649634]

[124] Monacelli F, Rosa G. Cholinesterase inhibitors: cardioprotection in Alzheimer's disease. J Alzheimers Dis 2014; 42(4): 1071-7.
[PMID: 25024324]

[125] Gill SS, Mamdani M, Naglie G, *et al.* A prescribing cascade involving cholinesterase inhibitors and anticholinergic drugs. Arch Intern Med 2005; 165(7): 808-13.
[http://dx.doi.org/10.1001/archinte.165.7.808] [PMID: 15824303]

[126] Gray SL, Anderson ML, Dublin S, *et al.* Cumulative use of strong anticholinergics and incident dementia: a prospective cohort study. JAMA Intern Med 2015; 175(3): 401-7.
[http://dx.doi.org/10.1001/jamainternmed.2014.7663] [PMID: 25621434]

[127] Torvinen-Kiiskinen S, Taipale H, Tanskanen A, Tiihonen J, Hartikainen S. Concomitant use of acetylcholine esterase inhibitors and urinary antispasmodics among Finnish community-dwelling persons with Alzheimer disease. J Clin Psychopharmacol 2014; 34(6): 722-7.
[http://dx.doi.org/10.1097/JCP.0000000000000218] [PMID: 25207860]

[128] Montastruc F, Rouanet S, Gardette V, Rousseau V, Bagheri H, Montastruc JL. Atropinic burden of prescriptions forms in patients with Alzheimer disease: a cross-sectional study in a French PharmacoVigilance Database. Eur J Clin Pharmacol 2015; 71(7): 891-5.
[http://dx.doi.org/10.1007/s00228-015-1869-0] [PMID: 25991052]

[129] Farlow MR, Grossberg GT, Sadowsky CH, Meng X, Velting DM. A 24-week, open-label extension study to investigate the long-term safety, tolerability, and efficacy of 13.3 mg/24 h rivastigmine patch in patients with severe alzheimer disease. Alzheimer Dis Assoc Disord 2015; 29(2): 110-6.
[PMID: 25437301]

[130] Pariente A, Sanctussy DJ, Miremont-Salamé G, Moore N, Haramburu F, Fourrier-Réglat A. Factors associated with serious adverse reactions to cholinesterase inhibitors: a study of spontaneous reporting. CNS Drugs 2010; 24(1): 55-63.
[http://dx.doi.org/10.2165/11530300-000000000-00000] [PMID: 20030419]

[131] Vilalta-Franch J, Lopez-Pousa S, Calvo-Perxas L, Garre-Olmo J. Psychosis of Alzheimer disease: prevalence, incidence, persistence, risk factors, and mortality 2013.
[http://dx.doi.org/10.1016/j.jagp.2013.01.051]

[132] Morris JC, Cyrus PA, Orazem J, *et al.* Metrifonate benefits cognitive, behavioral, and global function in patients with Alzheimer's disease. Neurology 1998; 50(5): 1222-30.
[http://dx.doi.org/10.1212/WNL.50.5.1222] [PMID: 9595967]

[133] Holmes C, Wilkinson D, Dean C, *et al.* The efficacy of donepezil in the treatment of neuropsychiatric symptoms in Alzheimer disease. Neurology 2004; 63(2): 214-9.
[http://dx.doi.org/10.1212/01.WNL.0000129990.32253.7B] [PMID: 15277611]

[134] Cummings J, Lai TJ, Hemrungrojn S, *et al.* Role of Donepezil in the Management of Neuropsychiatric Symptoms in Alzheimer's Disease and Dementia with Lewy Bodies. CNS Neurosci Ther 2016; 22(3): 159-66.
[http://dx.doi.org/10.1111/cns.12484] [PMID: 26778658]

[135] Hirsch C. Continued use of antipsychotic drugs increased long-term mortality in patients with Alzheimer disease. Evid Based Med 2009; 14(4): 115.
[http://dx.doi.org/10.1136/ebm.14.4.115] [PMID: 19648431]

[136] Musicco M, Palmer K, Russo A, *et al.* Association between prescription of conventional or atypical antipsychotic drugs and mortality in older persons with Alzheimer's disease. Dement Geriatr Cogn Disord 2011; 31(3): 218-24.
[http://dx.doi.org/10.1159/000326213] [PMID: 21474930]

[137] Liu CS, Ruthirakuhan M, Chau SA, Herrmann N, Carvalho AF, Lanctôt KL. Pharmacological Management of Agitation and Aggression in Alzheimer's Disease: A Review of Current and Novel Treatments. Curr Alzheimer Res 2016; 13(10): 1134-44.

[http://dx.doi.org/10.2174/1567205013666160502122933] [PMID: 27137221]

[138] Thinakaran G, Koo EH. Amyloid precursor protein trafficking, processing, and function. J Biol Chem 2008; 283(44): 29615-9.
[http://dx.doi.org/10.1074/jbc.R800019200] [PMID: 18650430]

[139] Mattson MP. Cellular actions of beta-amyloid precursor protein and its soluble and fibrillogenic derivatives. Physiol Rev 1997; 77(4): 1081-132.
[PMID: 9354812]

[140] Buxbaum JD, Oishi M, Chen HI, *et al.* Cholinergic agonists and interleukin 1 regulate processing and secretion of the Alzheimer beta/A4 amyloid protein precursor. Proc Natl Acad Sci USA 1992; 89(21): 10075-8.
[http://dx.doi.org/10.1073/pnas.89.21.10075] [PMID: 1359534]

[141] Bailey JA, Ray B, Greig NH, Lahiri DK. Rivastigmine lowers Aβ and increases sAPPα levels, which parallel elevated synaptic markers and metabolic activity in degenerating primary rat neurons. PLoS One 2011; 6(7): e21954.
[http://dx.doi.org/10.1371/journal.pone.0021954] [PMID: 21799757]

[142] Beach. Immunotoxin lesion of the cholinergic nucleus baslis causes Ab deposition:towards a physiologic animal model of Alzheimer's disease. Curr Med Chem - Immun Endoc & Metab Agents. 2003;3:233-43

[143] Beach TG, Walker DG, Potter PE, Sue LI, Fisher A. Reduction of cerebrospinal fluid amyloid beta after systemic administration of M1 muscarinic agonists. Brain Res 2001; 905(1-2): 220-3.
[http://dx.doi.org/10.1016/S0006-8993(01)02484-2] [PMID: 11423097]

[144] Ye CY, Lei Y, Tang XC, Zhang HY. Donepezil attenuates Aβ-associated mitochondrial dysfunction and reduces mitochondrial Aβ accumulation in vivo and in vitro. Neuropharmacology 2015; 95: 29-36.
[http://dx.doi.org/10.1016/j.neuropharm.2015.02.020] [PMID: 25744714]

[145] Meunier J, Ieni J, Maurice T. The anti-amnesic and neuroprotective effects of donepezil against amyloid beta25-35 peptide-induced toxicity in mice involve an interaction with the sigma1 receptor. Br J Pharmacol 2006; 149(8): 998-1012.
[http://dx.doi.org/10.1038/sj.bjp.0706927] [PMID: 17057756]

[146] Noh MY, Koh SH, Kim Y, Kim HY, Cho GW, Kim SH. Neuroprotective effects of donepezil through inhibition of GSK-3 activity in amyloid-beta-induced neuronal cell death. J Neurochem 2009; 108(5): 1116-25.
[http://dx.doi.org/10.1111/j.1471-4159.2008.05837.x] [PMID: 19077054]

[147] Romberg C, Mattson MP, Mughal MR, Bussey TJ, Saksida LM. Impaired attention in the 3xTgAD mouse model of Alzheimer's disease: rescue by donepezil (Aricept). J Neurosci 2011; 31(9): 3500-7.
[http://dx.doi.org/10.1523/JNEUROSCI.5242-10.2011] [PMID: 21368062]

[148] Meunier J, Ieni J, Maurice T. Antiamnesic and neuroprotective effects of donepezil against learning impairments induced in mice by exposure to carbon monoxide gas. J Pharmacol Exp Ther 2006; 317(3): 1307-19.
[http://dx.doi.org/10.1124/jpet.106.101527] [PMID: 16551835]

[149] Rosini M, Simoni E, Minarini A, Melchiorre C. Multi-target design strategies in the context of Alzheimer's disease: acetylcholinesterase inhibition and NMDA receptor antagonism as the driving forces. Neurochem Res 2014; 39(10): 1914-23.
[http://dx.doi.org/10.1007/s11064-014-1250-1] [PMID: 24493627]

[150] Castro A, Martinez A. Targeting beta-amyloid pathogenesis through acetylcholinesterase inhibitors. Curr Pharm Des 2006; 12(33): 4377-87.
[http://dx.doi.org/10.2174/138161206778792985] [PMID: 17105433]

[151] Muñoz-Torrero D. Acetylcholinesterase inhibitors as disease-modifying therapies for Alzheimer's disease. Curr Med Chem 2008; 15(24): 2433-55.

[http://dx.doi.org/10.2174/092986708785909067] [PMID: 18855672]

[152] Salloway S, Mintzer J, Weiner MF, Cummings JL. Disease-modifying therapies in Alzheimer's disease. Alzheimers Dement 2008; 4(2): 65-79. [http://dx.doi.org/10.1016/j.jalz.2007.10.001] [PMID: 18631951]

[153] Raschetti R, Albanese E, Vanacore N, Maggini M. Cholinesterase inhibitors in mild cognitive impairment: a systematic review of randomised trials. PLoS Med 2007; 4(11): e338. [http://dx.doi.org/10.1371/journal.pmed.0040338] [PMID: 18044984]

[154] Parnetti L, Amici S, Lanari A, Romani C, Antognelli C, Andreasen N, *et al.* Cerebrospinal fluid levels of biomarkers and activity of acetylcholinesterase (AChE) and butyrylcholinesterase in AD patients before and after treatment with different AChE inhibitors. Neurological sciences : official journal of the Italian Neurological Society and of the Italian Society of Clinical Neurophysiology 2002; 23(Suppl 2): S95-6.

[155] Parnetti L, Chiasserini D, Andreasson U, *et al.* Changes in CSF acetyl- and butyrylcholinesterase activity after long-term treatment with AChE inhibitors in Alzheimer's disease. Acta Neurol Scand 2011; 124(2): 122-9. [http://dx.doi.org/10.1111/j.1600-0404.2010.01435.x] [PMID: 20880294]

[156] Chalmers KA, Wilcock GK, Vinters HV, *et al.* Cholinesterase inhibitors may increase phosphorylated tau in Alzheimer's disease. J Neurol 2009; 256(5): 717-20. [http://dx.doi.org/10.1007/s00415-009-5000-2] [PMID: 19240967]

[157] Schneider LS, Insel PS, Weiner MW. Treatment with cholinesterase inhibitors and memantine of patients in the Alzheimer's Disease Neuroimaging Initiative. Arch Neurol 2011; 68(1): 58-66. [http://dx.doi.org/10.1001/archneurol.2010.343] [PMID: 21220675]

[158] Sona A, Zhang P, Ames D, *et al.* Predictors of rapid cognitive decline in Alzheimer's disease: results from the Australian imaging, biomarkers and lifestyle (AIBL) study of ageing. International psychogeriatrics / IPA 2012; 24(2): 197-204.

[159] Geldmacher DS, Provenzano G, McRae T, Mastey V, Ieni JR. Donepezil is associated with delayed nursing home placement in patients with Alzheimer's disease. J Am Geriatr Soc 2003; 51(7): 937-44. [http://dx.doi.org/10.1046/j.1365-2389.2003.51306.x] [PMID: 12834513]

[160] Beusterien KM, Thomas SK, Gause D, Kimel M, Arcona S, Mirski D. Impact of rivastigmine use on the risk of nursing home placement in a US sample. CNS Drugs 2004; 18(15): 1143-8. [http://dx.doi.org/10.2165/00023210-200418150-00008] [PMID: 15581384]

[161] Knopman D, Schneider L, Davis K, *et al.* Long-term tacrine (Cognex) treatment: effects on nursing home placement and mortality, Tacrine Study Group. Neurology 1996; 47(1): 166-77. [http://dx.doi.org/10.1212/WNL.47.1.166] [PMID: 8710072]

[162] Lu PH, Edland SD, Teng E, Tingus K, Petersen RC, Cummings JL. Donepezil delays progression to AD in MCI subjects with depressive symptoms. Neurology 2009; 72(24): 2115-21. [http://dx.doi.org/10.1212/WNL.0b013e3181aa52d3] [PMID: 19528519]

[163] Dobransky T, Rylett RJ, Fu AL, *et al.* A model for dynamic regulation of choline acetyltransferase by phosphorylation. J Neurochem 2005; 95(2): 305-13. [http://dx.doi.org/10.1111/j.1471-4159.2005.03367.x] [PMID: 16135099]

[164] Diniz BS, Pinto JA Jr, Gonzaga ML, Guimarães FM, Gattaz WF, Forlenza OV. To treat or not to treat? A meta-analysis of the use of cholinesterase inhibitors in mild cognitive impairment for delaying progression to Alzheimer's disease. Eur Arch Psychiatry Clin Neurosci 2009; 259(4): 248-56. [http://dx.doi.org/10.1007/s00406-008-0864-1] [PMID: 19224111]

[165] Ferris S, Nordberg A, Soininen H, Darreh-Shori T, Lane R. Progression from mild cognitive impairment to Alzheimer's disease: effects of sex, butyrylcholinesterase genotype, and rivastigmine treatment. Pharmacogenet Genomics 2009; 19(8): 635-46. [http://dx.doi.org/10.1097/FPC.0b013e32832f8c17] [PMID: 19617863]

[166] Sobów T, Kłoszewska I. Cholinesterase inhibitors in mild cognitive impairment: a meta-analysis of randomized controlled trials. Neurol Neurochir Pol 2007; 41(1): 13-21. [PMID: 17330176]

[167] Russ TC, Morling JR. Cholinesterase inhibitors for mild cognitive impairment 2012.http://www.ncbi.nlm.nih.gov/pubmed/22972133 [http://dx.doi.org/10.1002/14651858.CD009132.pub2]

[168] Fitzpatrick-Lewis D, Warren R, Ali MU, Sherifali D, Raina P. Treatment for mild cognitive impairment: a systematic review and meta-analysis. CMAJ Open 2015; 3(4): E419-27. [http://dx.doi.org/10.9778/cmajo.20150057] [PMID: 26770964]

[169] Saunders AM, Strittmatter WJ, Schmechel D, *et al.* Association of apolipoprotein E allele epsilon 4 with late-onset familial and sporadic Alzheimer's disease. Neurology 1993; 43(8): 1467-72. [http://dx.doi.org/10.1212/WNL.43.8.1467] [PMID: 8350998]

[170] Whitehair DC, Sherzai A, Emond J, *et al.* Influence of apolipoprotein E varepsilon4 on rates of cognitive and functional decline in mild cognitive impairment. Alzheimers Dement 2010; 6(5): 412-9. [http://dx.doi.org/10.1016/j.jalz.2009.12.003] [PMID: 20813342]

[171] Lehmann DJ, Johnston C, Smith AD. Synergy between the genes for butyrylcholinesterase K variant and apolipoprotein E4 in late-onset confirmed Alzheimer's disease. Hum Mol Genet 1997; 6(11): 1933-6. [http://dx.doi.org/10.1093/hmg/6.11.1933] [PMID: 9302273]

[172] Gallucci M, Spagnolo P, Aricò M, Grossi E. Predictors of response to cholinesterase inhibitors treatment of alzheimer's disease: Date mining from the TREDEM registry. J Alzheimers Dis 2016; 50(4): 969-79. [http://dx.doi.org/10.3233/JAD-150747] [PMID: 26836164]

[173] Roberts JS, Karlawish JH, Uhlmann WR, Petersen RC, Green RC. Mild cognitive impairment in clinical care: a survey of American Academy of Neurology members. Neurology 2010; 75(5): 425-31. [http://dx.doi.org/10.1212/WNL.0b013e3181eb5872] [PMID: 20679636]

[174] Kobayashi H, Ohnishi T, Nakagawa R, Yoshizawa K. The comparative efficacy and safety of cholinesterase inhibitors in patients with mild-to-moderate Alzheimer's disease: a Bayesian network meta-analysis. Int J Geriatr Psychiatry 2016; 31(8): 892-904. [http://dx.doi.org/10.1002/gps.4405] [PMID: 26680338]

[175] Guillozet AL, Smiley JF, Mash DC, Mesulam MM. Butyrylcholinesterase in the life cycle of amyloid plaques. Ann Neurol 1997; 42(6): 909-18. [http://dx.doi.org/10.1002/ana.410420613] [PMID: 9403484]

[176] Arendt T, Brückner MK, Lange M, Bigl V. Changes in acetylcholinesterase and butyrylcholinesterase in Alzheimer's disease resemble embryonic development--a study of molecular forms. Neurochem Int 1992; 21(3): 381-96. [http://dx.doi.org/10.1016/0197-0186(92)90189-X] [PMID: 1303164]

[177] Lahiri DK, Farlow MR. Differential effect of tacrine and physostigmine on the secretion of the beta-amyloid precursor protein in cell lines. J Mol Neurosci 1996; 7(1): 41-9. [http://dx.doi.org/10.1007/BF02736847] [PMID: 8835781]

[178] Shaw KT, Utsuki T, Rogers J, *et al.* Phenserine regulates translation of beta -amyloid precursor protein mRNA by a putative interleukin-1 responsive element, a target for drug development. Proc Natl Acad Sci USA 2001; 98(13): 7605-10. [http://dx.doi.org/10.1073/pnas.131152998] [PMID: 11404470]

[179] Furukawa-Hibi Y, Alkam T, Nitta A, *et al.* Butyrylcholinesterase inhibitors ameliorate cognitive dysfunction induced by amyloid-β peptide in mice. Behav Brain Res 2011; 225(1): 222-9. [http://dx.doi.org/10.1016/j.bbr.2011.07.035] [PMID: 21820013]

[180] Pearce BD, Potter LT. Effects of tetrahydroaminoacridine on M1 and M2 muscarine receptors.

Neurosci Lett 1988; 88(3): 281-5.
[http://dx.doi.org/10.1016/0304-3940(88)90224-8] [PMID: 3386874]

[181] Summers WK, Tachiki KH, Kling A. Tacrine in the treatment of Alzheimer's disease. A clinical update and recent pharmacologic studies. Eur Neurol 1989; 29 (Suppl. 3): 28-32.
[http://dx.doi.org/10.1159/000116478] [PMID: 2693104]

[182] Summers WK, Koehler AL, Marsh GM, Tachiki K, Kling A. Long-term hepatotoxicity of tacrine. Lancet 1989; 1(8640): 729.
[http://dx.doi.org/10.1016/S0140-6736(89)92246-0] [PMID: 2564541]

[183] Romero A, Cacabelos R, Oset-Gasque MJ, Samadi A, Marco-Contelles J. Novel tacrine-related drugs as potential candidates for the treatment of Alzheimer's disease. Bioorg Med Chem Lett 2013; 23(7): 1916-22.
[http://dx.doi.org/10.1016/j.bmcl.2013.02.017] [PMID: 23481643]

[184] Osman W, Mohamed T, Sit VM, Vasefi MS, Beazely MA, Rao PP. Structure-activity relationship studies of benzyl-, phenethyl-, and pyridyl-substituted tetrahydroacridin-9-amines as multitargeting agents to treat Alzheimer's disease. Chem Biol Drug Des 2016; 88(5): 710-23.
[http://dx.doi.org/10.1111/cbdd.12800] [PMID: 27282589]

[185] Hebda M, Bajda M, Więckowska A, *et al.* Synthesis, molecular modelling and biological evaluation of novel heterodimeric, multiple ligands targeting cholinesterases and amyloid beta. Molecules 2016; 21(4): 410.
[http://dx.doi.org/10.3390/molecules21040410] [PMID: 27023510]

[186] Dgachi Y, Ismaili L, Knez D, *et al.* Synthesis and biological assessment of racemic benzochromenopyrimidinimines as antioxidant, cholinesterase, and aβ1-42 aggregation inhibitors for alzheimer's disease therapy. ChemMedChem 2016; 11(12): 1318-27.
[http://dx.doi.org/10.1002/cmdc.201500539] [PMID: 26804623]

[187] Sun Q, Peng D-Y, Yang S-G, Zhu X-L, Yang W-C, Yang G-F. Syntheses of coumarin-tacrine hybrids as dual-site acetylcholinesterase inhibitors and their activity against butylcholinesterase, Aβ aggregation, and β-secretase. Bioorg Med Chem 2014; 22(17): 4784-91.
[http://dx.doi.org/10.1016/j.bmc.2014.06.057] [PMID: 25088549]

[188] Peng D-Y, Sun Q, Zhu X-L, *et al.* Design, synthesis, and bioevaluation of benzamides: novel acetylcholinesterase inhibitors with multi-functions on butylcholinesterase, Aβ aggregation, and β-secretase. Bioorg Med Chem 2012; 20(22): 6739-50.
[http://dx.doi.org/10.1016/j.bmc.2012.09.016] [PMID: 23041347]

[189] Christie JE, Shering A, Ferguson J, Glen AI. Physostigmine and arecoline: effects of intravenous infusions in Alzheimer presenile dementia. Br J Psychiatry 1981; 138: 46-50.
[http://dx.doi.org/10.1192/bjp.138.1.46] [PMID: 7023592]

[190] Drachman DA, Glosser G, Fleming P, Longenecker G. Memory decline in the aged: treatment with lecithin and physostigmine. Neurology 1982; 32(9): 944-50.
[http://dx.doi.org/10.1212/WNL.32.9.944] [PMID: 6287359]

[191] Haddad LM, Shannon MW, Winchester JF. Clinical Management of poisoning and drug overdose. Philadelphia: Harcourt 1998.

[192] Dawson AH, Buckley NA. Pharmacological management of anticholinergic delirium - theory, evidence and practice. Br J Clin Pharmacol 2016; 81(3): 516-24.
[http://dx.doi.org/10.1111/bcp.12839] [PMID: 26589572]

[193] Lieberman JA, Javitch JA, Moore H. Cholinergic agonists as novel treatments for schizophrenia: the promise of rational drug development for psychiatry. Am J Psychiatry 2008; 165(8): 931-6.
[http://dx.doi.org/10.1176/appi.ajp.2008.08050769] [PMID: 18676593]

[194] Raedler TJ, Bymaster FP, Tandon R, Copolov D, Dean B. Towards a muscarinic hypothesis of schizophrenia. Mol Psychiatry 2007; 12(3): 232-46.

[PMID: 17146471]

[195] Freedman R, Hall M, Adler LE, Leonard S. Evidence in postmortem brain tissue for decreased numbers of hippocampal nicotinic receptors in schizophrenia. Biol Psychiatry 1995; 38(1): 22-33. [http://dx.doi.org/10.1016/0006-3223(94)00252-X] [PMID: 7548469]

[196] Dean B, McLeod M, Keriakous D, McKenzie J, Scarr E. Decreased muscarinic1 receptors in the dorsolateral prefrontal cortex of subjects with schizophrenia. Mol Psychiatry 2002; 7(10): 1083-91. [http://dx.doi.org/10.1038/sj.mp.4001199] [PMID: 12476323]

[197] Crook JM, Tomaskovic-Crook E, Copolov DL, Dean B. Low muscarinic receptor binding in prefrontal cortex from subjects with schizophrenia: a study of Brodmann's areas 8, 9, 10, and 46 and the effects of neuroleptic drug treatment. Am J Psychiatry 2001; 158(6): 918-25. [http://dx.doi.org/10.1176/appi.ajp.158.6.918] [PMID: 11384900]

[198] Crook JM, Tomaskovic-Crook E, Copolov DL, Dean B. Decreased muscarinic receptor binding in subjects with schizophrenia: a study of the human hippocampal formation. Biol Psychiatry 2000; 48(5): 381-8. [http://dx.doi.org/10.1016/S0006-3223(00)00918-5] [PMID: 10978721]

[199] Meltzer HY, Deutch AY. Neurochemistry of Schizophrenia.Basic Neurochemistry. 6th ed. Philadelphia: Lippincott-Raven 1999; pp. 1053-72.

[200] Li Z, Bonhaus DW, Huang M, Prus AJ, Dai J, Meltzer HY. AC260584 (4-[3-(4-butylpiperidin-1- yl)-propyl]-7-fluoro-4H-benzo[1,4]oxazin-3-one), a selective muscarinic M1 receptor agonist, increases acetylcholine and dopamine release in rat medial prefrontal cortex and hippocampus. Eur J Pharmacol 2007; 572(2-3): 129-37. [http://dx.doi.org/10.1016/j.ejphar.2007.06.025] [PMID: 17628522]

[201] Davis KL, Berger PA, Hollister LE, Barchas JD. Cholinergic involvement in mental disorders. Life Sci 1978; 22(21): 1865-71. [http://dx.doi.org/10.1016/0024-3205(78)90472-1] [PMID: 27686]

[202] Friedhoff AJ, Alpert M. A dopaminergic-cholinergic mechanism in production of psychotic symptoms. Biol Psychiatry 1973; 6(2): 165-9. [PMID: 4709131]

[203] Tandon R. Cholinergic aspects of schizophrenia. Br J Psychiatry Suppl 1999; (37): 7-11. [PMID: 10211133]

[204] Tandon R, Greden JF. Cholinergic hyperactivity and negative schizophrenic symptoms. A model of cholinergic/dopaminergic interactions in schizophrenia. Arch Gen Psychiatry 1989; 46(8): 745-53. [http://dx.doi.org/10.1001/archpsyc.1989.01810080075010] [PMID: 2665688]

[205] Shekhar A, Potter WZ, Lightfoot J, *et al.* Selective muscarinic receptor agonist xanomeline as a novel treatment approach for schizophrenia. Am J Psychiatry 2008; 165(8): 1033-9. [http://dx.doi.org/10.1176/appi.ajp.2008.06091591] [PMID: 18593778]

[206] Kuehn BM. Link between smoking and mental illness may lead to treatments. JAMA 2006; 295(5): 483-4. [http://dx.doi.org/10.1001/jama.295.5.483] [PMID: 16449605]

[207] Simosky JK, Stevens KE, Freedman R. Nicotinic agonists and psychosis. Curr Drug Targets CNS Neurol Disord 2002; 1(2): 149-62. [http://dx.doi.org/10.2174/1568007024606168] [PMID: 12769624]

[208] Friedman JI. Cholinergic targets for cognitive enhancement in schizophrenia: focus on cholinesterase inhibitors and muscarinic agonists. Psychopharmacology (Berl) 2004; 174(1): 45-53. [http://dx.doi.org/10.1007/s00213-004-1794-x] [PMID: 15205878]

[209] Ribeiz SR, Bassitt DP, Arrais JA, Avila R, Steffens DC, Bottino CM. Cholinesterase inhibitors as adjunctive therapy in patients with schizophrenia and schizoaffective disorder: a review and meta-analysis of the literature. CNS Drugs 2010; 24(4): 303-17.

[http://dx.doi.org/10.2165/11530260-000000000-00000] [PMID: 20297855]

[210] Winteringham FP, Lewis SE. On the Mode of Action of Insecticides. Annu Rev Entomol 1959; 4(1): 303-18.
[http://dx.doi.org/10.1146/annurev.en.04.010159.001511]

[211] Casida JE, Durkin KA. Anticholinesterase insecticide retrospective. Chem Biol Interact 2013; 203(1): 221-5.
[http://dx.doi.org/10.1016/j.cbi.2012.08.002] [PMID: 22926007]

[212] Smallman BN, Mansingh A. The cholinergic system in insect development. Annu Rev Entomol 1969; 14: 387-408.
[http://dx.doi.org/10.1146/annurev.en.14.010169.002131] [PMID: 4302369]

[213] Eddelston M, Clark RF. Insecticides: Organic phosphorus compounds and carbamates. 9th ed. New York: McGraw-Hill Medical 2011; 2011: pp. 1450-63.

[214] Abrusow A. Regarding the structure of the phosphoic acids and their derivatives: IV. isomerization nad transition of the trivavelent phosphorus bond in place of the pentavalent. Chemisches Zentralblatt 1906; 77: 169.

[215] Balareff D. Untersuchungen über die Struktur der Pyrophosphorsäure. Zeitschrift für anorganische Chemie. 1914; 88(1): 133-50.
[http://dx.doi.org/10.1002/zaac.19140880111]

[216] Lange W, von Krueger G. On monofluoro-phosphoric acid. Ber Dtsch Chem Ges 1932; 65(9): 1598-601.
[http://dx.doi.org/10.1002/cber.19320650910]

[217] Gupta RC. Handbook of Toxicology of Chemical Warfare Agents. Gupta RC, editor. Burlington: Burlington : Elsevier Science; 2009.

[218] Struger J, Grabuski J, Cagampan S, Sverko E, Marvin C. Occurrence and distribution of carbamate pesticides and metalaxyl in southern ontario surface waters 2007-2010. Bull Environ Contam Toxicol 2016; 96(4): 429-31.
[http://dx.doi.org/10.1007/s00128-015-1719-x] [PMID: 26754544]

[219] Suratman S, Edwards JW, Babina K. Organophosphate pesticides exposure among farmworkers: pathways and risk of adverse health effects. Rev Environ Health 2015; 30(1): 65-79.
[PMID: 25741936]

[220] Pohanka M. Cholinesterases, a target of pharmacology and toxicology. Biomed Pap Med Fac Univ Palacky Olomouc Czech Repub 2011; 155(3): 219-29.
[http://dx.doi.org/10.5507/bp.2011.036] [PMID: 22286807]

[221] Colović MB, Krstić DZ, Lazarević-Pašti TD, Bondžić AM, Vasić VM. Acetylcholinesterase inhibitors: pharmacology and toxicology. Curr Neuropharmacol 2013; 11(3): 315-35.
[http://dx.doi.org/10.2174/1570159X11311030006] [PMID: 24179466]

[222] Sudakin DL, Power LE. Organophosphate exposures in the United States: a longitudinal analysis of incidents reported to poison centers. J Toxicol Environ Health A 2007; 70(2): 141-7.
[http://dx.doi.org/10.1080/15287390600755224] [PMID: 17365575]

[223] King AM, Aaron CK. Organophosphate and carbamate poisoning. Emerg Med Clin North Am 2015; 33(1): 133-51.
[http://dx.doi.org/10.1016/j.emc.2014.09.010] [PMID: 25455666]

[224] Wismer T, Means C. Toxicology of newer insecticides in small animals. Vet Clin North Am Small Anim Pract 2012; 42(2): 335-347, vii-viii. [vii-viii.].
[http://dx.doi.org/10.1016/j.cvsm.2011.12.004] [PMID: 22381183]

[225] Kapka-Skrzypczak L, Cyranka M, Skrzypczak M, Kruszewski M. Biomonitoring and biomarkers of organophosphate pesticides exposure - state of the art. Ann Agric Environ Med 2011; 18(2): 294-303.

[PMID: 22216802]

[226] Steenland K, Jenkins B, Ames RG, O'Malley M, Chrislip D, Russo J. Chronic neurological sequelae to organophosphate pesticide poisoning. Am J Public Health 1994; 84(5): 731-6. [http://dx.doi.org/10.2105/AJPH.84.5.731] [PMID: 8179040]

[227] Steenland K. Chronic neurological effects of organophosphate pesticides. BMJ 1996; 312(7042): 1312-3. [http://dx.doi.org/10.1136/bmj.312.7042.1312] [PMID: 8646032]

[228] Steenland K, Dick RB, Howell RJ, *et al.* Neurologic function among termiticide applicators exposed to chlorpyrifos. Environ Health Perspect 2000; 108(4): 293-300. [http://dx.doi.org/10.1289/ehp.00108293] [PMID: 10753086]

[229] Schrader G. Die Entwicklung neuer Insektizide auf Grundlage von Organischen Fluor- und Phosphorverbindungen. Verlag Chemie 1942; p. 62.

[230] Sidell FR, Borak J. Chemical warfare agents: II. Nerve agents. Ann Emerg Med 1992; 21(7): 865-71. [http://dx.doi.org/10.1016/S0196-0644(05)81036-4] [PMID: 1610046]

[231] Holstege CP, Kirk M, Sidell FR. Chemical warfare. Nerve agent poisoning. Crit Care Clin 1997; 13(4): 923-42. [http://dx.doi.org/10.1016/S0749-0704(05)70374-2] [PMID: 9330846]

[232] Szinicz L. History of chemical and biological warfare agents. Toxicology 2005; 214(3): 167-81. [http://dx.doi.org/10.1016/j.tox.2005.06.011] [PMID: 16111798]

[233] Barthold CL, Schier JG. Organic phosphorus compounds--nerve agents. Crit Care Clin 2005; 21(4): 673-689, v-vi. [v-vi.]. [http://dx.doi.org/10.1016/j.ccc.2005.05.010] [PMID: 16168308]

[234] McCOMBIE H, Saunders BC. Toxic organo-lead compounds. Nature 1947; 159(4041): 491-4. [http://dx.doi.org/10.1038/159491a0] [PMID: 20295226]

[235] Saunders BC, Stacey GJ. 138 Esters containing phosphorus Part IV Diisopropyl fluorophosphonate Journal of the Chemical Society. Resumed 1948; pp. 695-9.

[236] Tisdale WH, Flenner AL. Derivatives of dithiocarbamic acid as pesticides. Ind Eng Chem 1942; 34: 501-5. [http://dx.doi.org/10.1021/ie50388a031]

[237] Suchard J. Chemical Weapons, in Goldfrank's toxicologic emergencies. New York: McGraw-Hill Medical 2011; 2001: pp. 1735-49.

[238] Cannard K. The acute treatment of nerve agent exposure. J Neurol Sci 2006; 249(1): 86-94. [http://dx.doi.org/10.1016/j.jns.2006.06.008] [PMID: 16945386]

[239] Kassa J, Jun D, Kuca K. The reactivating and therapeutic efficacy of oximes to counteract Russian VX poisonings. Int J Toxicol 2006; 25(5): 397-401. [http://dx.doi.org/10.1080/10915810600846971] [PMID: 16940011]

[240] Munro N. Toxicity of the organophosphate chemical warfare agents GA, GB, and VX: implications for public protection. Environ Health Perspect 1994; 102(1): 18-38. [http://dx.doi.org/10.1289/ehp.9410218] [PMID: 9719666]

[241] Newmark J. The birth of nerve agent warfare: lessons from Syed Abbas Foroutan. Neurology 2004; 62(9): 1590-6. [http://dx.doi.org/10.1212/01.WNL.0000124519.85516.50] [PMID: 15136687]

[242] Morita H, Yanagisawa N, Nakajima T, *et al.* Sarin poisoning in Matsumoto, Japan. Lancet 1995; 346(8970): 290-3. [http://dx.doi.org/10.1016/S0140-6736(95)92170-2] [PMID: 7630252]

[243] Okumura T, Takasu N, Ishimatsu S, *et al.* Report on 640 victims of the Tokyo subway sarin attack.

Ann Emerg Med 1996; 28(2): 129-35.
[http://dx.doi.org/10.1016/S0196-0644(96)70052-5] [PMID: 8759575]

[244] Namba T. Cholinesterase inhibition by organophosphorus compounds and its clinical effects. Bull World Health Organ 1971; 44(1-3): 289-307.
[PMID: 4941660]

[245] Namba T, Nolte CT, Jackrel J, Grob D. Poisoning due to organophosphate insecticides. Acute and chronic manifestations. Am J Med 1971; 50(4): 475-92.
[http://dx.doi.org/10.1016/0002-9343(71)90337-8] [PMID: 4324629]

[246] Leikin JB, Thomas RG, Walter FG, Klein R, Meislin HW. A review of nerve agent exposure for the critical care physician. Crit Care Med 2002; 30(10): 2346-54.
[http://dx.doi.org/10.1097/00003246-200210000-00026] [PMID: 12394966]

[247] Eddleston M, Eyer P, Worek F, *et al.* Differences between organophosphorus insecticides in human self-poisoning: a prospective cohort study. Lancet 2005; 366(9495): 1452-9.
[http://dx.doi.org/10.1016/S0140-6736(05)67598-8] [PMID: 16243090]

[248] Dassanayake T, Weerasinghe V, Dangahadeniya U, *et al.* Cognitive processing of visual stimuli in patients with organophosphate insecticide poisoning. Neurology 2007; 68(23): 2027-30.
[http://dx.doi.org/10.1212/01.wnl.0000264423.12123.f0] [PMID: 17548553]

[249] Dassanayake T, Weerasinghe V, Dangahadeniya U, *et al.* Long-term event-related potential changes following organophosphorus insecticide poisoning. Clin Neurophysiol 2008; 119(1): 144-50.
[http://dx.doi.org/10.1016/j.clinph.2007.09.134] [PMID: 18042425]

[250] Yokoyama K. Our recent experiences with sarin poisoning cases in Japan and pesticide users with references to some selected chemicals. Neurotoxicology 2007; 28(2): 364-73.
[http://dx.doi.org/10.1016/j.neuro.2006.04.006] [PMID: 16730798]

[251] Yokoyama K, Araki S, Murata K, *et al.* Chronic neurobehavioral effects of Tokyo subway sarin poisoning in relation to posttraumatic stress disorder. Arch Environ Health 1998; 53(4): 249-56.
[http://dx.doi.org/10.1080/00039899809605705] [PMID: 9709988]

[252] Tochigi M, Umekage T, Otani T, *et al.* Serum cholesterol, uric acid and cholinesterase in victims of the Tokyo subway sarin poisoning: a relation with post-traumatic stress disorder. Neurosci Res 2002; 44(3): 267-72.
[http://dx.doi.org/10.1016/S0168-0102(02)00146-3] [PMID: 12413655]

[253] Gershon S, Shaw FH. Psychiatric sequelae of chronic exposure to organophosphorus insecticides. Lancet 1961; 1(7191): 1371-4.
[http://dx.doi.org/10.1016/S0140-6736(61)92004-9] [PMID: 13704751]

[254] Wesseling C, van Wendel de Joode B, Keifer M, London L, Mergler D, Stallones L. Symptoms of psychological distress and suicidal ideation among banana workers with a history of poisoning by organophosphate or n-methyl carbamate pesticides. Occup Environ Med 2010; 67(11): 778-84.
[http://dx.doi.org/10.1136/oem.2009.047266] [PMID: 20798019]

[255] Marrs TC. Organophosphate poisoning. Pharmacol Ther 1993; 58(1): 51-66.
[http://dx.doi.org/10.1016/0163-7258(93)90066-M] [PMID: 8415873]

[256] Costa LG. Current issues in organophosphate toxicology. Clin Chim Acta 2006; 366(1-2): 1-13.
[http://dx.doi.org/10.1016/j.cca.2005.10.008] [PMID: 16337171]

[257] Grob D, Harvey JC. Effects in man of the anticholinesterase compound sarin (isopropyl methyl phosphonofluoridate). J Clin Invest 1958; 37(3): 350-68.
[http://dx.doi.org/10.1172/JCI103615] [PMID: 13513766]

[258] Sidell FR. Soman and sarin: clinical manifestations and treatment of accidental poisoning by organophosphates. Clin Toxicol 1974; 7(1): 1-17.
[http://dx.doi.org/10.3109/15563657408987971] [PMID: 4838227]

[259] Karczmar AG. Acute and long lasting central actions of organophosphorus agents. Fundam Appl Toxicol 1984; 4(2 Pt 2): S1-S17.
[http://dx.doi.org/10.1016/0272-0590(84)90133-7] [PMID: 6144611]

[260] Jones HW Jr, Meyer BJ, Karel L. The relationship of cholinesterase inhibiting activity to the toxicity of some organic phosphorus compounds. J Pharmacol Exp Ther 1948; 94(3): 215-20.
[PMID: 18894879]

[261] Berry WK. Biochemical mechanisms involved in poisoning by anticholinesterases. Proc R Soc Med 1953; 46(10): 801-2.
[PMID: 13112187]

[262] Holmes R. Discussion on poisoning with anticholinesterases. Proc R Soc Med 1953; 46(10): 799-800.
[PMID: 13112184]

[263] Holmstedt B. Synthesis and pharmacology of dimethylamido-ethoxy-phosphoryl cyanide (tabun) together with a description of some allied anticholinesterase compounds containing the N-P bond. Acta Physiol Scand Suppl 1951; 25(90): 12-120.
[PMID: 14902517]

[264] Moore WK. Two cases of poisoning with di-isopropylfluorophosphonate. (D.F.P.). Br J Ind Med 1956; 13(3): 214-6.
[PMID: 13342378]

[265] Parkes MW, Sacra P. Protection against the toxicity of cholinesterase inhibitors by acetylcholine antagonists. Br J Pharmacol Chemother 1954; 9(3): 299-305.
[http://dx.doi.org/10.1111/j.1476-5381.1954.tb01685.x] [PMID: 13199249]

[266] McNAMARA BP, Koelle GB, Gilman A. The treatment of di-isopropyl fluorophosphate (DFP) poisoning in rabbits. J Pharmacol Exp Ther 1946; 88(1): 27-33.
[PMID: 20274522]

[267] Modell W, Krop S. Antidotes to poisoning by di-isopropyl fluorophosphate in cats. J Pharmacol Exp Ther 1946; 88(1): 34-8.
[PMID: 20274523]

[268] Heymans C. Les antidotes du di-isopropylfluoro-phosphonate. Arch Int Pharmacodyn Ther 1950; 81(2): 230-4.
[PMID: 15405459]

[269] Salerno PR, Coon JM. Durg protection against the lethal action of parathion. Arch Int Pharmacodyn Ther 1950; 84(2-3): 227-36.
[PMID: 14790868]

[270] Grob D, Garlick WL, Harvey AM. The toxic effects in man of the anticholinesterase insecticide parathion (p-nitrophenyl diethyl thionophosphate). Bull Johns Hopkins Hosp 1950; 87(2:1): 106-29.

[271] Wilson IB, Ginsburg B. A powerful reactivator of alkylphosphate-inhibited acetylcholinesterase. Biochim Biophys Acta 1955; 18(1): 168-70.
[http://dx.doi.org/10.1016/0006-3002(55)90040-8] [PMID: 13260275]

[272] Willems JL, Langenberg JP, Verstraete AG, *et al.* Plasma concentrations of pralidoxime methylsulphate in organophosphorus poisoned patients. Arch Toxicol 1992; 66(4): 260-6.
[http://dx.doi.org/10.1007/BF02307171] [PMID: 1514924]

[273] Wong L, Radic Z, Brüggemann RJ, Hosea N, Berman HA, Taylor P. Mechanism of oxime reactivation of acetylcholinesterase analyzed by chirality and mutagenesis. Biochemistry 2000; 39(19): 5750-7.
[http://dx.doi.org/10.1021/bi992906r] [PMID: 10801325]

[274] Worek F, Thiermann H, Szinicz L, Eyer P. Kinetic analysis of interactions between human acetylcholinesterase, structurally different organophosphorus compounds and oximes. Biochem Pharmacol 2004; 68(11): 2237-48.

[http://dx.doi.org/10.1016/j.bcp.2004.07.038] [PMID: 15498514]

[275] Dawson RM. Oximes in treatment of carbamate poisoning. Vet Rec 1994; 134(26): 687. [http://dx.doi.org/10.1136/vr.134.26.687-a] [PMID: 7941284]

[276] Buckley NA, Eddleston M, Szinicz L. Oximes for acute organophosphate pesticide poisoning. Cochrane Database Syst Rev 2005; (1): CD005085. [PMID: 15654704]

[277] Gunderson CH, Lehmann CR, Sidell FR, Jabbari B. Nerve agents: a review. Neurology 1992; 42(5): 946-50. [http://dx.doi.org/10.1212/WNL.42.5.946] [PMID: 1315942]

[278] Dirnhuber P, French MC, Green DM, Leadbeater L, Stratton JA. The protection of primates against soman poisoning by pretreatment with pyridostigmine. J Pharm Pharmacol 1979; 31(5): 295-9. [http://dx.doi.org/10.1111/j.2042-7158.1979.tb13504.x] [PMID: 37298]

[279] Solana RP, Gennings C, Carter WH Jr, *et al.* Evaluation of the efficacy of two carbamates, physostigmine and pyridostigmine, when used in conjunction for protection against organophosphate exposure. Fundam Appl Toxicol 1990; 15(4): 814-9. [http://dx.doi.org/10.1016/0272-0590(90)90197-R] [PMID: 2086320]

[280] Bajgar J, Fusek J, Kassa J, Kuca K, Jun D. Chemical aspects of pharmacological prophylaxis against nerve agent poisoning. Curr Med Chem 2009; 16(23): 2977-86. [http://dx.doi.org/10.2174/092986709788803088] [PMID: 19689278]

[281] Petroianu GA, Nurulain SM, Hasan MY, Kuča K, Lorke DE. Reversible cholinesterase inhibitors as pre-treatment for exposure to organophosphates: assessment using azinphos-methyl. J Appl Toxicol 2015; 35(5): 493-9. [http://dx.doi.org/10.1002/jat.3052] [PMID: 25186309]

[282] Bajgar J. Organophosphates/nerve agent poisoning: mechanism of action, diagnosis, prophylaxis, and treatment. Adv Clin Chem 2004; 38: 151-216. [http://dx.doi.org/10.1016/S0065-2423(04)38006-6] [PMID: 15521192]

[283] Henderson JD, Glucksman G, Leong B, *et al.* Pyridostigmine bromide protection against acetylcholinesterase inhibition by pesticides. J Biochem Mol Toxicol 2012; 26(1): 31-4. [http://dx.doi.org/10.1002/jbt.20410] [PMID: 21972196]

Frontiers in CNS Drug Discovery, 2017, *Vol. 3*, 240-249

SUBJECT INDEX

A

Atta-ur-Rahman & M. Iqbal Choudhary (Eds.)

B

C

D

E

F

G

H

I

K

L

M

N

O

P

Q

R

S

T

V

W

Made in the USA
Monee, IL
01 May 2026

49334981R00157